In Two Minds

In Two Minds

A casebook of psychiatric ethics

DONNA DICKENSON

and

BILL (KWM) FULFORD

with additional material by
JIM (JLT) BIRLEY

cartoons by
JONNY COWEE

Foreword by the editors
of *Psychiatric Ethics*
SIDNEY BLOCH, PAUL CHODOFF
and STEPHEN A. GREEN

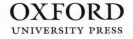

OXFORD
UNIVERSITY PRESS

OXFORD

UNIVERSITY PRESS

Great Clarendon Street, Oxford OX2 6DP

Oxford University Press is a department of the University of Oxford.
It furthers the University's objective of excellence in research, scholarship,
and education by publishing worldwide in

Oxford New York

Athens Auckland Bangkok Bogotá Buenos Aires Calcutta
Cape Town Chennai Dar es Salaam Delhi Florence Hong Kong Istanbul
Karachi Kuala Lumpur Madrid Melbourne Mexico City Mumbai
Nairobi Paris São Paulo Singapore Taipei Tokyo Toronto Warsaw

with associated companies in Berlin Ibadan

Oxford is a registered trade mark of Oxford University Press
in the UK and in certain other countries

Published in the United States
by Oxford University Press Inc., New York

British Library Cataloguing in Publication Data

Data available

Library of Congress Cataloguing in Publication Data
Dickenson, Donna Lee, 1946–
   In two minds: a casebook of psychiatric ethics/Donna Dickenson and
   Bill (K. W. M.) Fulford; with additional material by Jim (J.L.T.) Birley; and
   a foreword by Sidney Bloch, Paul Chodoff, and Stephen A. Green (editors
   of the sister volume to this book, Psychiatric ethics)
      p.cm.—(Oxford medical publications)
   Includes bibliographical references
   1. Psychiatric ethics—Case studies. I. Fulford, K. W. M.
   II. Psychiatric ethics. III. Title. IV. Series
   RC455.2.E8 D535 200   174'.2—dc21   00–064987

1 3 5 7 9 10 8 6 4 2
ISBN 0-19-26-28-58-5

Typeset by J&L Composition Ltd, Filey, North Yorkshire
Printed in Great Britain
on acid-free paper by
Biddles Ltd, Guildford & King's Lynn

Foreword

As editors of the third edition of *Psychiatric Ethics*, we are pleased to offer this foreword to our companion volume, *In Two Minds: A Casebook of Psychiatric Ethics*. Over the roughly twenty years since publication of the first edition of *Psychiatric Ethics*, a number of factors have spurred an ever-growing attention to the increasing influence of ethical issues on clinical practice. Prominent among these are a shift in the doctor–patient relationship from a paternalistic model to one primarily based in patient autonomy, the women's movement and its emphasis on possible violations of the psychiatrist–patient relationship, and changes in the economics of medical practice throughout the world (such as declining mental health care budgets and the rise of managed care) that significantly influence the distribution of health resources.

The growing influence of ethical issues on psychiatric practice has been marked by numerous publications in the form of journal articles and books, none of which has undertaken the detailed, systematic presentation of a series of case histories that illustrates the various phases of the clinical encounter as is now offered by Dickenson and Fulford in this rich, informative volume. They skilfully explore and explicate the ethical basis of clinical decision making in difficult (though surprisingly common) circumstances: what the authors regard as the 'real problems with which real people — patients, carers, and professionals — struggle in day-to-day practice in psychiatry'.

The book begins with a thoughtful recounting of the theory and skills required for ethical reasoning and problem solving in psychiatric treatment. The emphasis is on how many treatment decisions turn on an interplay between questions of value and questions of fact. Since psychiatry is a particularly value-laden discipline, the authors argue that ethical considerations regularly influence clinical decisions, as for example, when the value of individual autonomy must be weighed against the value of involuntary treatment. Most medical specialties are generally concerned with areas of human experience and behaviour in which the values of practitioners and patients are largely shared and, consequently, less adversarial. However, unlike other specialties, psychiatric practice greatly demands balancing diverse values, and requires mental health professionals to enhance their clinical expertise with a facility for ethical reasoning and problem solving. The task is demanding, often complex, and sometimes daunting; thankfully, *In Two Minds* provides clinicians with invaluable guidance towards this end.

Dickenson and Fulford provide keen insight into analysing and negotiating difficult, though common, clinical situations by exploring the theoretical underpinnings which guide reasoned treatment decisions. Each chapter — a carefully constructed discussion of the interplay between theory and clinical practice — is supplemented by a valuable reading guide, as well as a wealth of references which merit particular praise. The net result is a volume which reminds the reader that good clinical practice rests on the ability to reconcile sometimes conflicting values in a reasoned, systematic manner.

In Two Minds is a book to be consulted with profit by psychiatrists and other mental health professionals throughout the world and at all stages of practice.

Sidney Bloch, Paul Chodoff, and Stephen Green
(Editors of *Psychiatric Ethics*)

Preface

This book is a response to the practical challenges of psychiatric ethics. This is why it is a *case*book. It explores psychiatric ethics primarily through a series of case histories. In order to preserve confidentiality the cases are heavily disguised biographically and based on different stories drawn from different locations. The *problems* described are not philosophical inventions, however. They are all real problems with which real people — patients, carers, and professionals — struggle in day-to-day practice in psychiatry.

The clinical focus of the book is reflected in its structure. Thus, it begins with introductory chapters on the special features of psychiatric ethics (Chapter 1) and on ethical reasoning in clinical practice (Chapter 2). But the core of the book is a series of detailed case studies. These are organized into chapters covering each stage of the clinical encounter — basic concepts (Chapter 3), diagnosis (Chapter 4), aetiology (Chapter 5), treatment (Chapter 6), prognosis (Chapter 7), and the organization of services (Chapter 8). Each chapter starts with an introductory overview of the main ethical and philosophical issues arising in that area of practice and ends with a detailed guide to further reading. Every case study includes a commentary by a practitioner working in the field.

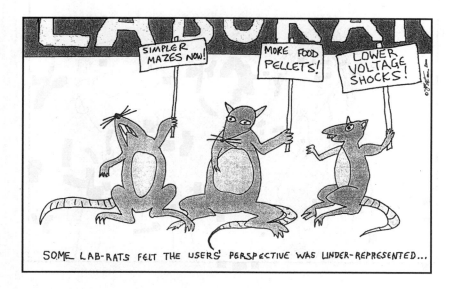

SOME LAB-RATS FELT THE USERS' PERSPECTIVE WAS UNDER-REPRESENTED...

The clinical chapters are followed by a section focusing on the practical aspects of teaching psychiatric ethics (Chapter 9) and on psychiatric research ethics (Chapter 10). In the final section, Jim Birley (Chapter 11), reflecting on the cases from his wide international experience, draws out the importance of an 'open society' for maintaining high standards of psychiatric care; and we conclude (Chapter 12) with a reflection on the significance of psychiatry as a 'window' on good practice in medicine generally.

The scope of the case studies which make up the central sections of the book may come as a surprise. Traditional bioethics, as it has developed mainly in response to the challenges of new medical technology, has been confined largely to issues of treatment choice. It covers problems such as patient autonomy, dual responsibility, and the distribution of resources. We will find that traditional bioethics can do useful work for us in psychiatry. A central theme of this book, however, is that ethical problems — defined generically as problems involving questions of value as well as questions of fact — are more pervasive and also deeper theoretically in psychiatry than in any other area of medicine.

Psychiatric ethics is difficult, therefore. It is difficult theoretically, and it is difficult practically. This should not lead to ethical paralysis, however! After

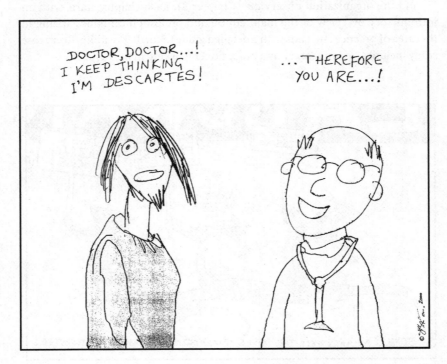

all, uncertainty is the norm in clinical practice. There is indeed nothing more dangerous in medicine than misplaced certainty, be it scientific or ethical. This is why our casebook is called *In Two Minds*. It is also why, although a *clinical* casebook, it draws on *philosophical* ideas more extensively than most standard textbooks of traditional bioethics. For the role of philosophy in medicine is not to provide ready-made answers but rather to give us a range of thinking skills which, in the pressures and perplexities of day-to-day practice, can help us to make up our minds in a clinically effective way. Such skills are important in any area of medicine. In psychiatry, they are the very basis of good clinical care.

Donna Dickenson
Bill Fulford
May 2000

About the authors

In Two Minds is the product of a long-term collaboration between its principal co-authors, Donna Dickenson and Bill Fulford. Donna Dickenson is Leverhulme Reader in Medical Ethics and Law, Imperial College, London. Apart from Case 4.3 and the commentaries on cases 5/1 and 5/2, Donna Dickenson wrote all the cases and case commentaries and the legal appendix. Bill Fulford is Professor of Philosophy and Mental Health, Department of Philosophy, University of Warwick and an Honorary Consultant Psychiatrist, Department of Psychiatry, University of Oxford. Bill Fulford wrote the introductory chapters 1 and 2, the introductions and reading guides to the clinical chapters 3 to 8, the chapters on education (9) and research (10), and the conclusions (chapter 12). Jim Birley is a past President both of the Royal College of Psychiatrists and of the British Medical Association. In chapter 11, on international aspects of psychiatric ethics, he draws on his experience as Honorary Chairman of the Geneva Initiative on Psychiatry. Jonny Cowee, the cartoonist, is a Senior Staff Nurse at the Warneford Hospital in Oxford and a recent MA graduate from Bill Fulford's programme in Philosophy, Ethics and Mental Health Practice at Warwick University.

Acknowledgements

The requirements of confidentiality mean that we are unable to thank individually the many colleagues, including users, informal carers, and professionals, who have made this book possible. We are indebted to those who have given us invaluable feedback on various sections of the book: Mark Bratton, Sue Chetwynd, Tony Colombo, Richard Ford, Mona Gupta, Tony Hope, Michael Rutter, and Tim Thornton. We are particularly grateful to Jennifer Radden for her detailed comments on the manuscript as a whole.

Our special thanks go to Michael Gelder who first suggested the need for a casebook in this most difficult of areas.

Some of the cases have been described elsewhere. We are grateful to Mike Jackson and the Johns Hopkins University Press for permission to reproduce Case 4.3. (First published in Jackson, M. and Fulford, K.W.M. (1997) 'Spiritual experience and psychopathology', *Philosophy, Psychiatry and Psychology*, **4/1**: 41–66.) A version of Case 6.3 was published by Donna Dickenson (1999) as 'Can children and young people consent to be tested for adult onset genetic disorders?', *BMJ*, **318**: 1063–5. Parts of Chapter 2 are based on materials from Module 2 of the distance learning version of Warwick University's MA/MSc in the Philosophy and Ethics of Mental Health. We are grateful to the members of the course team, Bill Fulford, Paul Sturdee, and Tim Thornton, for permission to reproduce them here.

Contents

Foreword *v*

Preface *vii*

Acknowledgements *xi*

Analytical table of contents *xv*

List of practitioner commentators *xxi*

Summary of reading guides *xxiv*

SECTION ONE **Introduction: the tools of the trade**

1 Theory and practice: the special features of psychiatric ethics *3*

2 Thinking skills: ethical reasoning and problem solving in psychiatric ethics *19*

SECTION TWO **Case studies in the clinical encounter**

3 Basic concepts: your myth or mine? *53*

CASE 3.1 Elizabeth Orton: does she have a mental illness at all? *58*

Practitioner commentary *65*

CASE 3.2 Tom Benbow: diagnosis and distributive justice *67*

Practitioner commentary *74*

4 Diagnosis: rationality, responsibility, and values in psychiatric classification *81*

CASE 4.1 Martin McKendrick: rational and irrational suicide *91*

Practitioner commentary *96*

CASE 4.2 Delia Jarrett: is the patient responsible for her behaviour? *98*

Practitioner commentary *105*

CASE 4.3 Simon Greer: schizophrenia or religious experience? *109*

Practitioner commentary *123*

5 Aetiology: causal and meaningful connections *133*

CASE 5.1 Jane Gillespie: agent and patient in depression *140*

Practitioner commentary *151*

CASE 5.2 Francesca Gindro: motivated self-deception or delusion? *155*

Practitioner commentary *166*

6 Treatment: trick or treat? *173*

   CASE 6.1 'Captain Ahab': dual role psychiatry *179*

   Practitioner commentary *186*

   CASE 6.2 Ida Harbottle: dementia, true wishes, and personal identity *188*

   Practitioner commentary *195*

   CASE 6.3 Robin and Alex: testing genetic testing *197*

   Practitioner commentary *208*

7 Prognosis: luck and judgement *219*

   CASE 7.1 Alan Masterson: clear and present danger? *226*

   Practitioner commentary *233*

   CASE 7.2 Philip Caversham: sense, nonsense, and supervision registers *237*

   Practitioner commentary *244*

8 Teamwork and the organization of services *253*

   CASE 8.1 Gilbert Ryan: tracking and tagging *259*

   Practitioner commentary *265*

   CASE 8.2 Sam Mason: the breakdown of a therapeutic alliance *267*

   Practitioner commentary *273*

SECTION THREE **Teaching and research**

9 Putting theory into practice: a sample teaching seminar *281*

10 The three Rs of research ethics *301*

SECTION FOUR **Wider perspectives**

11 Psychiatric ethics: an international open society (by Jim Birley) *327*

12 Conclusions: psychiatry first *335*

Notes *343*

Appendix: glossary of legal cases *347*

Alphabetical listing of all references *351*

Index *377*

Analytical table of contents

The book is divided into four main sections.

- **Section One** is introductory: it covers the scope and special features of psychiatric ethics (Chapter 1) and some of the main ways of reasoning about ethical problems (Chapter 2).

- **Section Two** is the longest section: it includes case histories taken from each of the main stages of the clinical encounter — basic concepts (Chapter 3), diagnosis (Chapter 4), aetiology (Chapter 5), treatment (Chapter 6), prognosis (Chapter 7), and teamwork and the organization of services (Chapter 8).

- **Section Three** looks at the practical applications of the case materials of Section II, in teaching (Chapter 9) and in writing/reviewing research ethics applications (Chapter 10).

- **Section Four** offers two overviews — of psychiatry in an international context (Chapter 11) and of the importance of psychiatric ethics for our understanding of good practice in medicine generally (Chapter 12).

- **Appendix** gives a glossary and guide to the legal cases referred to in the text.

SECTION ONE Introduction: the tools of the trade

This section outlines the scope of psychiatric ethics as both a practical and a theoretical discipline (Chapter 1). It then introduces the main ideas from ethical theory that will be used in the rest of the book (Chapter 2).

Chapter 1 Theory and practice: the special features of psychiatric ethics

The special features of psychiatric ethics are introduced. Psychiatric ethics is shown to be wider in scope than traditional bioethics, issues of value (as well as fact) arising in psychopathology and diagnosis as well as in treatment choice. It is also deeper philosophically in that it includes general philosophical problems such as personal identity, rationality, and determinism. Psychiatry is thereby no less scientific than other areas of medicine. Indeed, the proper role of ethics in psychiatry is to facilitate rather than frustrate good science. But what all this amounts to is that clinical problem solving in psychiatric ethics requires even sharper thinking skills than in other areas of bioethics.

Reading Guide — General introductions to philosophy; the philosophy of mind; the philosophy of science; the philosophy of psychiatry.

Chapter 2 Thinking skills: ethical reasoning and problem solving in psychiatric ethics

The thinking skills required for clinical problem solving in psychiatric ethics are introduced through an extended analysis of the case history of Mr Able, a man with depression who is treated on an involuntary basis under the Mental Health Act. The relevant skills are both generic and specific. Generic skills include good communication and an understanding of medical law; specific skills include the varieties of ethical reasoning — bioethical (for example, principles, casuistry, and perspectives), general ethical (deontological and utilitarian), and analytic (concerned with underlying conceptual issues). Ethical reasoning is not an algorithm for solving problems. It deepens understanding, improves communication, and helps us to act decisively in conditions of clinical uncertainty.

Reading Guide — General ethical theory; medical ethics and bioethics; psychiatric ethics; involuntary psychiatric treatment.

SECTION TWO Case studies in the clinical encounter

Traditional bioethics has concentrated on problems arising in treatment (consent, resource allocation, and so on). In psychiatry, as shown in Chapter 1, ethical problems (that is, problems involving judgements of value as well as of fact) arise at all stages of the clinical encounter. Hence, the case histories described and analysed in this section cover each stage of the clinical encounter, from basic concepts of mental disorder (Chapter 3) and diagnosis (Chapter 4), through aetiology (Chapter 5), to treatment (Chapter 6), prognosis (Chapter 7), and the organization of services (Chapter 8).

Chapter 3 Basic concepts: your myth or mine?

The debate in the 1960s and 1970s about the validity of mental illness was polarized between psychiatrists arguing that mental illness is *no* different from physical illness and antipsychiatrists holding that mental illness is *so* different from physical illness that it is really a moral rather than medical concept. The two cases described in this chapter show that the tension between these two models of mental disorder, although nowadays less overt, remains important in practice. A narrowly medical model of mental disorder is vulnerable to both overuse (Case 3.1, Elizabeth Orton) and underuse (Case 3.2, Tom Benbow). Some of the considerations that can help us to avoid either extreme are reviewed.

Reading Guide — Models of disorder; abusive uses of psychiatry; models of disorder and current practice.

Chapter 4 Diagnosis: rationality, responsibility, and values in psychiatric classification

Three of the many ways in which diagnosis may be ethically problematic in psychiatry are illustrated in this chapter, in relation to the rationality or otherwise of suicidal wishes (Case 4.1, Martin McKendrick), in the context of seriously irresponsible behaviour (Case 4.2, Delia Jarrett), and in distinguishing between psychosis and religious experience (Case 4.3, Simon Greer). Case 4.3 illustrates directly the central place of value judgements in the diagnosis of mental disorders.

Reading Guide — Responsibility; rationality; values in psychiatric classification and diagnosis.

Chapter 5 Aetiology: causal and meaningful connections

The title of this chapter consciously echoes an early paper by one of the founders of modern scientific psychiatry, Karl Jaspers, in which he spelled out the need for understanding meanings as well as attributing causes in psychiatry. We might think that with developments in neuroscience (brain scanning, the 'new' genetics, and so on) this is no longer true. Case 5.1, Jane Gillespie, shows that it is still true at least for depression. Case 5.2, Francesca Gindro, shows that it is still true for the psychotic disorders that Jaspers had in mind.

Reading Guide — Causes and meanings.

Chapter 6 Treatment: trick or treat?

As in other areas of medicine, involuntary psychiatric treatment (treatment without the patient's consent) is justified, essentially, on grounds of the patient's 'best interests'. Involuntary psychiatric treatment is covered in detail in Chapter 2. In this chapter we examine two particular kinds of problem which arise with the concept of best interests in psychiatry — problems of dual role (Case 6.1, Captain Ahab) and problems of establishing the patient's true wishes (Case 6.2, Ida Harbottle). Case 6.3 (Robin and Alex) illustrates the importance of these issues in child and adolescent psychiatry.

Reading Guide — Autonomy (recent approaches); capacity; competence and consent; personal identity.

Chapter 7 Prognosis: luck and judgement

The ongoing clinical responsibilities of psychiatrists in circumstances in which they have few powers of prediction, let alone control, raise some of the most contentious ethical issues in contemporary psychiatry. This chapter explores some of these issues. It draws in part on recent work in philosophy on what has become known as the 'paradox of moral luck' — that luck as well as judgement is endemic to responsible action in all areas of human activity.

Reading Guide — Predicting dangerous behaviour (ethical aspects); confidentiality; moral luck.

Chapter 8 Teamwork and the organization of services

Teamwork is an essential foundation of community psychiatric care. Besides offering a range of treatment skills, a well-functioning multidisciplinary team provides a range of value perspectives, essential for a balanced view of many of the ethical dilemmas described in earlier chapters. Here we describe two cases — one in which teamwork broke down; one in which it was at least partly successful.

Reading Guide — Professional ethics and the role of codes; resource issues.

SECTION THREE Teaching and research

This section pulls together some of the ideas developed in our case histories in relation to teaching (Chapter 9) and to research ethics (Chapter 10).

Chapter 9 Putting theory into practice: a sample teaching seminar

In this chapter we revisit our first case, Elizabeth Orton, in the context of a teaching seminar. This shows how the specifically ethical analysis of the problem given in Chapter 3 can be integrated with the other knowledge and skills required for problem solving at the clinical 'coalface'. Presented in the form of a seminar, the chapter doubles as one model for teaching psychiatric ethics.

Reading Guide — Sources and resources for teaching psychiatric ethics.

Chapter 10 The three Rs of research ethics

The 'three Rs' of research ethics, like the 'three Rs' at school, are reading, writing, and arithmetic. Presented in the form of an extended case study, this chapter aims to set out the skills required for reading and/or writing a research ethics application. The third R (arithmetic, or statistics) reminds us that ethical and technical aspects of good research design go hand in hand in psychiatry.

Reading Guide — Research ethics.

SECTION FOUR Wider perspectives

In this final section, the ideas and principles developed in the book are set in wider contexts — international (Chapter 11), and in relation to other areas of science and medicine (Chapter 12).

Chapter 11 **Psychiatric ethics: an international open society (by Jim Birley)**

Jim Birley draws on his wide international experience of clinical and public policy issues in psychiatry to draw out a number of lessons from the cases described in this book. The key theme that emerges is that good practice in psychiatry depends on the balance of different perspectives which is provided through an international 'open society'.

Chapter 12 **Conclusions: psychiatry first**

Because psychiatric ethics is more difficult than other areas of medical ethics, we have had to go 'beyond bioethics' in this book — in scope, in philosophical depth, in partnership with science, and, importantly, in integrating ethical reasoning with other clinical practice skills. In each of these areas psychiatry offers a 'window' on good practice in medicine as a whole.

List of practitioner commentators

CASE 3.1 Elizabeth Orton *Commentator:* **John Vile**

John Vile is a consultant in psychiatric rehabilitation and Senior Lecturer at the University of Kent, with a special interest in psychiatric ethics and the relationship of mental 'illness' to other psychological states.

CASE 3.2 Tom Benbow *Commentator:* **John Morgan**

John Morgan is currently working as Consultant Psychiatrist in Learning Disabilities and Medical Director of Oxfordshire Learning Disability NHS Trust. He has been interested in ethical issues in this field for several years and has written and lectured on this topic.

CASE 4.1 Martin McKendrick *Commentator:* **Sally Burgess**

Sally Burgess is a specialist registrar in psychiatry. She has published work on treatment outcomes for adolescents who attempt suicide and a clinician's perspective of bioethical issues relating to suicide, assisted suicide, and euthanasia in psychiatric patients.

CASE 4.2 Delia Jarrett *Commentator:* **David Osborn**

David Osborn is an MRC clinical research fellow and Honorary Specialist Registrar in General Adult Psychiatry working in London, whose clinical duties involve regular Mental Health Act assessment work. He also has an academic interest in competence/capacity and its relation to psychiatric conditions and diagnoses.

CASE 4.3 Simon Greer *Commentator:* **Mike Jackson**

Mike Jackson is a clinical psychologist in North Wales, specializing in cognitive therapy for psychoses. His doctoral research focused on the relationship between psychosis and spiritual experience, and the case of Simon is taken from this study.

CASE 5.1 Jane Gillespie *Commentator:* Jeremy Holmes

Jeremy Holmes is a consultant psychotherapist and psychiatrist in North Devon. He is currently Chair of the Psychotherapy Faculty of the Royal College of Psychiatrists. He is co-author, among many other texts, of *The Values of Psychotherapy*.

CASE 5.2 Francesca Gindro *Commentator:* Bob Hinshelwood

Bob Hinshelwood is a psychoanalyst, and currently Professor in the Centre for Psychoanalytic Studies, University of Essex, UK. He published *Therapy or Coercion: Does Psychoanalysis Differ from Brainwashing?* in 1997, and has a particular interest in the ethical implications of counter-transference in clinical work, and beyond.

CASE 6.1 Captain Ahab *Commentator:* Philip Robson

Philip Robson is Consultant Psychiatrist and Senior Clinical Lecturer in Oxford, and for ten years has run the regional drug dependency service. He is also active in research: the second edition of his book *Forbidden Drugs* was published by OUP in 1999.

CASE 6.2 Ida Harbottle *Commentator:* Julian Hughes

Julian Hughes is a consultant in old age psychiatry, Honorary Clinical Lecturer at Newcastle, and a research fellow at the Oxford Centre for Ethics and Communication in Health Care Practice (ETHOX). His recently completed PhD thesis at Warwick uses Wittgenstein's philosophy to understand dementia.

CASE 6.3 Robin and Alex *Commentator:* Hilary Henderson

Hilary Henderson is a consultant child psychiatrist. She gained experience in paediatrics, general practice, and rehabilitation prior to specializing in psychiatry, and has a long-standing interest in children and young people's resilience in adversity.

CASE 7.1 Alan Masterson *Commentator:* Gwen Adshead

Gwen Adshead is a consultant psychiatrist at the Traumatic Stress Clinic, Middlesex Hospital, and Consultant Forensic Psychotherapist at Broadmoor

Hospital. She has a Master's Degree in Medical Law and Ethics, and has a particular interest in how interpersonal relationships affect how we understand values and virtues, and how this in turn affects ethical reasoning. As a clinician and researcher, her work brings her regularly into contact with victims and perpetrators of violence.

CASE 7.2 Philip Caversham *Commentator:* Dominic Beer

Dominic Beer works as a senior lecturer and as Honorary Consultant Psychiatrist in a secure setting, with mentally ill patients who exhibit challenging and antisocial behaviours. His aim is to help patients modify the behaviour which has led them to be detained under the Mental Health Act, so that they can ultimately return to the community in a safe and supported way.

CASE 8.1 Gilbert Ryan *Commentator:* Catherine Oppenheimer

Catherine Oppenheimer is a consultant in old age psychiatry, and Medical Director of the Oxfordshire Mental Healthcare NHS Trust. She is particularly interested in long-term care and in ethical issues in old age.

CASE 8.2 Sam Mason *Commentator:* David Foreman

David Foreman is a senior lecturer in child and adolescent psychiatry with a particular interest in philosophical medical ethics. He has published papers both on the theory of consent in children, and on how consent is actually obtained in child and adolescent psychiatry clinics.

Summary of
reading guides

CHAPTER 1 – **Theory and Practice: The Special Features of Psychiatric Ethics**
- General introductions to philosophy
- The philosophy of mind
- The philosophy of science
- The philosophy of psychiatry

CHAPTER 2 – **Thinking Skills: Ethics and Psychiatry**
- General ethical theory
- Medical and bio-ethics
- Psychiatric ethics
- Involuntary psychiatric treatment

CHAPTER 3 – **Basic Concepts: Your Myth or Mine?**
- Models of disorder
- Abusive uses of psychiatry
- Models of disorder and current practice

CHAPTER 4 – **Diagnosis: Rationality, Responsibility, and Values in Psychiatric Classification**
- Responsibility
- Rationality
- Values in psychiatric diagnosis and classification

CHAPTER 5 – **Aetiology: Causal and Meaningful Connections**
- Causes and meanings

CHAPTER 6 – **Treatment: Trick or Treat?**
- Autonomy, capacity, competence and consent
- Autonomy: recent approaches
- Personal identity

CHAPTER 7 – **Prognosis: Luck and Judgement**
- Predicting dangerous behaviour (ethical aspects)
- Confidentiality
- Moral luck

CHAPTER 8 – **Teamwork and the Organisation of Services**
- Professional ethics and the role of codes
- Resource issues

CHAPTER 9 – **Putting Theory into Practice:**
A Sample Teaching Seminar
- Sources and resources for teaching psychiatric ethics

CHAPTER 10 – **The Three R's of Research Ethics**
- Research ethics

Introduction: the tools of the trade

Theory and practice: the special features of psychiatric ethics

Psychiatry is something of an ethical paradox[1]. It is deeply value-laden, so much so that its critics, like the American professor of psychiatry, Thomas Szasz, have argued that it is a moral rather than a medical discipline (Szasz 1960, 1987). Even some supporters regard it as a primitive or pre-scientific branch of medical science (Boorse 1975, 1976). Despite being so value-laden, however, psychiatry has been largely the 'blind spot' of bioethics, as one of us has described it elsewhere (Fulford 1993). There are important exceptions, of course, notably the sister volume to this book, Sidney Bloch, Paul Chodoff, and Stephen Green's *Psychiatric Ethics* (1999). The first edition of *Psychiatric Ethics*, published in 1981, was a trail-blazer for the subject.

Psychiatric Ethics is a scholarly textbook. This book by contrast is a *casebook*; it is concerned with practical problem solving. In order to meet the practical challenges of psychiatric ethics, however, we need to enlarge on the agenda of traditional bioethics. Whilst we draw extensively on bioethical sources, we also go beyond bioethics:

1 in the scope of the clinical topics with which we are concerned;

2 in the extent to which we draw on the philosophical theory underpinning ethics;

3 in the closeness of the relationships we find between ethical and scientific aspects of psychiatry; and

4 in the degree to which the skills of ethical reasoning, with which we are primarily concerned, have to be integrated with other practice skills as the basis of good clinical care.

We will look briefly at each of these extensions of traditional bioethics by way of setting the scene.

1 The scope of psychiatric ethics

Bioethics has developed primarily in response to the challenges of biotechnology (Fulford 1993). It has thus been concerned principally with issues of treatment choice in high-tech areas of medicine — transplant surgery (who gets the liver?), assisted reproduction (who gets the baby?), research ethics (who gets the placebo?), end-of-life issues (who gets to live?), the distribution of costly resources (who gets anything at all!).

These are important issues — literally important in that they turn on questions of *value*. One of the big issues for bioethics has been to shift the balance of health care decision making from the values of professionals, as the providers of health care, to the values of patients and carers, as the users of services. This shift, from paternalism as it used to be called (its 'pc' translation is 'parentalism') to patient autonomy, is a big issue for psychiatry too. Involuntary psychiatric treatment (who gets ECT whether they like it or not?) is ethically problematic precisely in that it involves a direct conflict of values between the patient and others. We will be looking at involuntary treatment in detail in Chapter 2. In psychiatry, though, values are important not just in treatment but in every part of the clinical process: in the personal and social values by which our basic concepts of mental disorder are (partly) defined; in the biases (particularly culture- and gender-based) built into the diagnostic process; in how we come to understand meaningful as well as causal explanations of people's experiences and behaviour (aetiology); and in judgements of dangerousness and other aspects of prognosis.

Whilst most bioethics books are arranged according to 'issues', the organization of this casebook reflects the pervasiveness of questions of value in psychiatry[2]. Thus our cases are organized around the stages of the clinical 'process': basic concepts — defining the proper scope of psychiatry (Chapter 3); diagnosis (Chapter 4); aetiology (Chapter 5); treatment (Chapter 6 and also covered in Chapter 2); prognosis (Chapter 7); and teamwork and the organization of services (Chapter 8). Chapter 9 revisits one of the cases discussed in Chapter 3 in the context of a teaching seminar and Chapter 10 examines a further case study in research ethics.

The pervasiveness of questions of value in psychiatry might seem to support the claims of those who believe that psychiatry is, at best a primitive branch of medical science, at worst a moral rather than a medical discipline. Closer inspection, however, shows that the value-ladenness of psychiatry reflects something deeply important about human beings, namely that in the areas of experience and behaviour with which psychiatry is concerned *human values are highly diverse.*

The theoretical basis for this way of understanding the relatively value-laden nature of psychiatry is to be found primarily in the work of the Oxford philosophers, R.M. Hare (1952 and 1963), J.O. Urmson (1950) and G.J. Warnock (1971), on the logical properties (the meanings and implications) of value terms. This may sound rather dull and dry! In fact, it has important practical implications for psychiatry[3]. We need not be concerned here with the details of this work. The link between human values and the value-laden nature of psychiatry follows straightforwardly from two broad points about value terms. We will describe these points briefly and then indicate their relevance to psychiatry.

1 *Value terms carry factual as well as evaluative meaning.* If I say of an apple that it is a 'good eating apple', this expresses the value judgement that the apple in question is good to eat. This is the evaluative meaning of 'good eating apple'. But in saying this I am also implying certain facts about the apple, that it is, say, clean-skinned, fairly sweet, and grub-free. These facts are the criteria by which I judge the apple in question to be a good eating apple. You can think of any number of examples along these lines. They all show that any value term, used in a real situation, carries two elements of meaning:

- an *evaluative element* (the value judgement expressed) and

- a *factual* element (the factual criteria for the value judgement).

2 *Value terms which express shared values may come to look like factual terms.* Most people like their eating apples to be clean-skinned, fairly sweet, and grub-free. In this sense our values in respect of eating apples are shared values; we have (broadly) the same factual criteria for what is a good eating apple. The result is that these factual criteria become stuck by association to the value term 'good' used of eating apples. 'Good eating apple' may thus end up being used to *describe* an apple as being clean-skinned, fairly sweet, and grub-free. This is quite different from cases in which our values are *not* shared. 'Good picture', for example, means very different things to different people. Therefore, there is no commonality of factual criteria for good pictures, there is no consistent factual meaning, and hence 'good' as applied to pictures remains an overtly value-laden value term.

We can see that 'good eating apple' is doing more than just describing an apple; it is also evaluating it as a good apple to eat. The point is that where our values are shared in this way, the association of the factual criteria with the use of the value term may be so strong that we forget about the evaluative meaning and focus on the factual meaning. This is how the value term ends up looking like a factual term — even though it is not. So the bottom line is that:

- *shared* values = *fact*-laden uses of value terms

- *diverse* values = *value*-laden uses of value terms

Now, what is the relevance of this to psychiatry? The broad point is that, in being relatively value-laden, psychiatry stands in relation to physical medicine much as 'good picture' stands in relation to 'good eating apple'. According to the medical model, you will recall, physical medicine is relatively value-free because it is more 'scientific'. According to antipsychiatry, psychiatry is rela-

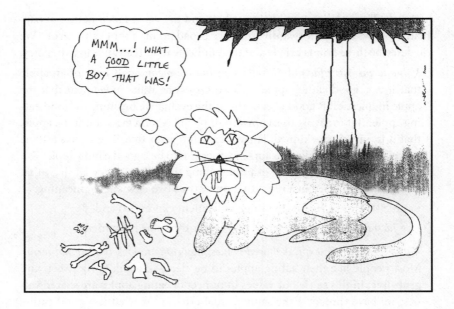

tively value-laden because it is a moral rather than a medical discipline. The 'Oxford' work on the logical properties of value terms suggests that both are wrong. As Fig. 1.1 shows, the difference between physical medicine and psychiatry in this respect is a direct reflection of the fact that *physical medicine* is concerned with areas of human experience and behaviour in which our values are (largely) *shared,* whereas *psychiatry* is concerned with areas of human experience and behaviour in which our values are (largely) *diverse.*

The language of science gives us a neat way of summing up the difference between physical medicine and psychiatry in this respect — whereas values are (largely) a *constant* in physical medicine, in psychiatry they are (largely) a *variable.*

Thus, a painful stubbed toe, nausea, collapse, paralysis, and so on, as conditions characteristically diagnosed in physical medicine, are all *bad* conditions for *anyone.* Here our values are shared. Hence the value judgements involved in diagnosing such conditions, although important in theory, can be and are ignored in practice because there is no disagreement over them. Hence physical medicine, in so far as it is concerned with such conditions, appears value-free. But psychiatry is concerned with areas of human experience and behaviour such as motivation, affect, wish, desire, and belief — areas in which our values are typically *not* shared and are indeed, characteristically and legitimately, *diverse.* Hence there is often disagreement over questions of value in psychiatry, though, as we will see in later chapters (for example,

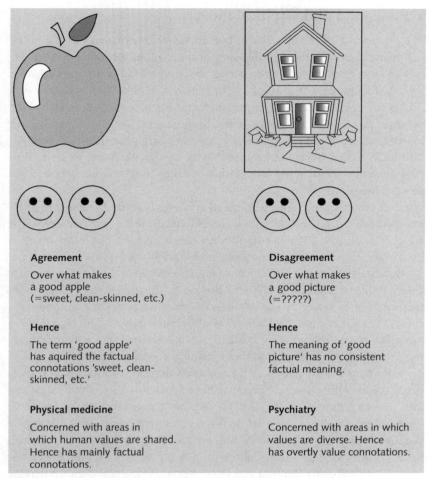

Agreement

Over what makes
a good apple
(=sweet, clean-skinned, etc.)

Hence

The term 'good apple'
has aquired the factual
connotations 'sweet, clean-
skinned, etc.'

Physical medicine

Concerned with areas in
which human values are shared.
Hence has mainly factual
connotations.

Disagreement

Over what makes
a good picture
(=?????)

Hence

The meaning of 'good
picture' has no consistent
factual meaning.

Psychiatry

Concerned with areas in which
values are diverse. Hence
has overtly value connotations.

Figure 1.1 Apples, pictures, physical medicine and pyschiatry. Most people agree that a good apple is one which is sweet, clean-skinned, etc. It is for this reason that the term 'good apple', although expressing a value judgement, conveys the *factual* meaning 'sweet, clean-skinned, etc'. But there is no corresponding agreement about what makes a good picture. Hence, in the absence of a stable factual meaning, the term 'good picture' remains clearly *value*-laden. It is for similar reasons that in health care, the term 'physical illness' is relatively fact-laden and 'mental illness' relatively value-laden (see also text).

case 4.3, Simon Greer), part of the problem is that such disagreements are often not recognized for what they are. In contrast to physical medicine, then, the value judgements involved in psychiatry *cannot* be ignored and psychiatry thus remains an overtly value-laden discipline.

2 Ethics and philosophical theory

The importance of the diversity of human values in psychiatry is one of the key themes that runs through this book and we will be returning to it repeatedly in later chapters. Given the pervasiveness of ethical issues in psychiatry, though, the question that arises is why bioethics should have neglected psychiatry for so long? Well, one important factor has been the dominance of the medical model (Fulford 1993). It has been assumed, by those involved in bioethics as much as in biomedicine, that psychiatry is an 'also ran' to physical medicine and hence that the problems, be they scientific or ethical, to which psychiatry is heir, will be solved in due time by techniques derived from physical medicine.

In fact though, whilst ethical problems are never easy to solve, those in physical medicine are relatively *tractable* compared with those in psychiatry which are of an altogether different magnitude. Consequently, in psychiatry we often have to dig deep into the philosophical underpinnings of ethics.

Involuntary treatment (to which we return in Chapter 2) is a case in point. The standard bioethical analysis of the ethical justification of involuntary treatment is in terms of loss of the capacities necessary for autonomous choice (Beauchamp and Childress 1994). This approach is based on paradigm examples drawn from physical medicine, such as unconscious patients requiring immediate life-saving procedures. Someone who is unconscious clearly does not have the capacities for making the voluntary and informed choices necessary for valid consent. The capacities approach is also helpful in psychiatry, up to a point — it works well for 'organic' conditions such as dementia, for example, in which there are well-defined impairments of the cognitive functions (orientation, memory, and so on). But the capacities approach breaks down altogether for other cases, notably the non-organic psychoses such as schizophrenia (Fulford and Hope 1993), for medical decision making involving children (Dickenson and Jones 1995), and for consent to psychotherapy (Hinshelwood 1997). The reason for this, as we will see in Chapter 2, is essentially that the concept of 'capacity', on which the standard bioethical analysis of involuntary treatment is based, although widely taken to be relatively transparent in physical medicine is often itself the very *nub* of the problem in psychiatry.

Time and again in this book, the tools of standard bioethics — principles, rights and duties, perspectives, casuistic (case-based) reasoning, and so forth — do much useful work for us. We will be introducing some of these bioethical tools in the next chapter. Their importance is not least because psychiatry, like physical medicine, is increasingly an area of technological advance — the new genetics, psychopharmacology, and dynamic brain imaging, for example, are all raising new ethical problems in psychiatry much as in other areas of medicine new ethical problems have been raised by, for example, assisted reproduction and transplant surgery (Gindro and Mordini 1998).

But in psychiatry, besides all the standard bioethical issues, we have a whole series of conceptual difficulties as well. 'Capacity', as just noted, is highly problematic in psychiatry. So too, however, are the concepts of 'rationality' and 'responsibility' (notably in forensic psychiatry), 'voluntariness' (as with obsessional symptoms, for example), 'intention' (as in hysteria), 'compulsion' (as in the addictions), 'personal identity' (as in dementia), 'true belief' (in delusion), and, not least, 'mental disorder' itself.

The special skill of philosophers is in working with concepts and with the meanings and implications of words and ideas which are problematic in one way or another. Besides making contributions from value theory, then, philosophers should be able to help us in psychiatry more generally with the conceptual difficulties underlying practical ethics. Indeed many of the concepts mentioned (intention, personal identity, and true belief, for instance) are already high on the philosophical agenda.

If philosophy is important to practical psychiatry, however, this is not to say that science is thereby *un*important. On the contrary, the purpose of this book is to 'add value' not to 'subtract facts'. In this respect, the model of medicine developed here and illustrated in Fig. 1.2 is quite different both from the traditional medical–scientific model and from antipsychiatry. The medical model, in so far as it construes the theoretical basis of medicine in 'purely' scientific terms, is a fact-only model[4]: ethics comes in, but only peripherally. Antipsychiatry, on the other hand, in so far as it construes mental disorders as moral rather than medical problems, is a value-only model. Work in the Oxford analytic tradition in ethics (the Hare–Urmson–Warnock work already referred to) gives us a balanced model — a 'fact + value' model — in which ethics is a partner to science. This brings us to the third respect in which psychiatric ethics goes beyond bioethics.

3 Ethics and science

Given the origins of bioethics as a response to biotechnology, it is perhaps not surprising that bioethicists have sometimes perceived themselves as a kind of ethical police force, safeguarding vulnerable patients from the predations of medical science. A respected bioethicist, at a recent meeting in the USA, defined their role as 'moral gatekeepers' (Fulford, personal communication). In bioethics, indeed, many of the big questions have been about setting limits — *what* should be allowed, *how far* should we go, *where* should we draw the line? Should a woman of 60 (or 55 or 50) be allowed to have a baby? Should we

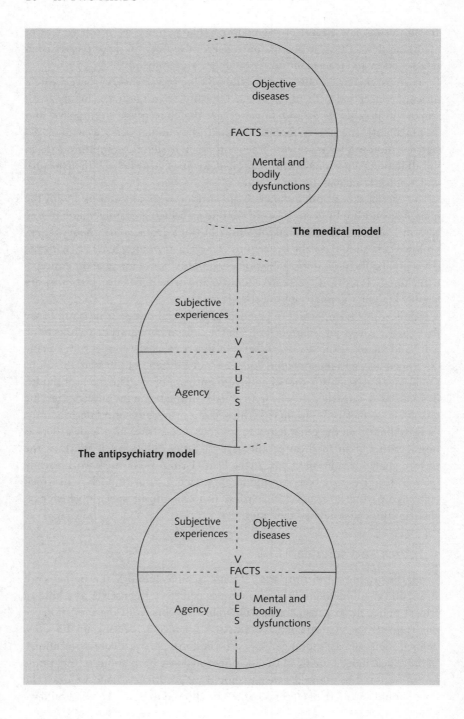

The medical model

The antipsychiatry model

wait 1 year (or 2 or 2½) before we switch off life support for a young person in a coma?

There is certainly a need for vulnerable people to be protected in some areas of psychiatry. Paul Chodoff's review of recent abuses of psychiatry provides sufficient evidence of this (Chodoff 1999). In psychiatry, though, what is needed from ethicists and philosophers is not so much policing as partnership. This follows directly from the diversity of human values in the areas with which psychiatry is concerned. If, as already noted, questions of value are 'part of the problem' in psychiatry, and if philosophers have a role to play in tackling such questions, then the relationship between practitioners and philosophers should be like that between practitioners and scientists. Psychiatrists need to work in partnership with biochemists, with pharmacologists, and so on, to help them solve problems in clinical practice and research. The diversity of values with which psychiatrists are concerned shows that they also need to work in partnership with philosophers and ethicists.

The 'ethical police' model has been particularly evident in research ethics. In research there is a clear need for independent review. As we will see in more detail in Chapter 10, this is because a key difference between research and clinical work lies in the degree of direct responsibility of doctors and researchers. In clinical work, everything a doctor does should normally be with the best interests of his or her particular patients in mind. Researchers, by contrast, are motivated primarily by the aim of advancing knowledge. Hence independent review, by a well-balanced research ethics committee, is an essential safeguard (for researchers as well as research subjects) against the general interest we all have in the advance of knowledge being allowed to subvert the interests of the individuals participating in research. But the role of the research ethics committee, nevertheless, should be as much to facilitate good research as to prevent bad, otherwise we may be in danger of killing the goose that lays the golden eggs! It would be a sad irony indeed if ethical concerns about the *misuses* of science in medicine ended up obstructing scientific *advance*. We have as much right to good science in psychiatry as in any other area of medicine.

4 Ethics and practice skills

The message of this chapter, and indeed of this book, is that psychiatry is a good deal more *complex* than other areas of medicine: we have to face questions

Figure 1.2 (opposite) A 'fact + value' model of psychiatry. The 'medical' model, emphasising the factual element in medicine, is a half-field view. The 'anti-psychiatry' model, emphasising the evaluative element (mental disorders being regarded as moral or life problems), is also a half-field view. Both models are thus not so much mistaken as blind to the importance of one or other element in the meanings of the medical concepts. In psychiatry good practice depends on being fully aware of both elements.

of value as well as questions of fact, head on; our everyday work raises deep conceptual difficulties, some of which (like 'voluntariness' and 'true belief') have occupied the sharpest intellects for over 2000 years; and scientifically, our research area — the higher mental functions — is at the very frontier of scientific difficulty.

One response to this, a maladaptive response, is to throw in the sponge. The renewed stigmatization of mental disorder, by press and politicians alike, is putting psychiatry at risk of developing a depressive posture of 'learned helplessness'! Another response, an adaptive response, is to develop new skills. The particular difficulty of clinical work in psychiatry means that our practice skills — the skills required to apply our expert knowledge in practice — have to be that much sharper than in other areas of medicine. All the genuinely scientific skills required for clinical problem solving (eliciting symptoms and signs, understanding causes, and so on) are as important in psychiatry as in any other branch of medicine. But the diversity of values and other conceptual difficulties, in the areas of experience and behaviour with which psychiatry is concerned, mean that a range of further skills are essential as well. Some of these are generic (summarized in Table 1.1); others are specific. They include the skills of ethical reasoning. It is to these that we turn in Chapter 2.

Table 1.1 Generic thinking skills important in psychiatry. Ethical reasoning is not separate from other clinical skills. It is a key practice skill which should be fully integrated with the wide range of thinking skills on which good clinical and research practice depend.

Awareness of
- different values/beliefs
- many paradigms of disorder
- value-ladenness of all aspects of practice (e.g. diagnosis)

Understanding of
- patients' perspectives
- other professionals

Tolerance of
- diversity
- complexity
- the unsolvable
- uncertainty

Knowledge of
- legal principles, ethical guidelines
- empirical findings (e.g. on communication skills)
- sources/resources

Reasoning skills including
- ability to analyse the ethical/conceptual aspects of practice, research, and teaching
- clear presentation of difficult ideas
- flexible, adaptive thinking (problem solving)
- critical appraisal of research design

References

Beauchamp, T.L. and Childress, J.F. (1994) *Principles of Biomedical Ethics* (4th edn). (1st edn, 1989). Oxford, Oxford University Press.

Bloch, S. and Chodoff, P. (1981) *Psychiatric Ethics* (1st edn). Oxford, Oxford University Press.

Bloch, S., Chodoff, P., and Green S.A. (1999) *Psychiatric Ethics* (3rd edn). Oxford, Oxford University Press.

Boorse, C. (1975) On the distinction between disease and illness. *Philosophy and Public Affairs*, 5: 49–68.

Boorse, C. (1976) What a theory of mental health should be. *Journal of Theory Social Behaviour*, 6:61–84.

Chodoff, P. (1999) Misuse and abuse of psychiatry: an overview. In *Psychiatric Ethics* (3rd edn) (ed. Bloch, S., Chodoff, P., and Green, S.), Chapter 4. Oxford, Oxford University Press.

Dickenson, D. and Jones, D. (1995) True wishes: The philosophy and developmental psychology of children's informed consent. *Philosophy, Psychiatry, and Psychology*, 2:287–304.

Fulford, K.W.M. (1989, reprinted 1995; 2nd edn forthcoming) *Moral Theory and Medical Practice*. Cambridge, Cambridge University Press.

Fulford, K.W.M. (1990) Philosophy and medicine: the Oxford connection. *British Journal of Psychiatry*, 157:111–15. Reprinted in translation in 1995 as 'Filosofin och läkekonsten: förbindelsen över Oxford' in *Begrepp om Hälsa. Filosofiska och etiska perspectiv på livskvalitet, hälsa och vård* (*Concepts of Health. Philosophical and Ethical Perspectives on Quality of Life, Health and Care*) (translated by Utbildning L.) (ed. Klockers, C. and Österman, B.), Chapter 7. Stockholm (Sweden), Liber Utbildning.

Fulford, K.W.M. (1993) Bioethical blind spots: four flaws in the field of view of traditional bioethics. *Health Care Analysis*, 1:155–62.

Fulford, K.W.M. and Bloch, S. (forthcoming). Psychiatric ethics: codes, concepts and clinical practice skills. In *New Oxford Textbook of Psychiatry* (ed. Gelder, M., Andreasen, N., and Lopez–Ibor, J.), Chapter 17. Oxford, Oxford University Press.

Fulford, K.W.M. and Hope, R.A. (1993) Psychiatric ethics: a bioethical ugly duckling? In *Principles of Health Care Ethics* (ed. Gillon, R. and Lloyd, A.), Chapter 58. Chichester (England): John Wiley and Sons.

Gindro, S. and Mordini, E. (1998) Ethical, legal and social issues in brain research. *Current Opinion in Psychiatry*, 11:575–80.

Hare, R.M. (1952) *The Language of Morals*. Oxford University Press.

Hare, R.M. (1963) Descriptivism. *Proceedings of the British Academy*, 49:115–34. Reprinted in 1972 in *Essays on the Moral Concepts*. London, The Macmillan Press Ltd.

Hinshelwood, R.D. (1995) The social relocation of personal identity as shown by psychoanalytic observations of splitting, projection and introjection. *Philosophy, Psychiatry, and Psychology,* **2**:185–204.

Szasz, T.S. (1960) The myth of mental illness. *American Psychologist,* **15**: 113–18.

Szasz, T.S. (1987) *Insanity: The Idea and Its Consequences.* Chichester (England): John Wiley and Sons.

Urmson, J.O. (1950) On grading. *Mind,* **59**:145–69.

Warnock, G.J. (1971) *The Object of Morality.* London, Methuen & Co. Ltd.

Reading Guide

After a long period of mutual neglect there has been a recent flood of books and articles on philosophy and psychiatry. Besides ethics, the main contributors to the philosophy of psychiatry are philosophy of mind and philosophy of science, although many other areas of philosophy are also relevant. We include here introductory readings on the philosophy of mind, the philosophy of science, and the philosophy of psychiatry. Ethics is covered in the Reading Guide at the end of the next chapter. Further reading on particular philosophical areas relevant to psychiatry will be given in later chapters (for example, personal identity in Chapter 6).

General introductions to philosophy

A very readable brief introduction to philosophy is *What does it all mean? A Very Short Introduction to Philosophy* (1987) by Thomas Nagel. This covers the main themes in modern philosophy for the 'complete beginner' in 100 pages! Slightly more extended is Martin Hollis' *Invitation to Philosophy* (1985) — simultaneously lively and deep, no mean achievement. Anthony O'Hear's *What Philosophy Is* (1985) gives a more formal account. An edited volume with contributions from a wide range of philosophers on each of the main problems of philosophy (free will, mind and body, and so on; also two articles on political philosophy) is *Key Themes in Philosophy* (1989), edited by A. Philips Griffiths. A companion volume providing an introduction to classic texts is *Philosophers Ancient and Modern* (1986), edited by Godfrey Vesey. A highly readable introduction to recent French philosophy is Eric Matthew's *Twentieth-Century French Philosophy* (1996).

An excellent set of succinct 'lecture notes' covering each of the main areas of modern philosophy (philosophy of science, philosophy of mind, ethics, and so on) is given in William James Earle's *Introduction to Philosophy* (1992).

The philosophy of mind

Good general introductions to the philosophy of mind include *The Character of Mind* (1982) by Colin McGinn and *Philosophy of Mind: an Introduction* (1993) by George Graham.

The philosophy of science

Useful introductions to the philosophy of science include Anthony O'Hear's *An Introduction to the Philosophy of Science* (1989 and 1991) and Rom Harré's *Laws of Nature* (1993). A useful collection of classic papers on the philosophy of science is *The Philosophy of Science* (1991) edited by Richard Boyd, Philip Gasper, and J. D. Trout.

The philosophy of psychiatry

The philosophy of psychiatry includes any work in the interdisciplinary area between philosophy, psychiatry, and abnormal psychology. One of the founding fathers of philosophy of psychiatry was the philosopher–psychiatrist, Karl Jaspers. His *General Psychopathology* has recently been republished by The Johns Hopkins University Press (1997). Modern contributors to the field have been concerned, like Jaspers, with issues in psychopathology (Radden 1996; Spitzer *et al.* 1993; Wilkes, K.V. 1988); but other topics have included concepts of disorder (e.g. Fulford 1989), the scientific status of psychiatry (e.g. Reznek 1991), the nature of personal identity (e.g. Glover 1988), the relationship between psychiatry, philosophy of mind, and neuroscience (Hundert 1989), and so forth. Indeed there are few areas of philosophy which do not have rich interconnections with problems in clinical work or research in psychiatry. An illustrative collection is *Philosophy, Psychology and Psychiatry* (1995), edited by A. Phillips Griffiths. The introduction and first chapter of this book describe the historical context of the recent resurgence of cross-disciplinary work between psychiatry and philosophy (Fulford 1995*a* and *b*, see also, Fulford 2000).

A valuable edited collection covering many topics in the crossover area between psychiatry and the philosophy of mind is George Graham and G. Lynn Stephen's *Philosophical Psychopathology* (1994). A corresponding collection with a number of excellent articles broadly in the area of the philosophy of science is *Philosophical Perspectives on Psychiatry Diagnostic Classification* (1994), edited by J.Z. Sadler, O.P. Wiggins, and M.A. Schwartz.

Articles on the philosophy of psychiatry are appearing with increasing regularity in mainline journals in a number of disciplines including philosophy, bioethics, and psychiatry. Regular reviews of key areas appear in the 'History and Philosophy' section of *Current Opinion in Psychiatry* (published by

Lippincott Williams and Wilkins for the World Psychiatric Association). The international journal, *PPP— Philosophy, Psychiatry and Psychology* (published by the Johns Hopkins University Press) is dedicated to philosophy of psychiatry. *The Philosopher's Index*, which is the main literature database for philosophy (it is the philosopher's 'Medline'!), now includes 'Philosophy of Psychiatry' as a distinct subdiscipline alongside such topics such as jurisprudence, philosophy of law, and metaphysics.

Reading Guide: references

Boyd, R., Gasper, P., and Trout, J.D. (eds.) (1991) *The Philosophy of Science*. Cambridge (Mass.), The MIT Press.

Earle, W.J. (1992) *Introduction to Philosophy*. New York, McGraw–Hill.

Fulford, K.W.M. (1989, (reprinted 1995; 2nd edn forthcoming) *Moral Theory and Medical Practice*. Cambridge, Cambridge University Press.

Fulford, K.W.M. (1995a) Introduction: just getting started. Introduction to *Philosophy, Psychology, and Psychiatry* (ed. A. Phillips Griffiths). Cambridge, Cambridge University Press (for the Royal Institute of Philosophy).

Fulford, K.W.M. (1995b) Mind and madness: new directions in the philosophy of psychiatry. In *Philosophy, Psychology, and Psychiatry* (ed. A. Phillips Griffiths), Chapter 1. Cambridge, Cambridge University Press (for the Royal Institute of Philosophy).

Fulford, K.W.M. (2000a) Philosophy meets psychiatry in the twentieth century— Four looks back and a brief loof forward. In Louhiala, P., Stenman, S. (eds.): *Philosophy Meets Medicine*. Helsinki: Helsinki University Press; p. 116–34.

Fulford, K.W.M. (2000b) Disordered minds, diseased brains and real people in *Philosophy, Psychiatry and Psychopathy: Personal identity in mental disorder*. (ed. Heginbotham, C.), Chapter 4 Avebury Series in Philosophy in association with The Society for Applied Philosophy. Aldershot (England): Ashgate Publishing Ltd.

Fulford, K.W.M. and Bloch, S. (forthcoming). Psychiatric ethics: codes, concepts and clinical practice skills. In *New Oxford Textbook of Psychiatry* (ed. Gelder, M., Andreasen, N., and Lopez–Ibor, J.), Chapter 17. Oxford, Oxford University Press.

Glover, J. (1988) *I: The Philosophy and Psychology of Personal Identity*. London, The Penguin Group.

Graham, G. (1993) *Philosophy of Mind: An Introduction*. Oxford, Blackwell.

Graham, G. and Stephen, G.L. (1994) *Philosophical Psychopathology*. Cambridge (Mass.), The MIT Press.

Harré, R. (1993) *Laws of Nature*. London, Duckworth.

Hollis, M. (1985, reprinted 1992) *Invitation to Philosophy*. Oxford, Blackwell.

Hundert, E.M. (1989) *Philosophy, Psychiatry and Neuroscience*. Oxford, Clarendon Press.

Jaspers, K. (1913) *Allgemeine Psychopathologie*. Berlin, Springer. In translation in 1963 as *General Psychopathology* (translated by Hoenig, J. and Hamilton, M.W.). Manchester, Manchester University Press. New edition in 1997, with a new foreword by McHugh, P.R. Baltimore, The Johns Hopkins University Press.

Matthew, E. (1996) *Twentieth-Century French Philosophy*. Oxford, Oxford University Press.

McGinn, C. (1982) *The Character of Mind*. Oxford, Oxford University Press.

Nagel, T. (1987) *What Does It All Mean? A Very Short Introduction to Philosophy*, Oxford, Oxford University Press.

O'Hear, A. (1985) *What Philosophy Is*. Harmondsworth (England), Penguin.

O'Hear, A. (1989 and 1991) *An Introduction to the Philosophy of Science*. Oxford, Clarendon Press.

Phillips Griffiths, A. (ed.) (1995) *Philosophy, Psychology and Psychiatry*. Cambridge, Cambridge University Press (for the Royal Institute of Philosophy).

Phillips Griffiths, A. (ed.) (1989) *Key Themes in Philosophy*. Cambridge, Cambridge University Press.

Radden, J. (1996) *Divided Minds and Successive Selves: Ethical Issues in Disorders of Identity and Personality*. Cambridge (Mass.), The MIT Press.

Reznek, L. (1991) *The Philosophical Defence of Psychiatry*. London, Routledge.

Sadler, J.Z., Wiggins, O.P., and Schwartz, M.A. (ed.) (1994) *Philosophical Perspectives on Psychiatry Diagnostic Classification*. Baltimore, Johns Hopkins University Press.

Spitzer, M., Uehlein, F., Schwartz, M. A., and Mundt, C. (ed.) (1993) *Phenomenology, Language and Schizophrenia*. New York, Springer–Verlag.

Vesey, G. (ed.) (1986) *Philosophers Ancient and Modern*. Cambridge, Cambridge University Press.

von Wright, H.G. (1963) *The Varieties of Goodness*. London, Routledge and Kegan Paul. New York, The Humatics Press.

Wilkes, K.V. (1988) *Real People: Personal Identity Without Thought Experiments*. Oxford, Clarendon Press.

World Psychiatric Association, Geneva (1996) Declaration of Madrid. (Reproduced with a brief commentary in 1999 in *Psychiatric Ethics* (3rd edn) (Bloch, S., Chodoff P., and Green S.A.), Appendix — Codes of Ethics, pp. 511–31. Oxford, Oxford University Press.)

CHAPTER 2

Thinking skills: ethical reasoning and problem solving in psychiatric ethics

In Chapter 1 we found that the ethical problems we face in psychiatry are often a good deal trickier, both practically and theoretically, than those arising in other areas of medicine. We thus need sharper tools to tackle them effectively. The tools for ethical problem solving in medicine come from a variety of sources — psychology, social science, anthropology, political theory, law, and many other disciplines. We will be drawing on some of these later on in thinking about the cases in this book. Perhaps most important of all, though, are the thinking skills — the strategies for analysing and thinking through ethical problems — that we get from philosophy.

   In this chapter we illustrate some of the tools of ethical reasoning available from philosophy by working through a first clinical case, the story of Mr Able[1]. We will be using these and other ethical tools in the cases that follow in Chapters 3 to 8. Chapter 9 will offer an overview in the form of a teaching seminar. This will illustrate how ethical reasoning can be incorporated into teaching psychiatric ethics as a key component of the skills required for clinical problem solving in psychiatry.

CASE HISTORY The story of Mr Able

Mr Able, a 48-year-old bank manager, came to the casualty department of his local hospital complaining of burning pains in his face and head. He had a letter from his GP saying that she believed Mr Able had become seriously depressed. He admitted that he had had episodes of depression in the past and that during one of these he had made a sudden and nearly fatal suicide attempt. However (despite appearances) he denied any such feelings now.

   Mr Able refused to let the casualty officer call his wife. The casualty officer tried telephoning the GP but she was out 'on call'. He then got Mr Able's home number from Directory Enquiries and telephoned his wife. She was very concerned, being unaware that her husband had gone to see their GP. She confirmed what the GP's letter said, that over three to four weeks her husband had become gloomy and preoccupied and had lost interest in his work. But she added that on the last occasion when he had complained similarly of head and facial pains, he had made a sudden and nearly fatal suicide attempt. Mrs Able said she would come to the hospital but was very concerned that her husband should not be allowed to leave, at any rate not before she got there.

The casualty officer then called the duty psychiatrist. Mr Able was initially very guarded in what he said, but eventually admitted that he believed that he had advanced brain cancer. After a careful neurological examination, the psychiatrist explained to Mr Able that there were no signs of this, but Mr Able remained adamant. All he wanted was something for the pain. The psychiatrist then saw Mrs Able, who said that she was very much afraid that her husband was planning to kill himself. He was behaving as he had done before his previous suicide attempt. As Mr Able still insisted that he would not stay in hospital, it seemed to everyone at this stage that there was no option but to admit him under the Mental Health Act as an involuntary patient. He accordingly came into the ward and over a period of eight weeks made a full recovery on antidepressant therapy.

The aims of psychiatric ethical theory

Most psychiatrists struggle initially for a moment or two to think of this as an 'ethics case'. This is partly because when it comes to everyday practice, whether as professionals or as users of services, the ethical aspects of our work are generally very much in the background. At least in acute cases, like Mr Able's, this is as it should be. Otherwise we would indeed be in danger of what we called, in the Preface to this book, ethical paralysis!

All the same, the practical demands of our day-to-day work should not be allowed to blind us to its underlying ethical issues. Thus, while Mr Able's case may at first glance *appear* ethically uncomplicated, it is certainly far from being ethically uncontestable. The use of involuntary treatment in a case like this would be contested by radical antipsychiatry (for example, Szasz 1960). The British social psychiatrist John Wing, responding to radical antipsychiatry, described the refusal of involuntary treatment for suicidally depressed patients as 'morally repellent' (Wing 1978, p. 244). Perhaps it is. But exactly when involuntary treatment is appropriate is not always clear. In a case vignette study which included a shortened version of Mr Able's case, psychiatrists were split 50:50 over whether involuntary treatment was appropriate (Fulford and Hope 1993). And the theoretical issues involved in resolving this split vote — in deciding what to do in cases like Mr Able's — are deep indeed.

We reviewed some of the ethical issues raised by involuntary treatment in the last chapter. We compared the problems raised specifically by involuntary psychiatric treatment with the ethically and conceptually more straightforward cases of involuntary treatment encountered in physical medicine (as in cases of unconsciousness, for example). In this chapter, we consider a number of ways of thinking about these issues which, though derived from philosophy, are particularly helpful in resolving clinical problems in everyday clinical work and research.

But what should count as 'helpful' here? Most ethics books take it for granted that exposure to ethical theory will improve practice. Yet their specific educational aims are usually left unstated. In their article 'Medical education: patients, principles and practice skills' (1993), Tony Hope and Bill Fulford outlined four practical objectives which they identified originally as the goals of a course in practice skills for medical students in Oxford. The overall aim of the course was to improve the skills of *application* of medical knowledge. This is what 'practice skills' is all about. Doctors have to learn a huge body of facts, but the skills of applying that knowledge in practice has usually been left to a process of learning by apprenticeship — in other words, following the consultant around the ward! The practice skills approach aims to bring together the ethical, legal, and communication skills necessary to apply our medical knowledge successfully in our everyday clinical work. Within this overall aim, it has four specific objectives:

1 to increase awareness;

2 to change attitudes;

3 to increase knowledge; and

4 to improve thinking skills.

Increasing awareness

Being aware of an ethical issue is usually the first step towards doing something about it. Yet as we saw in Mr Able's case, even with an area like involuntary psychiatric treatment which is notoriously ethically problematic, the ethical issues may not be 'up front' when we are confronted with an acute problem in the context of everyday clinical work.

Ethical issues, once we take a moment to reflect upon them, are often more or less visible. But sometimes they are not. What about Mr. Able? The most obvious ethical problems in Mr Able's case were to do with consent: he didn't want treatment (for depression); everyone else thought he needed it. But what about confidentiality? Was the casualty officer right to call Mr Able's wife? He might have been negligent if he had not done so; but this *is* a breach of confidentiality, even if ethically justified. A first aim of ethics training must therefore be to raise awareness of the ethical issues implicit in everyday practice.

Changing attitudes

As an educational objective, this is more contentious. The question of which attitudes should be encouraged is itself an ethical issue! In most ethics teaching it is assumed that health care practitioners should be non-judgemental and patient-centred in their approach to their work. These attitudes are not incompatible with holding strong *personal* views on matters such as abortion, for example. But they are not value-neutral, either. They represent a liberal ethic which requires respect for other people's values. In some cases, therefore, where personal and professional values clash, a health care practitioner may feel that a patient should get help from someone else.

Changing attitudes has been discussed recently as an educational objective in the context of a renewed interest in 'virtue ethics'. The virtues are dispositions to think and to act in certain ethically approved ways. Hence virtue ethics is concerned with what sort of person it is right to be rather than what sort of things it is right to do. William May, of the Southern Methodist University in Galveston, Texas, has discussed the virtues on which health care should concentrate in 'The virtues in a professional setting' (1994). Building on the Scottish philosopher Alasdair MacIntyre's rehabilitation of the virtues in his *After Virtue* (1985), William May lists a large number of 'health care virtues'. Many of these we take for granted, assuming they will be acquired through apprenticeship as part of our training in the health care professions. Justice, beneficence, and so forth might come within this category. Other virtues, although less obvious, are clearly important, at least in mental health. From May's list, perseverance and humility, for example, were essential to the proper management of Mr Able's depression. The casualty officer concerned showed just these virtues in this case. Had he been less conscientious, or had he adopted a more high-handed attitude, things might have turned out very differently.

Increasing knowledge

This is a neglected but increasingly important aspect of ethics, especially in mental health. Traditionally, ethical reasoning has been based on more or less tacit intuitions about what people want, feel, fear, and so forth. It has been widely assumed, first, that we can judge accurately what other people want, and, second, that we can judge accurately what other people would regard as satisfying their wants. These assumptions are, at best, optimistic. In the area of mental health, at least, people in general and health care practitioners in particular perform rather badly on both counts (Rogers *et al.* 1993).

The importance of basing ethical thinking as far as possible on knowledge has led to a growth in 'empirical ethics'. This has taken a number of forms, from greater use of narrative (Parker and Dickenson, 2000, pp. 269–311), through the use of ethnographic and other methods derived from medical anthropology (for example, Ersser 1995), to psychological studies (for example, work on the effects of counselling in the context of genetic testing for Huntington's disease — see Case 6.3), and, most important of all, to direct assessment of the needs of users and carers (Marshall 1994). The value of the latter is well illustrated by Peter Campbell's article 'What we want from crisis services' (1996). As Campbell indicates, what is important to service users is often very different from what is important to service providers.

That it should be necessary at all to point out the need for basing ethical thinking on facts, rather than on presuppositions about what people want, is a sobering thought. It is not really so surprising, however, that professionals should be relatively blind to the values of their clients. After all, to be a professional is to have expert knowledge — this is part of what it is to *be* a professional (Fulford 1994). A professional's expertise is both *general* (where particular people's values are highly individualistic) and itself *driven by* particular values (of the individual professional and of the profession as a whole). This combination means that professionals, by their very nature, are inclined to draw unwarranted conclusions about their client's values. In mental health, this is aggravated by the fact that, as we saw in Chapter 1, it differs from other areas of health care precisely in that it is concerned with areas of experience and behaviour in which people's values are *particularly* diverse.

Improving thinking skills

This whole chapter is mainly concerned with thinking skills. Some people are surprised that we can reason about ethical issues; they feel that ethics is a matter of personal opinion, ultimately no more subject to rational agreement or disagreement than, say, taste in food. We could leave it at that if there were neither dilemmas nor disagreements; and it is certainly true that in reasoning about ethical issues we may come to an impasse. Before we reach the point of impasse, however, there are a number of different ways in which we can try to think through ethical issues. We will be looking at these in the remainder of this chapter. They cover:

1 law and ethics;

2 bioethical approaches;

3 general ethical theory; and

4 other areas of philosophy.

As already noted, at the end of this chapter we will think about how theory and practice fit together. In Chapter 9, after we have considered our series of cases, we will illustrate in more detail how the skills derived from ethical and philosophical theory can be built into the general practice skills required for good clinical care.

Law and ethics

Mental health law provides a framework for clinical practice in psychiatry and it will probably have figured strongly in your thinking about Mr Able. In the UK, the Mental Health Act 1983 is the main legislation relevant to Mr Able; very similar legislation exists in the USA and in most European countries (Fulford and Hope 1996). This mental health legislation directly reflects two core ethical intuitions about involuntary treatment and thus usually requires two conditions to be fulfilled for such treatment (of a fully conscious adult patient of normal intelligence, like Mr Able):

• *Condition 1* — the patient must be suffering from a mental disorder

• *Condition 2* — there must be a risk to the patient or others arising from the disorder

In Section 2 of the Mental Health Act 1983 (Admission for Assessment), condition 1 is expressed as '...[the patient is] suffering from mental disorder of a nature or degree which warrants the detention of the patient in a hospital for assessment (or for assessment followed by medical treatment) for at least a limited period'; and condition 2 is expressed as '...[the patient] ought to be so detained in the interests of his own health or safety or with a view to the protection of other persons'.

So the Mental Health Act 1983 provides a framework for deciding what to do in a case like Mr Able's. Indeed, if you are a mental health professional and were not at least aware of the relevance of the Act, you would be at risk of a negligence claim! The difficulty though is whilst such legislation covers the cases most people would intuitively treat, it covers a great many other cases as well: mental health legislation is so broadly drawn that it is massively over-comprehensive. Besides people like Mr Able, the Mental Health Act 1983 would cover *anyone* with a mental disorder (condition 1) who is at risk to themselves or others (condition 2).

The natural response to this is to say 'OK, but it's not 'mental disorder + risk' as such that is relevant ethically. What is required for involuntary treatment is *serious* mental disorder and/or *serious* risk.' The difficulty with this response though is to define just what 'serious' should mean. In the bioethical literature on involuntary treatment in general physical medicine, 'serious' is widely taken to mean immediately life-threatening. But if we apply this sense of 'serious' to psychiatric cases, we move from an over-comprehensive criterion to one which is not comprehensive enough! 'Immediately life-threatening' excludes cases that most people would intuitively treat (including possibly Mr Able, since his risk of suicide was not 'immediate'), and it includes others (such as psychopathic disorder) that most people would *not* treat.

The problem of defining 'serious' was examined by the Butler Committee (Butler 1975), set up by the UK Government to review the whole question of the treatment of the mentally disordered in law in the run up to the Mental Health Act 1983. The Butler Committee was concerned primarily with mental illness as a legal excuse ('mad v. bad'), but essentially the same considerations arise for involuntary treatment ('mad v. sad'). The Committee identified the relevant sense of 'serious' with the traditional psychopathological concept of psychosis. As indicated in Fig. 2.1, which represents an ethical map of psychopathology, psychotic disorders have been widely recognized as the core or paradigm case of mental disorder involving loss of responsibility. Psychotic disorders correspond in this respect with lay notions of madness and legal concepts of insanity (Fulford 1987). As such, the central place of psychotic disorders has deep historical roots (Robinson 1996) and it is identifiable in many different cultures around the world (Wing 1978). The problem though, as the Butler Committee recognized, is that psychosis is difficult to define. Their solution was thus to circumscribe the relevant category of 'severe mental disorder' by reference to a defined list of specific and readily identifiable symptoms (such as delusion and hallucination) by which the psychotic disorders are categorized.

We will be returning several times in this book to the ethical and conceptual problems surrounding the psychopathological concepts of delusion, hallucination, and so forth. For now though, the point is that the Butler solution — the Butler Committee's list of specific psychotic symptoms — gives a good 'fit' with practice (Fulford and Hope 1993). Mr Able had at least one psychotic symptom (a delusion of brain cancer). Furthermore, the importance of such symptoms to clinical decisions about involuntary treatment has been shown both by questionnaire studies (Fulford 1993) and by empirical research on the kind of cases actually treated on an involuntary basis, or regarded as legally not responsible, in practice (for example, Sensky *et al.* 1991 and Walker 1967). Given this correlation

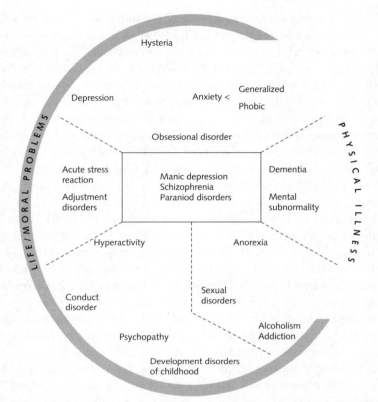

Fig. 2.1 An ethical map of psychopathology. This figure represents some of the key ethical features of mental disorders. It illustrates, 1) the wide diversity of mental disorders, 2) the central conceptual and ethical place of functional psychotic disorders, and 3) the way in which psychopathology forms a bridge between physical illnesses and moral or life problems. Any proposed philosophical theory of the concept of mental disorder has to explain these three features of psychopathology.

between involuntary psychiatric treatment and the psychopathological criterion of 'psychosis', it seems likely that the concept of 'psychosis' does indeed correspond with the relevant ethical sense of 'serious'.

Despite this good fit, however, this part of the Butler report was excluded from the Mental Health Act. The approach finally adopted was to provide a wide legal criterion ('mental disorder' — condition 1) and to leave it to professionals to apply the criterion in an appropriately focused way. This 'wide legal net + narrow professional use' approach has been adopted in most mental health legislation. In a recent European study, only Denmark was found to specify psychotic disorder, and even Denmark added a catch-all phrase 'or similar mental states' (Fulford and Hope 1996, Table 6). Thus legal definitions leave the problem of deciding when involuntary treatment is ethically justified with the practitioner. This is where bioethics comes in.

Bioethics and psychiatry

There are two main approaches to ethical reasoning in the standard bioethics literature — *principles* and *casuistry*. In addition, the Oxford psychiatrist and ethicist, Tony Hope, has emphasized the importance of *perspectives* (Hope and Fulford 1993). We will consider each of these approaches briefly, thinking about Mr Able, and looking at their strengths and weaknesses specifically in mental health ethics.

Principles

The principles approach was developed originally at Georgetown University in the USA by the philosopher Tom Beauchamp and the theologian James Childress in their *Principles of Biomedical Ethics* (1989). In the UK the approach has been taken up and extended by the former Professor of Medical Ethics at Imperial College in London, Raanan Gillon. His *Philosophical Medical Ethics* (1985) helped to introduce bioethics into British medicine and remains a valuable introduction to the subject.

The four principles are:

1 **Autonomy** (respecting the patient's wishes)

2 **Beneficence** (doing good)

3 **Non-maleficence** (avoiding harm)

4 **Justice** (in particular, treating equal problems equally)

These are prima facie principles. That is, they are all prima facie relevant to ethical issues in health care and have to be balanced one against another in particular cases. There are no general rules for balancing principles; it is according to our intuitions about their relative importance in a given case.

Critics of the principles approach often say that it is too algorithmic — you feed in the problem, crank through the principles, and get out an answer. However, such mechanical uses of the principles approach would be quite wrong. In their book, Beauchamp and Childress themselves carefully spell out that this would be a gross misuse of principles reasoning.

Casuistry

The principles approach is 'top-down': it tackles ethical problems by applying general theory (that is, the four principles) to particular cases. The casuistic approach is 'bottom-up': it starts from particular cases. Where there is a dilemma or disagreement, casuistry asks two questions:

1 what *changes* to the case would make it clearer what to do, and

2 what *related* cases would be either more or less problematic ethically.

Thus in Mr Able's case, a relevant casuistic variant would be the extent of the risk of suicide: if there were less evidence of suicide risk, this would (for most people) reduce the ethical justification for involuntary treatment, and vice versa. Similarly, one might imagine Mr Able presenting in the same way but without a family dependent on him.

Historically, casuistry has had a bad reputation. It became associated with a Jesuitical practice of moulding cases to fit one's own beliefs and wishes. The term was rehabilitated recently by two American philosophers, Albert Jonsen and Stephen Toulmin, in their seminal book, *The Abuse of Casuistry* (1988). This was inspired by their experience on an American Government committee — the President's Commission on Bioethics. They noted that on many ethical issues, the members of the Commission often agreed on *what* ought to be done in a given case, even though they disagreed about *why*. This, they argued, showed the irrelevance of theory. The way to reason about ethical issues is not to apply general theories but to look carefully at the details of particular cases.

A valuable introduction to casuistry is the American philosopher Tom Murray's article, 'Medical ethics, moral philosophy and moral tradition' (1994). In this he contrasts casuistry with principles reasoning (or more generally, deductive reasoning) and sets it in the context of recent work on moral tradition. He notes that casuistry has sometimes been viewed by ethicists as a competitor to the four principles, even as a more 'advanced' ethical method. In the detail and complexity of real-life cases, he argues, *immersion in* and *interpretation of* moral theory, are inescapable. To these, the moral traditions of a culture are an essential resource.

In both these respects, then, ethical reasoning in health care must look to casuistic, bottom-up approaches, rather than theory-led, top-down approaches. But is this a recipe for rigid conservatism, for the endorsement and perpetuation of received values? We will return to the dangers of rigid conservatism in mental health shortly. The point that will emerge is that in mental health ethics, the two approaches — casuistry and principles — are often complementary.

Perspectives

The perspectives approach emphasizes the importance in ethical reasoning of the different points of view of all those concerned in a given case. This includes, centrally, the patient; but it also includes relatives, carers, doctors, nurses, and other professionals. The status of perspectives is rather different from the other two approaches: it is not a distinct form of ethical reasoning. It is rather a way of emphasizing the importance of different perspectives in *any* form of ethical reasoning, including principles and casuistry. How, for example, can the principle of beneficence be applied if we do not understand what someone wants? How, on the other hand, in reasoning casuistically, can the circumstances of a case be varied in an ethically relevant way without understanding what is significant from a particular person's point of view?

The perspectives approach is a relative newcomer on the bioethical scene. This is essentially because, as we noted in Chapter 1, it has been assumed that what people want is more or less transparent. In some cases this may be true — for example, with abortion or transplant surgery, many of the ethical issues arise from clear *conflicts* of perspectives. In Mr Able's case, similarly, there was a clear conflict between his perspective (that he did not believe he needed treatment for depression) and everyone else's perspective (that he did). However, perspectives may be all too readily misunderstood. There is a particular danger of such misunderstandings in mental health because, as we also saw in Chapter 1, people's values are inherently more diverse in this area.

Advantages and disadvantages of the three approaches

In practice, especially in mental health, the three approaches — principles, casuistry, and perspectives —are often usefully combined. However, it is important to be aware of their strengths and weaknesses.

The principles approach

The principles approach is intuitively straightforward. It also reflects many of the ideas that people fall back on naturally when faced with ethical issues in health care. This was shown, for example, by David Robertson's combined empirical and conceptual study of ethical decision making in old-age psychiatry (Robertson 1996).

The principles approach can be especially helpful in broadening our understanding of a case. In relation to the four practical objectives of ethical teaching already outlined, it can:

1 increase awareness (by forcing us to think about more than one aspect of a case);

2 change attitudes (by showing that a particular approach may be biased towards, say, beneficence at the expense of patient autonomy);

3 point to knowledge that may be lacking (this ties in with perspectives especially);

4 improve thinking skills (by giving us a well-structured way of analysing the pros and cons in a given case).

The main danger with the principles approach is that it can suggest that ethical issues may be solved, like mathematical or scientific problems, in a clear-cut way. In fact, as we noted a moment ago, this would be to misunderstand the approach (remember that prima facie principles have to be weighed intuitively); but it is a danger, nonetheless, especially when the principles approach is used on its own.

Casuistry

Casuistry was developed in part as a response to the misuse of 'principalism'. Based, as it is, directly on cases, it has the great advantage of practical relevance. Reasoning about cases is something that all practitioners are familiar with in other clinical contexts, and this kind of reasoning can often lead to agreement.

One problem with casuistry is that it can be overly loose and unstructured. A more significant difficulty, especially with the importance of different value perspectives in mental health, is the danger of reinforcing prejudices. Casuistic reasoning only 'goes through' to agreement where the perspectives of those concerned are in fact shared. But in the case of mental health, as has repeatedly been noted in earlier sections, values are often *not* shared. We return to this point later in this chapter in relation to involuntary treatment.

Perspectives

Perspectives is the most patient-centred of the three approaches. It is especially important as the basis of good communication — an essential requirement for good practice in health care.

There are no significant disadvantages to being sensitive to people's perspectives (to their values and beliefs). But unlike principles and casuistry, the perspectives approach, in itself, gives us no method of *reasoning* ethically, no way of deciding what ought to be done. It provides essential *data* for ethical and other aspects of clinical decision making; but it has to be linked up to a substantive theory of some kind if it is to give grounds for action.

A related theoretical danger with the perspectives approach is relativism — an underlying assumption that 'anything goes'. But it is of the essence of the professional relationship that, as against simple consumerism, there has to be a *balance* of values (Fulford 1995*b*). So perspectives are essential (especially in mental health, because of the diversity of people's values in this area) but they are not sufficient.

Each of the three main methods of bioethical reasoning thus offers strengths and weaknesses. But how do these work out specifically in relation to mental health? We will consider this question by looking at how each of these approaches helps us to understand the issues raised by involuntary psychiatric treatment.

The four principles and involuntary psychiatric treatment

The principles approach, in giving us an open framework within which to explore the ethical aspects of treatment decisions, looks promising as a basis for resolving issues raised by involuntary psychiatric treatment. In their book, Beauchamp and Childress take the key ethical issue in involuntary treatment to be a balancing of the principle of autonomy (respecting the patient's wishes) with that of beneficence (the professional's responsibility to act in the patient's best interests). The argument runs thus. Normally, the best guide to anyone's best interests is their express wishes. In the past, however, in a 'doctor knows best' model, it was the doctor who decided what was in a patient's best interests. More recently, this 'paternalistic' approach has given way to a recognition of the importance of patient autonomy. Most people, even so, recognize cases (young children, for example) in which a person's express wishes are not the most reliable guide to their best interests. Hence we cannot simply substitute a 'patient knows best' principle for the old 'doctor knows best' approach. There will always be cases where 'best interests' and 'express wishes' are in conflict, and it is this conflict, interpreted by Beauchamp and Childress in terms of beneficence and autonomy, which is at the heart of the ethical dilemmas and difficulties presented by involuntary treatment.

This then leads naturally into an account of involuntary *psychiatric* treatment. Mental illness, Beauchamp and Childress argue, to the extent that it involves people becoming irrational, impairs the capacities required for making fully autonomous choices. Hence this is one of the situations in which the principle of beneficence may outweigh that of autonomy. Of course, not *all* irrationality impairs autonomous choice sufficiently, or in the relevant way, to justify involuntary treatment. After all, we are all irrational at times! Beauchamp and Childress thus suggest a series of criteria that must be satisfied if a choice is to be considered genuinely autonomous. Such a choice must be:

1 intentional

2 made with understanding

3 free from external controlling influences (that is, uncoerced).

In addition, though, the subject must have the cognitive capacities for autonomous choice, in particular for coherent thought and deliberation. Correspondingly therefore, if one or more of these criteria is not satisfied, a person's choices are not fully autonomous and involuntary psychiatric treatment may be justified.

So far so good. But, and this is a crucial 'but', do these criteria really fit what actually happens in practice? Do they reflect the decisions about involuntary treatment which, most people would argue, are ethically justified? Beauchamp and Childress discuss a case of dementia. Here their cognitive criteria of capacity fit the case rather well, the defining characteristic of dementia being impaired cognitive capacities. But what about Mr Able? His behaviour was clearly intentional; he had understanding; and he was free from coercion. So involuntary treatment could not be justified by these criteria. And so far as his cognitive capacities were concerned, he was thinking coherently and with deliberation. Depression, it is true, produces an affective 'colouring' of cognition (everything looks gloomy when you are feeling sad). This is a subtle effect, however, on which to base so radical a treatment. Of course, Mr Able had a delusion (of brain cancer). But delusion, although the core symptom of psychotic disorder, is not associated with any as yet identified cognitive disturbance (for a recent review, see Garety and Freeman, 1999).[2]

The 'failure of fit' between involuntary treatment of functional psychotic disorders and the Beauchamp and Childress criteria does not mean that the principles approach, as such, is wrong. Involuntary treatment is appropriately analysed, up to a point, in terms of a balancing act between beneficence and autonomy. Nor does the failure of fit, in itself, show that the underlying analysis of rationality offered by Beauchamp and Childress is wrong. On the contrary, the analysis really *does* fit many cases of involuntary treatment, in general medicine, and even in psychiatry (such as Beauchamp and Childress' own case of dementia). The point is that the analysis fails to fit the *full range* of diverse cases represented by involuntary *psychiatric* treatment.

Why should there be this remarkable failure of fit between a (sophisticated) bioethical account of involuntary psychiatric treatment and the psychopathological reality? One reason is identified by Fulford and Hope (1993) in their analysis of Beauchamp and Childress' account of rationality. The key, they argue, is that Beauchamp and Childress have failed to recognize the importance of value judgements in psychiatric diagnosis (as well as in treatment choice). In this, Beauchamp and Childress, along with many others in bioethics, identify with the so-called 'medical' model, in which diagnosis in general is assumed to be value-free[3]. Whilst Beauchamp and Childress show that values are indeed involved in judgements of rationality, they conclude from this, not that value judgements are thereby involved in psychiatric diagnosis, but that value judgements (and hence judgements of rationality) are outside the scope of medicine. Such judgements, they reason, bring in 'moral *rather than* [our italics] medical considerations'.

Casuistry and the values of the majority

Of course, there is a good deal more to judgements of rationality and irrationality, and hence to diagnoses of mental disorder, than merely a negative value judgement. We return to the role of values in psychiatric diagnosis in Chapter 4. But if we accept, for the moment, that values are integral, rather than external, to medical judgements of rationality, and hence to decisions about involuntary psychiatric treatment, this would seem to suggest that casuistry, embedded as it is in moral tradition, will give us a better basis for analysing the ethical issues in this area.

Casuistry, however, brings with it its own dangers for mental health. Indeed, as the American bioethicist Loretta Kopelman (1994) has pointed out, these dangers are generated by the very reliance of casuistry on values. Thus, the power of casuistry, what makes it 'go through', is a *shared value system*. Jonsen and Toulmin's original observation, you will recall, was that the members of the President's Commission on Bioethics agreed on what ought to be done despite their different theories about why it should be done. Their agreement on what *ought* to be done thus reflected a common value system. But it is this reliance on a shared (if implicit) value system which makes casuistry, if used in isolation, potentially dangerous in mental health. For the key difference between mental health and many other areas of health care, to which we have returned several times, is, precisely, that in mental health people's values are often *diverse*.

This is well illustrated by Mr Able. There is a clear sense in which the very *problem* of involuntary treatment is a problem of conflicting values: Mr Able did not want psychiatric treatment; everyone else (doctors, social workers, relatives, and so on) believed that he needed treatment. A merely casuistic approach, therefore, cannot but fail to impose the values of the majority on the minority (the patient). In this situation, the Jonsen and Toulmin observation of everyone agreeing on what ought to be done is, at best, hazardously extended to mental health, for it carries with it unavoidable risks of abusive practices arising through conflicts of values. And the hazards are greatly increased when the relevant values are hidden behind a mask of scientific objectivity. This was a factor, for example, in the abusive uses of psychiatry in the USSR (Fulford *et al.* 1993) and Nazi Germany (Chodoff 1999). It is also, though more subtly, a factor in the less high-profile but equally damaging abuses so widely experienced by psychiatric patients in cross-cultural psychiatry (see several chapters in Bhui and Olajide 1998).

Although a powerful method of ethical reasoning in mental health, casuistry thus needs to be used in conjunction with other more transparent and discursive methods. To rely merely on casuistic reasoning is as likely to endorse as to prevent abusive practice in mental health, to the extent that it imposes one group's or person's values on others.

When applied to involuntary psychiatric treatment, both the principles approach and casuistry bring out the central place of values. The principles approach, useful as it is for resolving issues about involuntary treatment with some kinds of mental disorder (such as dementia), fails with the functional disorders (as in the case of Mr Able) essentially because, in adopting a medical model, it excludes values. Casuistry includes values — its very power as a method of ethical reasoning being derived from shared value systems. But this means that, given the *essentially divergent* values characteristic of mental health, casuistry carries with it serious risks of abuse through the imposition of majority values on the minority.

Perspectives and the values of the patient

If values are central, this brings us back to the importance of perspectives in mental health ethics. Tony Hope introduced the term 'perspectives' as a distinct aspect of ethical reasoning in his work on the Oxford Practice Skills Course for medical students (Hope *et al.* 1996). Practice skills combine ethical and legal reasoning with communication skills in a problem-based approach to medical ethics education. The communication aspect of this approach emphasizes the central role of perspectives, for perspectives highlight the importance of the values not just of professionals in mental health care, but also of users, of carers, and of others involved in non-clinical roles.

There is now a substantial literature illustrating how the user's perspective may differ from those of professionals. We noted some of this work earlier, in particular the remarkable book by Anne Rogers, David Pilgrim, and Ron Lacey — *Experiencing Psychiatry: Users' Views of Services* (1993). This book describes the results of a survey carried out by the authors on behalf of the patients' advocacy group, MIND (now called The National Association for Mental Health). (Chapter 6 is concerned with users' views of treatment.) We might expect, on an antipsychiatry model of the relationship between professionals and patients, outright rejection of drug therapy, especially where this is part of involuntary treatment. In fact, what Rogers, Pilgrim, and Lacey found was that many users are *not* against drug treatment. The Schizophrenia Fellowship has argued, similarly, that psychiatrists are too *reluctant* to use the Mental Health Act because of the pressures on 'beds'. What is important though, as Peter Campbell's (1996) personal account also brings out, is to recognize that in any form of treatment there will always be a range of issues which are vitally important from the user's

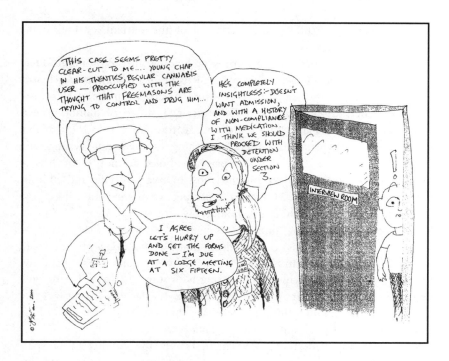

perspective as an *individual with a unique set of values*. These issues are often needlessly ignored in the *way* decisions about treatment are actually made. (The importance of the side-effects of drugs, in particular, is often largely neglected.)

The need to recognize different values has been repeatedly emphasized by users in mental health care (for example, Campbell 1996). As the cartoon above illustrates, the unequal power relationship between users and providers of services means that users often feel unable to express their concerns. Such concerns are, in many cases, not about whether to take a particular treatment or medication, for example, or even whether involuntary treatment may or may not be justified, but rather about the extent to which *the values of the individual concerned* are built into the way in which decisions about these important issues are made.

However, even perspectives are no panacea for psychiatric ethics. The problem with perspectives, you will recall, is a danger of relativism — of 'anything goes'. In fact, 'anything goes' does *not* follow from acknowledging the central place of values in the conceptual structure of medicine. We will return to this later. But in the case of involuntary psychiatric treatment, if casuistry carries a risk of the majority values being imposed on the patient, perspectives carries the opposite risk — of the patient's values being imposed on the majority.

The perspectives approach, if unsupported by other methods of ethical reasoning, thus fails on the centrally important issue of involuntary psychiatric treatment. The essential difficulty here stems directly from the place of psychotic disorders as the paradigm for ethically justified involuntary treatment (see p. 25 and Fig. 2.1). The defining feature of such disorders is that from the patient's perspective there is nothing psychiatrically wrong with them. This is captured by the core psychopathological notion of 'loss of insight'. In psychotic disorders, insight is lost in a very specific and ethically relevant sense (Fulford 1993). From the perspective of someone who is psychotically ill, there is nothing psychologically wrong *with them*. The problem lies either with something that is being *done to them* (for example, with persecutory delusions) or something that *they have done* (for example, with delusions of guilt). In Mr Able's case, from everyone else's perspective there was something psychiatrically wrong with him (he was suffering with depression). But from Mr Able's own perspective what was wrong was that he had a brain tumour: this was a disease that was doing things *to* him, causing him facial pain and threatening his life.

We may, along with the antipsychiatrists, see the conflict of perspectives involved in loss of insight as sufficient justification for avoiding involuntary treatment altogether. But this avoids rather than resolves the problem; it neither explains nor explains away, but simply rejects, the widespread ethical intuition that in cases like Mr Able's, involuntary treatment is not only justified but ethically obligatory.

General ethical theory and psychiatric ethics

All three methods of bioethical reasoning are therefore important in mental health: principles for the open framework of discursive argument they can help to supply; casuistry for the power of case-based reasoning to attach ethical arguments to the realities of day-to-day care; and perspectives for the focus they give to the essential place of the values of the individuals concerned. None is sufficient though, in itself, to deal with the difficult questions raised by mental health ethics. This brings us to the role of general ethical theory. Although further from the coalface of practice, ethical theory offers a range and depth of argument which underpins the more pragmatic tools of bioethics.

Philosophical ethical theory comes in two main varieties, *substantive* and *analytic*. Substantive theories are concerned with the most general kinds of consideration that are relevant to establishing ethical conclusions. Analytic philosophical ethics is concerned with the meanings and implications of value terms and hence with the logical form of ethical argument. We will return shortly to the role of analytic ethics in psychiatry.

The two most widely used forms of substantive ethical theory are *duty-based* (or *deontological*) and *consequentialist.*

- **Duty-based ethics.** Duty-based ethical theories, as the name implies, seek to define duties which are incumbent upon people no matter what the consequences might be. Duties are closely linked with rights and responsibilities and with law. Thus, in Mr. Able's case, the professionals could be said to have a *duty* to treat him under the Mental Health Act. This duty arises from the *rights* of the patient (and others) to protection, and the *responsibility* of the professionals to provide such protection. If they fail in this they could be held negligent in law, and so on.

- **Consequentialist ethics** seek to base ethical conclusions on the consequences of various possible courses of action. The most familiar consequentialist ethic is utilitarianism, the slogan for which is the well-known 'the greatest good of the greatest number'. In Mr Able's case, consequentialist arguments for treating him under the Mental Health Act include his future happiness, avoiding the tragedy for his family of suicide, and so forth.

Both kinds of substantive theory lie behind and underpin bioethical reasoning. The principles approach is perhaps closest to duty-based ethics. Mr Able had a 'right' to treatment which the professionals had a 'duty' to give — hence the principle of beneficence. Equally though, Mr Able's right to 'bodily integrity' would normally stand in the way of medical treatment against his wishes — hence the principle of autonomy. Consequences, on the other hand, are closer to casuistry than to perspectives. Reasoning casuistically, for instance, earlier in this chapter, it was relevant for us to imagine Mr Able's case without suicide risk because suicide, as a consequence of failing to treat him on an involuntary basis, would be so disastrous an outcome for his family. Similarly though, even if involuntary treatment is ethically justified in principle, the research by Rogers, Pilgrim, and Lacey (already referred to) showed clearly that its outcome in practice will depend crucially on whether or not it is carried through with an understanding of Mr Able's particular perspective.

The bioethical territory is not sharply divided between duties and consequences, however. Autonomy, as a principle, is justified not only deontologically but also by the good outcomes of respecting people's wishes (the principle of non-maleficence is *primarily* justified by the importance in medicine of avoiding *bad* outcomes). Conversely, casuistic reasoning must have regard to duties; and the duties that individuals recognize are crucial to their perspectives. The two substantive theories, moreover, are often complementary. The Oxford philosopher R.M. Hare makes this point specifically in relation to medical ethics in his *Medical Ethics, Can the Moral Philosopher Help?* (1993).

Duties, consequences, and psychiatric ethics

There are advantages and disadvantages of both kinds of substantive ethical theory for mental health ethics. The deontological approach is valuable especially where it is necessary to protect the rights of vulnerable groups (such as the mentally ill). As the British lawyer Jonathan Montgomery notes, rights (with their corresponding duties) can provide important protections against other people's vested interests, and indeed their well-intentioned interference (Montgomery 1995). But rights *talk* is not enough. Too often rights are prescribed, particularly by politicians, as a substitute for providing what people really need — Montgomery cites the UK's Patients' Charter as a case in point. Rights, therefore, need legal teeth. But the danger of this, as Montgomery goes on to describe, is that genuine care can all too easily become tied up in bureaucratic knots. So, patient-centredness in health care requires rights with teeth, but a balance must be maintained with the professional's freedom of right action.

However, consequences are not without their problems. Consequences force us to look squarely at the facts, but they leave us exposed to the ever-present danger of the 'abuse of casuistry' — of the facts being fitted to suit what we would *like* to be done rather than what *ought* to be done.

An illustration of the strengths and weaknesses of using utilitarianism in health care ethics is given in the use of QALYs in resource allocation. QALYs aim to make the balance of utilities more objective by basing resource allocation on the expressed utilities of the parties to the decision-making process. Thus, a QALY is a 'Quality-Adjusted Life Year'. It is calculated by asking a sample of people to rank different diseases and disabilities for 'quality or life'. This gives a measure of seriousness which can then be weighted by duration. The resulting figures allow (in principle) the cost of a year of healthy life to be calculated.

All this seems fair and equal. But the difficulty with balancing utilities in this way is that it necessarily disadvantages minorities. The Oxford philosopher Roger Crisp has pointed out that this is crucial in mental health (Crisp 1994). Mental disorders are common enough, but *serious* mental disorder is relatively uncommon. The 'public image' of mental disorders is also unglamorous; it is much easier to raise votes for eye disease, for example, or cancer research. Hence mental disorder will not attract the 'sympathy vote' in the same way as, say, heart disease. But the needs of the seriously mentally ill are no less acute for all that. This then is an 'abuse of consequences' writ large, for it expresses what the majority would like to be done to the exclusion of what ought to be done for minorities. The mentally ill, already disadvantaged, are thus further disadvantaged in any 'one-QALY, one-vote' system.

But perhaps the most serious difficulty with the QALY approach is a difficulty with all utilitarian calculations — that of imaginative identification with other people's (or our own future) states. The utility of a year with, say, cancer, as measured by someone suffering from the disease, may be very different from what anyone without the disease would imagine. Indeed, as we noted earlier, sociological work in this area suggests that actual and imagined utilities *will* be very different.

This is not to say that QALY thinking is all wrong. After all, squaring health service budgets and balancing needs with resources across a wide spectrum of very different conditions is impossibly difficult. We need all the help we can get with health economics, which is the area for which QALYs were originally devised. But QALY thinking, without the counterbalancing of rights to protect the needs of disadvantaged minorities, leads to serious injustices.

Analytic ethics and linguistic analysis

Analytic ethics, as we have just noted, is concerned with the meanings of moral and other value words. It has been given a hard time recently in philosophy. Philosophers, concerned to be seen to be contributing directly to practical issues, have turned away from questions of meaning to questions of substance. But in psychiatric ethics this is a false dichotomy. Indeed, as we saw in Chapter 1, part of what makes psychiatry so difficult as a clinical discipline is precisely that questions of meaning (that is, conceptual problems, as we called them in Chapter 1) are often no less important practically than questions of substance (that is, empirical problems).

This is well illustrated by involuntary psychiatric treatment. The ethical justification of Mr Able's involuntary treatment turned, centrally, not on the facts but on how the facts were interpreted or understood. It was not enough that, as a matter of fact, he was at risk of suicide. It would not have been enough that he was at risk of suicide as a result of being sad. It would not have been enough even that he was at risk of suicide as a result of being sad on the basis of a false belief (that he had brain cancer). The critical ethical consideration was that his false belief was properly understood to be a delusion and hence that he was correctly interpreted as being *psychotically mentally ill*. We return later (in Case 5.2) to the conceptual difficulties involved here. But the point for now is that it is how Mr Able's experience and behaviour is conceptualized which is ethically crucial. And as we noted earlier, similar issues arise in the 'mad/bad' questions of forensic psychiatry.

In psychiatric ethics, then, there is no divorce between substantive ethical issues and conceptual issues (questions of meaning). This was the point we reached at the end of the last chapter. Combined with the recognition of the importance of values in psychiatry, this leads to a whole series of practically important consequences about the role of the patient in psychiatry and of the multidisciplinary team, not just in treatment (as in traditional bioethics) but at all stages of the clinical process, from diagnosis right through to prognosis and to wider issues about the organization and delivery of mental health care.

We pick up on these practical consequences in later chapters. For now, though, the remaining question for this chapter is that if philosophy is important to us in psychiatry, alongside science, how should we go about converting theory into practice?

Learning and doing

The key point to remember about philosophy is that, not unlike clinical medicine, it is as much a matter of skills as of knowledge. The relevant skills in the case of philosophy are thinking skills. Some of these skills are generic (see Table 1.1 in Chapter 1); others are specific skills of ethical reasoning, as outlined in this chapter. In either case, the trick in turning theory into practice is to separate learning from doing, the acquisition of a new skill from its deployment in everyday clinical work and research. Thus, if you come across a way of analysing ethical issues which you feel would be useful, try it out first simply as an exercise when there is nothing practical hanging on the outcome, and reflect on its success or failure. Repeating this a couple of times will then allow you to use the new skill in a natural and unselfconscious way when it is needed in practice.

The Oxford philosopher R.M. Hare (1981) has written about the relationship between theory and practice in ethics in terms of different levels of moral reasoning. Hare distinguishes two main levels. Level 1 is the level of *everyday action*: at this level, to be effective we have to be unselfconscious and decisive. Hence it is our ethical intuitions which must guide us at level 1. Level 2, by contrast, is a level of *critical reflection* on practice. This includes ethical reasoning in terms of principles, casuistry, perspectives, and so forth as applied to particular cases in particular clinical contexts. Hare distinguishes both these, as concerned with questions of substance, from the logical enquiries of analytic ethics — though as we have seen, this distinction is difficult to sustain in psychiatry.

Hare's level 1 reasoning, in that it involves more or less spontaneous responses to ethical problems in the heat of the moment, is related to the virtues (that is, dispositions to think and to act ethically — see p. 22). There has been considerable interest in virtue ethics in relation to medical education. William May's article, noted earlier, explores the aims of medical education in terms of such traditional virtues as fidelity, truthfulness, and so on (May 1994). Level 1 is also the practical level at which training in 'practice skills' (the skills of *applying* medical knowledge) takes place.

Level 2 reasoning, though — the level of reflection on practice — is no less important practically. It is essential to reflect sometimes on practice if we are to continue to develop as practitioners. Level 2 reasoning, broadened to include analytic ethics, and indeed other relevant areas of philosophy, is the level at which we will be mainly working in this book. In the cases that follow, we set out and explore a wide range of practical issues drawing on ethical theory and in some cases other areas of philosophy. We do not, as such, offer 'solutions'. This is not the role of ethical analysis. Its role is rather to deepen understanding and thus, through improved thinking skills, to help us act decisively in the conditions of uncertainty which are characteristic of psychiatry as a clinical discipline.

References

Beauchamp, T.L. and Childress, J.F. (1989; 4th edn 1994) *Principles of Biomedical Ethics*. Oxford, Oxford University Press.

Bhui, K. and Olajide, D. (ed.) (1999) *Mental Health Service Provision for a Multi-Cultural Society*. London, W.B. Saunders Ltd.

Boorse C. (1975) On the distinction between disease and illness. *Philosophy and Public Affairs*, 5: 49–68.

Butler, the Rt. Hon. Lord (1975) *Report of the Committee on Mentally Abnormal Offenders, Cmnd., 6244*. London, Her Majesty's Stationery Office.

Campbell, P. (1996) What we want from crisis services. In *On Speaking Our Minds: Anthology* (ed. Read, J. and Reynolds, J.), pp. 180–4. London, MacMillan Press Ltd. (for The Open University).

Chodoff, P. (1999) Misuse and abuse of psychiatry: an overview. In *Psychiatric Ethics* (3rd edn) (ed. Bloch, S., Chodoff, P., and Green, S.), Chapter 4. Oxford, Oxford University Press.

Crisp, R. (1994) Quality of life and health care. In *Medicine and Moral Reasoning* (ed. Fulford, K.W.M., Gillett, G., and Soskice, J.), Chapter 13. Cambridge, Cambridge University Press.

Ersser, S. (1995) Ethnography and the development of patient-centred nursing. In *Essential Practice in Patient-Centred Care* (ed. Fulford, K.W.M., Ersser, S., and Hope, T.), Chaper 4. Oxford, Blackwell Science.

Fulford, K.W.M. (1987) Insanity. In *Dictionary of Philosophy and Psychology* (ed. Harré, R. and Lamb, D.). Oxford, Blackwells.

Fulford, K.W.M. (1993) Value, action, mental illness and the law. In *Action and Value in Criminal Law* (ed. Shute, S., Gardner, J., and Horder, J.), pp. 279–310. Oxford, Oxford University Press.

Fulford, K.W.M. (1989, reprinted 1995; 2nd edn forthcoming) *Moral Theory and Medical Practice*. Cambridge, Cambridge University Press.

Fulford, K.W.M. (1991) The concept of disease. In *Psychiatric Ethics* (2nd edn) (ed. Bloch, S. and Chodoff, P.), Chapter 6. Oxford, Oxford University Press.

Fulford, K.W.M. (1993) Thought insertion and insight: disease and illness paradigms of psychotic disorder. In *Phenomenology, Language and Schizophrenia* (ed. Spitzer, M., Uehlein, F., Schwartz, M.A., and Mundt, C.). New York, Springer–Verlag.

Fulford, K.W.M. (1994) Medical education: knowledge and know-how. In *Ethics and the Professions* (ed. Chadwick, R.), Chapter 2. Aldershot (England), The Avebury Press.

Fulford, K.W.M. (1995*a*) Psychiatry, compulsory treatment and a value-based model of mental illness. In *Introducing Applied Ethics* (ed. Almond, B.), Chapter 10. Oxford, Blackwell.

Fulford, K.W.M. (1995*b*) Concepts of disease and the meaning of patient-centred care. In *Essential Practice in Patient-Centred Care* (ed. Fulford, K.W.M., Ersser, S., and Hope, T.), Chapter 1. Oxford, Blackwell Science.

Fulford, K.W.M., Smirnoff, A.Y.U., and Snow. E. (1993) Concepts of disease and the abuse of psychiatry in the USSR. *British Journal of Psychiatry,* **162**:801–10. Reprinted in 1996 in *Medical Ethics* (ed. Downie, R.S.), volume in *The International Research Library of Philosophy* series (series ed. J. Skorupski). Aldershot (England), Dartmouth.

Fulford, K.W.M. and Hope, R.A. (1993) Psychiatric ethics: a bioethical ugly duckling? In *Principles of Health Care Ethics* (ed. Gillon, R. and Lloyd, A.), Chapter 58. Chichester (England), John Wiley and Sons.

Fulford, K.W.M. and Hope, T. (1996) Informed consent in psychiatry: comparative assessment of Section 5 of the National Reports — Report for Biomed 1 project (published as Control and Practical Experience).In *Informed Consent in Psychiatry: European Perspectives on Ethics, Law and Clinical Practice* (ed. Koch, H.-G., Reiter–Theil, S., and Helmchen, H.), pp. 349–77. Baden–Baden, Nomos Verlagsgesellschaft.

Garety, P.A. and Freeman, D. (1999) Cognitive Approaches to Delusions: a Critical Review of Theories and Evidence. *British Journal of Clinical Psychology,* 38, pp. 113–154.

Gillon, R. (1985) *Philosophical Medical Ethics*. Chichester (England), John Wiley and Sons.

Hare, R.M. (1981) *Moral Thinking: Its Levels, Method and Point.* Oxford, Clarendon Press.

Hare, R.M. (1993) Medical ethics, can the moral philosopher help? In *Essays on Bioethics,* pp. 1–14. Oxford, Clarendon Press.

Hope, R.A. and Fulford, K.W.M. (1993) Medical education: patients, principles and practice skills. In *Principles of Health Care Ethics* (ed. Gillon, R.), Chapter 59. Chichester (England), John Wiley and Sons.

Hope, T., Fulford, K.W.M., and Yates, A. (1996) *Manual of the Oxford Practice Skills Project.* Oxford, Oxford University Press.

Jonsen, A.R. and Toulmin, S. (1988) *The Abuse of Casuistry: a History of Moral Reasoning.* Berkeley, University of California Press.

Kopelman, L.M. (1994) Case method and casuistry: the problem of bias. *Theoretical Medicine,.* 15(1):21–38.

MacIntyre, A. (1985) *After Virtue: A Study in Moral Theory.* London, Duckworth.

Marshall, M. (1994) How should we measure need? Concept and practice in the development of a standardised assessment schedule. *Philosophy, Psychiatry, and Psychology,* 1:27–36. (Commentaries by Crisp, R. and Morgan, J., 37–40.)

May, W. F. (1994) The virtues in a professional setting. In *Medicine and Moral Reasoning* (ed. Fulford, K.W.M., Gillett, G.R., and Soskice, J.M.), Chapter 6. Cambridge, Cambridge University Press.

Montgomery, J. (1995) Patients first: the role of rights. In *Essential Practice in Patient-Centred Care* (ed. Fulford, K.W.M., Ersser, S., and Hope, T.), Chapter 9. Oxford, Blackwell Science.

Murray, T. H. (1994) Medical Ethics, Moral Philosophy and Moral Tradition. In *Medicine and Moral Reasoning* (ed. Fulford, K.W.M., Gillett, G.R., and Soskice, J.M.), Chapter 8. Cambridge, Cambridge University Press.

Parker, M., and Dickenson, D. (2000) *The Cambridge Medical Ethics Workbook.* Cambridge, Cambridge University Press.

Robinson, D. (1996) *Wild Beasts and Idle Humours.* Cambridge (Mass.), Harvard University Press.

Robertson, D.W. (1996) Ethical theory, ethnography and differences between doctors and nurses in approaches to patient care. *Journal of Medical Ethics,* 22:292–9.

Rogers, A., Pilgrim, D., and Lacey, R. (1993) *Experiencing Psychiatry: Users' Views of Services.* London, The Macmillan Press.

Sensky, T., Hughes, T., and Hirsch, S. (1991) Compulsory psychiatric treatment in the community, part 1. A controlled study of compulsory community treatment with extended leave under the Mental Health Act: special characteristics of patients treated and impact of treatment. *British Journal of Psychiatry,* 158:792.

Szasa, T.S. (1960) The myth of mental illness. *American Psychologist,* 15:113–18.

Walker, N. (1967) *Crime and Insanity in England*. Edinburgh, Edinburgh University Press.

Wing, J.K. (1978) *Reasoning about madness*. Oxford, Oxford University Press.

Reading Guide

This Reading Guide covers introductions to ethical theory, to medical ethics, and to psychiatric ethics, including the links between ethical reasoning and clinical thinking skills. We have also included further general reading on the main clinical topic considered in this chapter — involuntary psychiatric treatment. Involuntary treatment raises a wide range of more specialized ethical issues, such as consent and confidentiality, and we return to each of these in later chapters.

General ethical theory

Among many excellent introductions to ethics, D.D. Raphael's *Moral Philosophy* (1994) is brief and very readable. It includes a guide to further reading for both classic and modern sources. Mary Warnock's *Ethics since 1900* (1978), although out of print, remains an exceptionally clear introduction to each of the main ethical theories noted in this chapter. Her more recent *The Uses of Philosophy* (1992) illustrates the value of clear ethical reasoning in a range of public policy issues (including some in medicine). R.M. Hare's *Sorting Out Ethics* (1997) offers a brief but authoritative introduction to each of the main philosophical theories of ethics. Hare aims to provide us with a clear map to guide us through the 'moral maze'.

A recent comprehensive and very readable introduction is James Rachels' *The Elements of Moral Philosophy* (1999). Brenda Almond and Don Hill's *Applied Ethics* (1991) is a lively edited collection with articles on personal relationships, medicine, crime and punishment, economics, war, and environmental ethics. Geoffrey Warnock's *Contemporary Moral Philosophy* (1967) gives a clear and non-partisan introduction to the issues in the debate about the logical relationship between facts and values. Chapters 2, 3, and 4 of Fulford's *Moral Theory and Medical Practice* (1989) explore implications of this debate for our understanding of the concepts of illness and disease (as mixed fact–value concepts) in medicine and psychiatry.

For a clear summary of Kantian, consequentialist, and virtue ethics, organized as an extended debate, see *Three Methods of Ethics* by Marcia W. Baron, Philip Petit, and Michael Slote (1997). A useful by-product of reading the book is that it gives a good sense of how philosophers conduct discussion, and of how to construct an argument. The collected introductory essays by notable philosophers in *A Companion to Ethics*, edited by Peter Singer (1993), are clear and accurate; the book also has the great advantage of expanding the usual range of topics in ethics into new and exciting areas.

Medical ethics and bioethics

An introductory text in medical ethics, which has the advantage of also being an interactive guide for self-study, is Michael Parker and Donna Dickenson's *The Cambridge Workbook in Medical Ethics* (2000). Mental health and mental illness are among the subjects covered, in a chapter of their own. *The Cambridge Workbook* also introduces new approaches beyond principlism and casuistry, particularly from Europe rather than the USA. Grant Gillett's *Reasonable Care* (1989) is an entertainingly written introduction drawing on much case material. The BMA's *Medical Ethics Today* (1993) is a comprehensive and detailed introduction to each of the main areas of medical ethics and includes relevant legal guidance.

The classic account of the principles approach to medical ethics is Tom Beauchamp and James Childress' *Principles of Biomedical Ethics* (1989). Raanan Gillon's *Philosophical Medical Ethics* (1985) offers a brief and very clear account of the principles approach. A large edited collection of articles on all aspects of the principles approach is his *Principles of Health Care Ethics* (1994). This includes an article by Tony Hope and Bill Fulford (1994) describing the relationship between ethical reasoning and communication skills in medicine.

The 'practice skills' approach to medical ethics teaching, which combines ethics, law, and communication skills, is described in *The Oxford Practice Skills Manual* (Hope, Fulford, and Yates 1996). An early case study drawing out the perspectives of all those involved in a vivid and highly readable way is *In That Case: Medical Ethics in Everyday Practice* (1982) by Alastair Campbell (a philosopher) and Roger Higgs (a GP).

Narrative ethics has recently come into prominence as part of narrative-based (in contrast to evidence-based) medicine: see Anne Hudson Jones' article 'Narrative in medical ethics', which was published as part of a series on narrative approaches to medicine in the *BMJ* (1999). Carl Elliott's collection of essays, *A Philosophical Disease,* illustrates the value of storytelling in biomedical ethics. Similarly, communitarian ethics is providing a valuable new resource (see, eg, Mike Parker's work, 1996 and 1999).

Core texts in medical law include Ian Kennedy and Andrew Grubb, *Principles of Medical Law* (1998); Jonathan Montgomery, *Health Care Law* (1997); Margaret Brazier, *Medicine, Patients and the Law* (1992); and J.K. Mason and R.A. McCall–Smith, *Law and Medical Ethics* (1999).

Psychiatric ethics

The first edition of the sister volume to this book, *Psychiatric Ethics* (Bloch and Chodoff 1981), was one of the trail-blazers for the otherwise relatively neglected area of psychiatric ethics. The third edition (Bloch, Chodoff, and Green 1999) includes chapters on each of the main areas of ethical concern in psychiatry and we note these at relevant points in later chapters. Also important in establishing the subject was Michael Moore's *Law and Psychiatry: Rethinking the Relationships* (1984) and Alan Stone's *Law, Psychiatry and Morality* (1984). Useful early reviews defining the subject include those by L. Kopelman (1989), R.A. Hope (1990), and D.J. Anzia with J. La Puma (1991).

A series of case histories with careful ethical and legal analysis from an American perspective is given in *A Casebook in Psychiatric Ethics*, published for the Group for the Advancement of Psychiatry (1990). Rem B. Edward's *Psychiatry and Ethics* (1982) is a valuable edited collection of classic articles.

The practical and theoretical links between ethical codes, concepts of disorder, and communication skills in psychiatric ethics, are described in Fulford and Bloch's article 'Codes, concepts, and clinical practice skills' in the *New Oxford Textbook of Psychiatry* (forthcoming). R.A. Hope's *Ethics and Psychiatry* (1994) gives an excellent succinct overview.

Literature reviews covering particular areas of ethical concern in psychiatry are published regular in the 'History and philosophy' and other sections of *Current Opinion in Psychiatry*. Articles on psychiatric ethics appear in *The Journal of Applied Philosophy, Theoretical Medicine,* and *The Journal of Medicine and Philosophy*. Most bioethics journals publish articles on psychiatric ethics, in particular *The Journal of Medical Ethics*. A series of annotated ethical case studies has been published in *The Psychiatric Bulletin* (published by the Royal College of Psychiatrists). *PPP —Philosophy, Psychiatry and Psychology* publishes articles which build on philosophical theory to illuminate problems in psychiatric ethics: see, for example, Pat Bracken (1995) and Eric Mathews (1995) on Michel Foucault and critical psychiatry; Hinshelwood (1995 and 1997) on personal identity and the ethics of psychotherapy; and the special issue on 'Suicide and psychiatric euthanasia' (1998; volume 5, 2).

Involuntary psychiatric treatment

Roger Peele and Paul Chodoff — Chapter 20 in Bloch, Chodoff, and Green's *Psychiatric Ethics* (1999) — give an excellent overview of the ethical issues raised by involuntary psychiatric treatment particularly in the context of deinstitutionalization. For an outline treatment of the ethical and conceptual issues underlying involuntary treatment in psychiatry, see Bill Fulford's 'Psychiatry, compulsory treatment and the value-based model of mental health' — Chapter 10 in *Introducing Applied Ethics* (1995), edited by

B. Almond. An example of empirical work supporting the central place of psychiatric disorders in the justification of involuntary psychiatric treatment is 'Compulsory psychiatric treatment in the community, part 1, [etc.]' by Sensky, Hughes, and Hirsch (1991).

A solid philosophical underpinning of the justification for involuntary treatment in terms of risk to others and self can be found in Joel Feinberg's *Harm to Self: The Moral Limits of the Criminal Law* (1986). Feinberg's Chapter 2 includes a nuanced treatment of autonomy in its various forms.

For related topics, see later Reading Guides, especially models of disorder and abuse of psychiatry (Chapter 3), responsibility (Chapter 4), autonomy, capacity, competence, and consent (Chapter 6), confidentiality (Chapter 7), and teamwork (Chapter 8).

Reading Guide: references

Almond, B. (ed.) (1995) *Introducing Applied Ethics.* Oxford, Blackwell Publishers.

Almond, B. and Hill, D. (1991) *Applied ethics: moral and metaphysical issues in contemporary debate.* London, Routledge.

Anzia, D.J. and La Puma, J. (1991) An annotated bibliography of psychiatric medical ethics. *Academic Psychiatry,* 15:1–7.

Baron, M.W., Petit, P., and Slote, M. (1997) *Three Methods of Ethics.* Oxford, Blackwell.

Beauchamp, T.L. and Childress, J.F. (1989) *Principles of Biomedical Ethics* (1st edn). Oxford, Oxford University Press.

Bloch, S., Chodoff, P., and Green, S.A. (1999) *Psychiatric Ethics* (3rd edn). Oxford, Oxford University Press.

BMA (1993) *Mental Ethics Today: Its Practice and Philosophy.* London, BMA.

Bracken, P.J. (1995) Beyond liberation: Michael Foucault and the notion of a critical psychiatry. *Philosophy, Psychiatry, and Psychology,* 2:1–14.

Brazier, M. (1992) *Medicine, Patients and the Law.* London, Penguin Books.

Campbell, A.B. and Higgs, R. (1982) *In That Case: Medical Ethics in Everyday Practice.* London, Darton, Longman and Todd.

Edwards, R.B. (ed.) (1982) *Psychiatry and Ethics: Insanity, Rational Autonomy, and Mental Health Care.* New York, Prometheus Books.

Elliott, C. (1999) *A Philosophical Disease: Bioethics, Culture and Identity.* Routledge.

Fulford, K.W.M. (1989, reprinted 1995; 2nd edn forthcoming) *Moral Theory and Medical Practice.* Cambridge, Cambridge University Press.

Fulford, K.W.M. (1995) Psychiatry, compulsory treatment and a value-based model of mental illness. In *Introducing Applied Ethics* (ed. Almond, B.), Chapter 10. Oxford, Blackwell.

Fulford, K.W.M. and Bloch, S. (forthcoming). Psychiatric ethics: codes, concepts and clinical practice skills. In *New Oxford Textbook of Psychiatry* (ed. Gelder, M., Andreasen, N., and Lopez–Ibor, J.), Chapter 17. Oxford, Oxford University Press.

Feinberg, J. (1986) *Harm to Self: The Moral Limits of the Criminal Law.* Oxford, Oxford University Press.

Gillett, G. (1989) *Reasonable Care.* Bristol (England), The Bristol Press.

Gillon, R. (1985) *Philosophical Medical Ethics.* Chichester (England): John Wiley and Sons.

Gillon, R. and Lloyd, A. (eds) (1994) *Principles of Health Care Ethics.* Chichester (England): John Wiley and Sons.

Hare, R.M. (1997) *Sorting out Ethics.* Oxford, Oxford University Press.

Hinshelwood, R.D. (1995) Commentary on 'Psychoanalysis. Science, and common-sense'. *Philosophy, Psychiatry, and Psychology, 2/2*:115–18.

Hinshelwood, R.D. (1997) Primitive mental processes: psychoanalysis and the ethics of integration. *Philosophy, Psychiatry, and Psychology, 4/2*:121–44.

Hope, R.A. (1990) Ethical philosophy as applied to psychiatry. *Current Opinion in Psychiatry, 3*: 673–6.

Hope, R.A. (1990) Ethics and psychiatry. In *Essential Psychiatry* (ed. Rose, N.D.B.), Chapter 4. Oxford, Blackwells.

Hope, R.A., and Fulford, K.W.M. (1993) Medical Education: Patients, Principles and Practice Skills. Ch 59 in Gillon R., ed., *Principles of Health Care Ethics.* Chichester (England): John Wiley and Sons.

Hope, T., Fulford, K.W.M., and Yates, A. (1996). *The Oxford Practice Skills Course: Ethics, Law and Communication in Health Care Education.* Oxford, Oxford University Press.

Hudson Jones, A. (1999) Narrative in medical ethics. *BMJ, 318*:253–6.

Kennedy, I. and Grubb, A. (1998) *Principles of Medical Law.* Oxford, Oxford University Press.

Kopelman, L.M. (1989) Moral problems in psychiatry. In *Medical Ethics* (ed. Veatch, R.). Massachusetts, Jones and Bartlett Publishing Company.

Mason, J.K. and McCall–Smith, R.A. (1999) *Law and Medical Ethics* (5th edn). London, Butterworth–Heinemann.

Mathews, E. (1995) Moralist or therapist? Foucault and the critique of psychiatry. *Philosophy, Psychiatry, and Psychology, 2*:19–30.

Montgomery, J. (1997) *Health Care Law.* Oxford, Oxford University Press.

Moore, M. (1984) *Law and Psychiatry: Rethinking the Relationships.* Cambridge, Cambridge University Press.

Parker, M. (1996) Communitarianism and its problems. *Cogito, 10*:3.

Parker, M. (1999) *Ethics and Community in the Health Care Professions.* London, Routledge.

Parker, M. and Dickenson, D. (2000) *The Cambridge Medical Ethics Workbook*. Cambridge, Cambridge University Press.

Rachels, J. (1999) *The Elements of Moral Philosophy*. McGraw–Hill.

Raphael, D.D. (1994) *Moral Philosophy* (2nd edn). Oxford, Oxford University Press.

Sensky, T., Hughes, T., and Hirsch, S. (1991) Compulsory psychiatric treatment in the community, part 1. A controlled study of compulsory community treatment with extended leave under the Mental Health Act: special characteristics of patients treated and impact of treatment. *British Journal of Psychiatry*, **158**:792.

Singer, P. (ed.) (1993) *A Companion to Ethics* (2nd edn). Oxford, Blackwell.

Stone, A.A. (1984) *Law, Psychiatry, and Morality*. Washington, American Psychiatric Press.

Warnock, G.J. (1967) *Contemporary Moral Philosophy*. London and Basingstoke, The Macmillan Press Ltd.

Warnock, M. (1978) *Ethics Since 1900* (3rd edn). Oxford, Oxford University Press.

Warnock, M. (1992) *The Uses of Philosophy*. Oxford, Blackwell Publishers.

Case studies in the clinical encounter

SECTION TWO

Case studies in the clinical encounter

CHAPTER 3

Basic concepts: your myth or mine?

Achieving a balance between medical and moral conceptions of mental disorder is central to good practice in psychiatry

An important characteristic of modern mental health practice is the variety of ways in which mental distress and disorder are understood (Colombo 1997). These 'models of disorder' range along a spectrum from medical (or biological) conceptions of mental *illness* (according to which mental disorders are caused by distinct pathological lesions in the brain and hence are no different in principle from bodily illnesses), through various psychological models (for example, behavioural, psychoanalytic, family dynamic), to overtly moral models. According to the latter, mental disorders are, in one way or another, either problems of living for which those concerned are responsible, or labels imposed by society to justify the control of deviance.

We return to the practical importance of this variety of models in Chapter 8 in connection with the teamwork which is fundamental to effective community care. In this chapter we will be concerned particularly with the medical and moral models. As we saw in Chapter 1, these are in a sense antithetical, in that the medical model construes mental disorders essentially as matters of fact, while the moral model construes them essentially as matters of value. The message of the present chapter is that important as the medical model has been in generating new and more effective treatments, we need to strike a balance between it and the moral model in coming to an appropriate understanding of mental distress and disorder in a given case.

The two cases that we consider illustrate some of the ways in which both overusing (as in Case 1, Elizabeth Orton) and underusing (as in Case 2, Tom Benbow) the medical model may be equally abusive. In the first case a psychiatrist finds himself under pressure from Social Services to see a mother (Elizabeth Orton) who has rejected her child. He feels that he is being asked to take on a socially coercive rather than genuinely medical role. The second case (Tom Benbow) is an alternative example of imbalance: a diagnosis of mental disorder is inappropriately withheld from a learning-disabled man who is thus denied medical help. These cases bring out a number of the factors driving such abuses, notably the differential distribution of psychiatric diagnoses by age and gender, and the availability of resources.

The different models of disorder have generated an extensive theoretical literature (see Reading Guides to this chapter and to Chapter 8). The tension between medical and moral conceptions in this literature was most transparent in the debate in the 1960s and 1970s between psychiatrists, defending a hardline medical model, and various schools of antipsychiatry (see Fulford 1998, for review). Antipsychiatrists believed that the medical model, if not abusive in intent, was abusive in effect. Treating mental distress and disorder as diseases, they argued, invalidated the meaningful human experiences they represented. Properly understood, mental disorders were, variously, a product of being 'labelled' mad (Scheff 1963; Rosenhan 1973), a sane reaction to an insane society (Laing 1960), or, merely, a construct devised by society as a means of controlling deviance (Cooper 1967; Foucault 1973). Hence those suffering from mental disorders were not *patients*, the passive victims of a disease process, but moral *agents*, citizens with rights who remain responsible for their actions and capable of actively tackling their problems. As the Professor (now Emeritus Professor) of Psychiatry at Syracuse University, Thomas Szasz, famously put it, 'mental illness is a myth'; mental disorders are real enough, but they are 'problems of living', not diseases (Szasz 1960).

Moral and medical models of mental disorder, although the focus of the psychiatry versus antipsychiatry debate, both have long histories. Critics of psychiatry have sometimes argued that the concept of mental illness is a modern invention. The French historian and philosopher, Michel Foucault, regarded it as a product of the Industrial Revolution, driven by the needs of the work ethic of the time (Foucault 1973). In fact, the idea that some forms of mental disorder are generically linked with bodily diseases can be traced back, at least in Western civilization, to classical times (Kenny 1969). A moral conception was dominant in the early Christian world; but Islamic medicine adopted a medical model. Similarly in subsequent periods, we see the medical model sometimes dominant (for example, the later Middle Ages, the eighteenth century) and at others, the moral model (for example, the Renaissance and Reformation witch hunts). Both kinds of model have reflected prevailing theories, on the one hand of disease, on the other of moral agency; but the essential tension between 'patient' and 'agent' is evident throughout.

With the rise of the 'new' neurosciences — brain imaging, genetics, neuropharmacology, and so forth — many have come to believe that antipsychiatry, and with it the moral conception of mental disorder, is dead. Historically, this would make the many alternatives to the medical model advanced in the 1960s and 1970s a last-ditch stand against the final triumph of the medical model! Closer examination, though, shows that far from being dead, the antipsychiatry of the 1960s and 1970s has been absorbed into the mainstream in the form of the different models represented by different professionals in multidisciplinary teams. Mental health practice now is, at its best, multiperspectival (McHugh and Slaveney 1983), social and psychological factors being given equal weight with biological. The moral model, too, emphasizing the *agency* of those with mental disorders, is more rather than less evident than it was. Its influence is apparent, for example, in the emphasis on patient autonomy in mainstream medical ethics (the principle of autonomy reflecting respect for the agency of the patient), in the growing importance of cognitive–behavioural treatments (the aim of which is to restore agency through the acquisition of new skills of self-management), and, most significant of all, in the ever-increasing authority of the user's voice, at all levels from overall priority setting through to day-to-day clinical care.

In the present state of psychiatry, medical and moral models, although not sharply distinct, are both represented in all aspects of clinical care — hence the need to strike the right balance between them in a given case. Push the balance too far towards an exclusively medical model, and psychiatry slides from a properly medical role into coercive functions: a headline example of the medicalization of deviance occurred in the USSR, where political dissidents were diagnosed as suffering from schizophrenia on the basis of 'delusions of reformism' (Bloch and Reddaway 1997). But push the balance too far towards an exclusively moral model, refuse to recognize *any* mental distress as disease, and we end up denying the resources of medicine to those who most desperately need them. In the early days of community care, for example, an overemphasis on respect for the autonomy of those with long-term mental illness resulted in the most severely ill falling through the net because they were unable to initiate contact with relevant services (Clinical Standards Advisory Group 1995).

How then do we strike the right balance? Theoretically, this is very difficult. The distinction between the medical and moral models centres, as we saw earlier in connection with the psychiatry versus antipsychiatry debate, on the distinction between patients and agents. This in turn involves or is closely connected with some deeply problematic concepts — volition, intention, and meaning; freedom and determinism; and, not least, the mind–brain problem! These concepts are important to psychiatry. The significance of meanings in psychopathology was highlighted by no less a figure than Karl Jaspers (Jaspers 1913); and Jaspers' concerns have recently become a renewed focus of research interest with developments in artificial intelligence and the neurosciences (Bolton and Hill 1996, see Chapter 5). Volition and intention, similarly, are important elements in attributions of rationality and responsibility which, as we saw in Chapter 2, are at the heart both of the justification of involuntary psychiatric treatment and of the status of mental illness as a legal excuse ('mad versus sad' and 'mad versus bad' issues, respectively).

We return to some of these concepts in later chapters. As we will see, problematic as they are theoretically, we cannot avoid being concerned with them in practice. This is part of what makes psychiatry intellectually as well as clinically challenging. In everyday practice, though, there are a number of well-recognized factors which can push the overall balance between moral and medical models one way or the other. A driving factor in our first case is social disapproval. Elizabeth Orton rejected her child. This seems so unnatural we feel 'she must be mad'. Those concerned with her did not actually use this expression, but the thought behind it is implicit in their assumption that she should be referred to (and indeed required to see) a psychiatrist. In our second case, Tom Benbow, a driving factor was the lack of resources available for offering him appropriate medical treatment. This was pushing those concerned against regarding him as mentally ill. This is why the case is titled 'Diagnosis and distributive justice'. Distributive justice means treating equal problems equally. Ethical problems of resource allocation have been widely discussed in bioethics in terms of distributive justice. In psychiatry, diagnosis, too, can be a concern of distributive justice.

Both these factors — social disapproval and lack of resources — are likely to become increasingly important in psychiatry over the next few years. The public mood, aggravated by a press which is often hostile to psychiatrists and their patients alike, is of disaffection with 'community care'. The demand is for a swing back to a more overtly medical model, in which psychiatrists take responsibility for people with mental disorders, in which they treat them with drugs, and in which they place them on Supervision Registers. Yet even as the demands on psychiatry increase, the resources available for all aspects of health care are ever more strained. The UK Government has recently announced substantial investment in mental health provision. This has been welcomed by professionals and user groups alike. But the current review of the Mental Health Act looks set to extend the powers of compulsion of psychiatrists, with proposed 'community treatment orders' and an obligation to 'treat' personality disorders as well as mental illnesses. This can hardly fail to increase the pressure on psychiatrists to avoid diagnosing mental disorder.

Those committed to a hard-line medical model tend to assume that the difficulties involved in diagnosing mental disorders will all be resolved by future advances in the neurosciences. There are theoretical arguments to suggest that this is wrong (we touch on these in Chapter 5). But history, at least, is against it, for scientific advance has often provoked an increase rather than a reduction in the influence of the moral model: the witch hunts of the seventeenth century, for example, were a product not of mediaeval Christianity but of

Renaissance science; and in the present century, the political abuse of psychiatry in the USSR was driven by a strongly medical model of mental disorder (Fulford *et al.* 1993).

We can speculate on the reasons for this. But the lesson of history is clear — scientific advance, far from removing the need for a balance between medical and moral models of mental disorder, may make it even more important to get the balance right in the future. Be that as it may, in the present stage of the development of psychiatry, the balance is essential. Achieving the right balance in practice is not easy; it depends on a range of knowledge and skills, and we return to these at several points in later chapters. Better understanding of different models is a first step (Colombo 1997). This can be built on anthropological, historical, and narrative sources. Good communication is essential: in Elizabeth Orton's case (Case 1), failure of communication between the psychiatrist and social workers was at the heart of the clinical dilemma. (We revisit this case in Chapter 9 in the context of a teaching seminar, exploring further the importance of communication to a practical resolution of the problem.) Patient advocacy may also be crucial. The mobilization of resources in a later case (Case 4.2, Delia Jarrett) followed representations on her behalf by MIND.

Finally, it is worth adding that besides the directly ethical issues involved in balancing moral and medical understandings of mental distress and disorder, differences of models may be an important factor blocking interagency co-operation (Colombo 1997; Perkins and Repper 1998). Such differences, though, if acknowledged and respected, can be helpful in providing a range of perspectives as the basis for a balanced approach to a given case. We noted the ethical importance of this aspect of interagency work in Chapter 2 in connection with involuntary treatment, and we will be returning to it at several points elsewhere in the book.

References

Bloch, S. and Reddaway, P. (1997) *Russia's Political Hospitals: The Abuse of Psychiatry in the Soviet Union.* London, Gollancz. (Also published in the USA in 1997 as *Psychiatric Terror.* New York, Basic Books.)

Bolton, D. and Hill, J. (1996) *Mind, Meaning and Mental Disorder: the Nature of Causal Explanation in Psychology and Psychiatry.* Oxford, Oxford University Press.

Colombo, A. (1997) *Understanding Mentally Disordered Offenders: a Multi-Agency Perspective.* Aldershot (England), Ashgate.

Cooper, D. (1967) *Psychiatry and Anti-Psychiatry.* London, Tavistock.

CSAG (1995) *Report of the Clinical Standards Advisory Group on Schizophrenia (Volume 1).* London, HMSO.

Foucault, M. (1973) *Madness and Civilization: a History of Insanity in the Age of Reason*. New York, Randon House.

Fulford, K.W.M. (1998) Mental illness. In *Encylopaedia of Applied Ethics* (ed. Chadwick, R.). San Diego, Academic Press.

Fulford, K.W.M., Smirnoff, A.Y.U., and Snow, E. (1993) Concepts of disease and the abuse of psychiatry in the USSR. *British Journal of Psychiatry*, **162**:801–10.

Jaspers, K. (1913) Causal and meaningful connexions between life history and psychosis. Reprinted in 1974 in *Themes and Variations in European Psychiatry* (ed. Hirsch, S.R. and Shepherd, M.), Chapter 5. Bristol, John Wright and Sons Ltd.

Kenny, A.J.P. (1969) Mental health in Plato's Republic. *Proceedings of the British Academy*, **5**: 229–53.

Laing, R.D. (1960) *The Divided Self*. London, Tavistock.

Laing, R.D. and Esterson, A. (1964) *Sanity, Madness and the Family*. London, Tavistock. (Also (1970) Harmondsworth, Penguin.)

McHugh, P.R. and Slaveney, P.R. (1983) *The Perspectives of Psychiatry*. Baltimore (USA), The Johns Hopkins University Press.

Perkins, R. and Repper, J. (1998) *Dilemmas in Community Mental Health Practice: Choice or Control*. Aberdeen, Radcliffe Medical Press.

Rosenhan, D. (1973) On being sane in insane places. *Science*, **179**:250–8.

Scheff, T. J. (1963) The role of the mentally ill and the dynamics of mental disorder: a research framework. *Sociometry*, **26**:436–53.

Szasz, T.S. (1960) The myth of mental illness. *American Psychologist*. **15**:113–18.

CASE 3.1

Elizabeth Orton — does she have a mental illness at all?

Synopsis A 35-year-old solicitor asks for help from Social Services after finding herself shaking her ten-month-old baby. She had postnatal depression but now appears normal, though she continues to insist that she does not want the baby. She would have her baby adopted except that her husband is strongly opposed to this. She agrees to see a psychiatrist under protest when threatened with her baby being put into care.

Key dilemma Is this social control or medical treatment?

Main topics Abuse of psychiatry; danger of overuse of concept of mental disorder; distinction between medical treatment and social coercion.

Other topics Involuntary treatment; values in attribution of 'mental illness' and of 'risk' in Mental Health Act; gender bias in attribution of mental illness; components of attribution of agency (failure to bond in mothers more 'pathological' than in fathers); dual role of psychiatrist (protection of patient versus protection of others, including family of the patient); importance of facts (likely outcome of failure to bond); teamwork (between Social Services and mental health); practical options; communication skills (involvement of patient); autonomy; risk assessment and responsibility; clinical confidentiality; iatrogenic harm.

Elizabeth Orton is a 35-year-old solicitor, with a ten-month-old baby, Anthony. She has a congenital hip malformation which has required numerous surgical procedures and sometimes confinement to a wheelchair, although at present her mobility is quite good. Her delivery, however, was by Caesarean section, and afterwards she suffered some postnatal depression. Although there are now no clinical signs of depression, she continues to insist that she does not want the baby. Her 50-year-old husband, Tim, who is semi-retired, does most of the child care outside the hours when Anthony attends a day nursery, but recently he was away for six nights. During that time Elizabeth telephoned her health visitor for help, upset because she had shaken the baby.

The health visitor alerted Social Services, who (together with the police) have the statutory responsibility for investigating cases of suspected child abuse, and the child protection machinery was set in motion. Anthony was placed on the Child Protection Register. When the baby is not at his day nursery, Tim or another designated person must be with the baby; Elizabeth is no longer allowed to care for him on her own. She has also been required by Social Services to agree to see a psychiatrist. If she does not accept psychiatric treatment, she has been told that Anthony may well be taken into care — to which Tim is deeply opposed.

Elizabeth insists that she is perfectly willing to have the baby taken away from the home, but that she fears her marriage would not survive. In a way she would be happier if the baby could be adopted immediately: what she dreads is the social embarrassment, her husband's grief, and the uncertainty of the child's long-term future if a series of short-term fostering placements are arranged. So she is co-operating very minimally with the requirement of psychiatric treatment, which she calls 'emotional blackmail.' At the most recent interagency child protection case conference, however, it was decided to keep Anthony at home, on the at-risk register, and to continue the requirement of psychiatric care for Elizabeth, in the hope that she will develop more 'normal' maternal feelings.

The consultant psychiatrist treating Elizabeth, Daniel Isaacs, feels caught in an extremely awkward position. He has developed a reasonably good therapeutic relationship with Elizabeth, because, he thinks, she feels he is the only one who is concentrating on her rather than on the baby. He does not actually believe that Elizabeth has any form of mental illness. Although his opinion was sought at the case conference, he thought that this finding was not very welcome. In addition, he had doubts about whether he should have revealed confidential clinical information about Elizabeth in that setting. (Elizabeth and Tim were also invited to attend, but chose not to.) Dr Isaacs also got himself into hot water by pointing out that in his experience, fathers who posed a threat of violence to their children were not usually asked to seek psychiatric treatment, so long as the mother was there to protect the child. 'Probably not,' he was told, 'although the child would still be on the at-risk register. But could we please concentrate on the child's best interests, and leave gender politics out of this?'

'Treating' Elizabeth poses a particular problem for the psychiatrist: is there any illness there to treat? This is a troublesome instance of a general problem which renders psychiatry ethically controversial — treating the unwilling patient who may not have a psychiatric disorder at all. But we need to break that problem down into two separate quandaries: treatment without consent, and the value status of psychiatric diagnoses. Although these two key questions interweave throughout the case study, it is important to bear in mind that they are conceptually separate.

Treatment without the patient's consent is prima facie wrong, and it may lead to a legal action of battery. But although this is the general context in which we need to consider the case of Elizabeth, it is too rough a sketch of what actually happens in practice. Other areas of medical practice may sometimes treat those unable to give informed consent to treatment (for example, the comatose patient); but the law is increasingly developing ways of getting around this problem, allowing at least a simulacrum of consent (for example, by the use of advance directives). Against this attempt to seek out the wishes of those who might be presumed incapable of expressing wishes, we have a case in which an articulate woman, clearly able to express a wish, is being forced to accept treatment — an action she views as 'emotional blackmail'. The difficulty is especially acute because psychotherapy would be the only indicated treatment, but how can psychotherapy be given to unwilling subjects? Treating an unwilling patient promises little success; psychotherapy usually fails if the patient does not wish to change. (Karasu 1991). And whereas 'psychotherapy is, more than anything, about helping people to choose' (Holmes and Lindley 1989, p. 123), one choice is already forbidden to Elizabeth: her current rejection of the baby.

If there can be any ethical justification for imposing treatment on the unwilling patient, the argument most often advanced depends on improving autonomy, to which the patient can be expected to give retrospective consent. This is a utilitarian justification, hinging on an expected future benefit which will outweigh the present infringement of autonomy. Even such radical courses as ECT and psychosurgery without consent have ironically been supported on the grounds that they will improve the patient's chances of acting as an autonomous agent afterwards (Kleinig 1985; Komrad 1993; Sherlock 1983). There are many reasons for scepticism about this argument, not least the Kantian one that it makes the patient a means to the end of his or her own autonomy (Dickenson 1991, p. 104). But even proponents of this view would be dismayed if greater autonomy is not the goal, and in this case it seems that it is not.

What the clinicians are asked to produce in Elizabeth's case is in a sense a decrease in autonomy — a greater willingness to accept the socially conditioned role of motherhood. Even though the baby's needs were being provided adequately by the father (with the important exception of the period in which Elizabeth had to cope on her own, when the shaking incident occurred), Elizabeth still has to 'be Mother.' Treatment is intended to produce more 'normal' maternal feelings, but is that a proper role for psychiatry, any more than producing more compliant citizens was a proper role for Soviet psychiatrists? In Victorian England, too, excessive sexual activity was classified as the disease of 'spermatorrhoea'. Again, however, there was no disease there to treat — no matter how undesirable the social consequences might have appeared to some.

Here we move into the domain of the second question — the value status of a psychiatric diagnosis. This case highlights the value-laden nature of psychiatric diagnosis, and its capacity for misuse. It is not merely that the diagnostic process is open to clinical error or inconsistency: psychiatric diagnosis is itself an ethical problem (Reich 1991). This argument has become more familiar through the use of a diagnosis of schizophrenia to control social dissent, as in the USSR during the 1980s. Elizabeth's case is not so blatant an example, but it does touch on the boundary between psychiatric illness and social nonconformity. That the maternal role is socially conditioned, and that it differs from the father role, is shown by Social Services' admission to Dr Isaacs that if it were the father who had shaken the child, he would not be asked to seek psychiatric treatment. So no, we cannot leave gender politics out of it; gender politics is already in it. But there is an important difference between Elizabeth's absence of 'normal' maternal feelings and the improper use of psychiatric diagnosis and treatment in Soviet Russia or Victorian England — the apparent consequence, shaking the baby. Whilst excessive sexual activity might be viewed as self-harm at most, and dissent from the Soviet regime was in fact praiseworthy, no one would deny that the risk to Anthony must be taken seriously.

Treating Elizabeth against her will may not be warranted in terms of increasing her own autonomy, but it could be justified in terms of risk to Anthony. The same is true of breaches of clinical confidentiality. After all, the UK General Medical Council guidance notes on confidentiality (1995) recognize that 'disclosures may be necessary in the public interest where a failure to disclose information may expose the patient, or others, to risk of death or serious harm' (General Medical Council 1995, Section 18). The case of W v Egdell (1990) established that although a duty of confidentiality was suggested between psychiatrist and patient, not only by equity but by implied contract, the duty to protect allowed the psychiatrist to override confidentiality by passing on information designed to prevent risk to the public from a patient in a secure hospital unit. In the USA, the Tarasoff decision (1974) established that 'protective privilege ends where public peril begins'.

Although the possibility that her confidentiality will be breached may undermine Elizabeth's willingness to trust Daniel Isaacs and impede the clinical encounter between doctor and patient, we might feel that this is the necessary price to pay for Anthony's safety. It is true that the clinician's duty of care to the patient is muddied by his responsibility towards Social Services, but perhaps he has a wider responsibility than simply the duty of care to the patient. Indeed, it has been argued that one thing that sets psychiatry apart from other clinical disciplines is that balancing individual versus social responsibilities is not a rare event, but an everyday occurrence (Bloch and Chodoff 1991, p. 10). Perhaps a realist might advise Daniel Isaacs simply to accept that his function in this case is to control Elizabeth's potential for violence towards Anthony — to control through treatment if possible, but if not, simply to control. 'Much of professional practice has an important social control function, and mental health practitioners are in part political actors' (Mechanic 1981, p. 46). Although the requirements of clinical work demand faith that one is helping patients, perhaps it is more honest to recognize the power aspect in the clinical encounter (Brody 1992). That power would be legitimized into rightful authority, in this case, by considerations of the baby's safety.

But who decides what constitutes an unacceptable level of risk to Anthony? If we could be certain that 'coercive' treatment of Elizabeth would leave Anthony 100 per cent safe, we might be willing to allow it — or at least a philosophical utilitarian might be. But with questions of risk we are always looking at probabilistic assessment, at degrees of risk rather than absolute safety. Here, too, values and gender bias enter play a part. Comparison with Case 7.1 in this book provides dramatic, though not conclusive, evidence that women who depart from 'normal' maternal feelings are thought to pose more of a risk than men who commit much more dangerous actions against their children. Systematic, though not deliberate, underrating of the risk men pose to children and conversely, overestimation of the risk posed by women has been identified more generally in social work practice (O'Hagan and Dillenburger 1995). More speculatively, we might question whether men's potential for violence is simply taken as a fact of nature, whereas women's is seen as a suitable case for treatment. This is not to condone or excuse what Elizabeth did, but only to set it in context.

Even though Tim is providing good care for Anthony, and even though he or another designated person is always required to be present when Elizabeth is with the baby, there is still too much risk for comfort, Social Services conclude. But are they simply transferring the responsibility for a bad outcome — even at this low level of probability — from themselves to Dr Isaacs? What magic wand can he wave to ensure that the level of risk to Anthony drops to zero? And is his assessment of the risk Elizabeth poses to Anthony necessarily any more reliable? In one study of risk assessment in psychiatry, 60 per cent agreement among a group of assessors was achieved in only four out of sixteen cases (Montandon and Harding 1984), although recent studies indicate some improvement (Taylor 1995).

The question is whether Dr Isaacs can 'cure' Elizabeth so that she no longer poses any risk to her child. This is not just a matter of Elizabeth's individual clinical mental state; for example, whether or not her call to the health visitor actually did reflect maternal concern, on which Dr Isaacs can try to build. Nor is it just a purely clinical matter of what kind of therapy to offer: this is a case about whether to offer therapy at all. 'In discussing problems concerning the use of therapy in coercive contexts, it is vital to distinguish the question of whether it is right to offer therapy at all in such contexts from the question of whether particular types of therapy are justifiable' (Holmes and Lindley 1989, pp. 168–9). In this case there is thus a broader issue about the role of psychiatry in society and the meaning of mental illness.

Does Elizabeth have a mental illness? One need not be a fully paid-up member of the antipsychiatry school (for example, Szasz 1961 and 1963) to doubt whether 'mental illness' has any meaning in this case. Uncertainty about whether Elizabeth's overt lack of love for her baby is an illness reflects a more general societal uncertainty about the scope and powers of psychiatry, and in particular about whether the disease model of psychiatric illness is valid. This medical paradigm of psychiatry includes, among other components:

- the **Causal Thesis**: a subclass of abnormal behaviour is caused by disease.
- the **Identification Thesis**: scientific methodology enables us to identify diseases.
- the **Epistemological Thesis**: scientific methodology enables us to discover the causes and cures for these diseases.
- the **Teleological Thesis**: psychiatry's goal is the prevention and treatment of mental diseases.

- the **Guardianship Thesis**: having a serious mental illness entitles the psychiatrist to act against the patient's will (Reznek 1991, p. 12ff.)

But the medical paradigm assumes that disease status can be settled by facts, whereas 'it is our values that determine the disease status of a condition. Ethics precedes nosology' (Reznek 1991, p. 157). To take an example from physical illness rather than psychiatry, infection of the gastrointestinal tract by commensals has the same nature as many diseases, but because we view it as beneficial, it is not a disease — in fact, it prevents diarrhoea. 'It is because we value the consequences of this infection that we do not take it to be a disease' (Reznek 1991, p. 158). Does symmetrical logic apply? Is it because Social Services — perhaps rightly — fears the consequences of 'abnormal' absence of maternal feelings that it takes Elizabeth to have a mental illness?

Yet, broadly speaking, it is only on a medical model of mental illness that Elizabeth can rightfully be treated without her genuine consent — taking us back to the first of our two issues. The Mental Health Act 1983 for England and Wales does authorize treatment on the basis of 'mental disorder,' meaning mental illness and any other disorder or disability of mind. But we cannot escape from the question of whether or not Elizabeth has a mental illness by taking refuge in the notion that she has a disorder of mind, because all the same arguments about the social, value-laden definition of disorder and abnormality still apply. Perhaps we might want to say that she is 'disabled' by her absence of maternal feelings; but this is a circular argument. She would probably reply that she is only disabled insofar as she is under restrictions imposed because she is seen as abnormal in her coldness towards Anthony. So we cannot use 'disability of mind' to justify those restrictions.

If Dr Isaacs is being treated as a means to a favourable child protection record for Social Services, Elizabeth is being used as a means to the end of Anthony's safety. Although she is not actually being detained in hospital, there is an element of forcing her to be somewhere she doesn't want to be — facing Dr Isaacs in a clinical session. And there is even a strong possibility of iatrogenic harm: no matter how conscientious and sensitive the clinician, enforced treatment may conceivably worsen Elizabeth's relationship with her baby. To the extent that diagnosis is a self-confirming hypothesis (Reich 1991), enforced treatment may leave Elizabeth more confirmed in her antipathy towards the baby than when therapy began.

But suppose all these arguments have been exhausted, and Dr Isaacs has no options except either to 'treat' Elizabeth or to hand her care over to another consultant who does not have the same objections. The second course may itself strike Dr Isaacs as ethically compromising; he would be ending the reasonably good therapeutic relationship which he has built up with Elizabeth, who might well regard transfer to someone else as yet more coercion. Yet how can he maintain the imperfect but important level of trust which he has built up if Elizabeth knows that her confidentiality can be breached at will? An additional difficulty is that if Dr Isaacs tells Social Services that Elizabeth refuses to allow details from the therapeutic encounter to be passed on, they may regard her silence as incriminatory.

One positive way forward would be to seek Elizabeth's permission before relaying any confidential information, and accepting whatever Elizabeth decides (Roth and Meisel 1977). Because clinician and patient have welded a reasonably good relationship, despite the inauspicious state of affairs, there is a good chance that Elizabeth will give an answer which also takes Daniel's responsibilities into account, not one rooted solely in defiance. So he needs to reveal something of his professional and ethical dilemma to Elizabeth, although that itself raises professional and ethical dilemmas about countertransference (Holmes and Lindley 1989, p 128). It might be thought inappropriate by some psychotherapists for Daniel to reveal his own responses to Elizabeth's situation; this may appear to be putting friendship before therapy. But so long as he limits his revelations to the professional and ethical strain put on him by having to treat a patient who does not need treatment, this objection should not pose a problem. By placing himself in Elizabeth's power, to the extent that he is open about the pressures on him to reveal confidential information, Daniel Isaacs can perhaps achieve the best result possible under the unhappy circumstances.

Practitioner commentary (CASE 3.1)

Dr John Vile Consultant Psychiatrist, Rehabilitation Services, East Kent Community NHS Trust

I found the case of Elizabeth Orton a fascinating one. In this commentary I offer some rather categorical views from the perspective of a working psychiatrist. The limits of space preclude a discussion of the 'grey areas' which, as the authors of this book show, are many indeed. In my view, however, there are key questions to ask in deciding how to proceed:

1 *Is there any reason to believe 'treatment' from Dr Isaacs will effect a change in Elizabeth to reduce the risk to her son?*

This should be the main criterion in determining whether treatment should be insisted on by Social Services as a condition for the child to remain with Elizabeth. An analogous situation might be where a short-sighted mother, who could not see well enough to care for her baby, might be required to get a pair of glasses. In this case the question would be whether the glasses would be effective. I believe the question of whether

Elizabeth has an 'illness' is, in her case, a side-issue. The aim of Social Services is only to ensure the well-being of the child as far as possible. In the case of the short-sighted mother, the question of whether the short-sightedness is an illness is not crucial. Treatment (especially in the case of psychotherapy) is often given in the absence of a recognized 'illness'.

2 *Is Elizabeth able to give informed consent for the 'treatment'?*

Clearly the answer is 'yes'. Her choice is clear (but not simple) — treatment, marriage, child, restrictions imposed by Social Services; or no child, no treatment, no marriage, no restrictions. This is not blackmail, but an aspect of her autonomy. At its most brutal, she must choose. In my experience, the agencies involved, such as Social Services and doctors, try to cushion the client from the responsibility of this sort of choice, by delaying the need for the decision and not emphasizing the client's autonomy. It is then that the client's autonomy is reduced. However, such postponement of a definite decision often allows those involved to have time for reflection and hence to come to a decision with which they will be happy in the long term.

3 *Has Elizabeth given valid consent?*

Because of the nature of psychotherapy consent is more complex than for other forms of treatment. It is not a matter simply of 'information and voluntariness'. It requires a real desire to change. Whether Elizabeth really desires to change will be a difficult judgement for Dr Isaacs to make.

To summarize, in my view the imposition of the requirement for psychotherapy by Social Services demands that the answers to the following three questions should be 'yes':

1 Will psychotherapy reduce the risk to the child?
2 Is Elizabeth able to give informed consent?
3 Does Elizabeth actually give informed consent in the form of a desire to change?

If any of these are answered 'no', then the imposition of the requirement of psychotherapy is both unlikely to be effective and, in my view, unethical since it amounts to the use of medical treatment as a form of social control.

References (CASE 3.1)

Bloch, S. and Chodoff, P. (1991) Introduction. In *Psychiatric Ethics* (2nd edn) (ed. Bloch, S. and Chodoff, P.), pp. 1–13. Oxford, Oxford University Press.

Brody, H. (1992). *The Healer's Power*. New Haven, Yale University Press.

Dickenson, D. (1991). *Moral Luck in Medical Ethics and Practical Politics*. Aldershot (Avebury), Gower Publishers.

General Medical Council (1995). *Confidentiality: Guidance from the General Medical Council*. London, General Medical Council.

Holmes, J. and Lindley, R. (1989). *The Values of Psychotherapy*. Oxford, Oxford University Press.

Karasu, T. (1991). Ethical aspects of psychotherapy. In *Psychiatric Ethics* (2nd edn) (ed. Bloch, S. and Chodoff, P.), pp. 135–66. Oxford, Oxford University Press.

Kleinig, J. (1985). *Ethical Issues in Psychosurgery*. London, George Allen and Unwin.

Komrad, M.S. (1993) A defence of medical paternalism: maximising patients' autonomy. *Journal of Medical Ethics*, **9/2**:38–44.

Mechanic, D. (1981). The social dimension. In *Psychiatric Ethics* (1st edn) (ed. S. Bloch and P. Chodoff), pp. 46–59. Oxford, Oxford University Press.

Montandon, G. and Harding, T. (1984) The reliability of dangerous assessments: a decision-making exercise. *British Journal of Psychiatry*, **144**:149.

O'Hagan, K. and Dillenburger, K. (1995). *The Abuse of Women within Childcare Work*. Buckingham, Open University Press.

Reich, W. (1991). Psychiatric diagnosis as an ethical problem. In *Psychiatric Ethics* (2nd edn) (ed. Bloch, S. and Chodoff, P.), pp. 101–34. Oxford, Oxford University Press.

Reznek, L. (1991). *The Philosophical Defence of Psychiatry*. London, Routledge.

Roth, L.H. and Meisel, A. (1977) Dangerousness, confidentiality, and the duty to warn. *American Journal of Psychiatry*, **126**:508–11.

Sherlock, R. (1983). Contribution to symposium on 'Consent, competence and ECT'. *Journal of Medical Ethics*, **9/3**.

Szasz, T. (1963). *Law, Liberty and Psychiatry*. New York, Macmillan.

Szasz, T. (1961) *The Myth of Mental Illness*. New York, Harper and Row.

Tarasoff *v* Regents of the University of California (1974), 118 California Reporter 129, 529, P 2d 553.

Taylor, P. (1995) Schizophrenia and the risk of violence. In *Schizophrenia* (ed. Hirsch, S. and Weinberger, D.), pp. 163–83. Oxford, Blackwell Science.

W *v* Egdell (1990) 1 All ER 835.

CASE 3.2

Tom Benbow — diagnosis and distributive justice

Synopsis A 53-year-old man, with mild to moderate learning disability, refuses consent of a manual evacuation of faeces under general anesthetic, this being the fifth occasion on which such treatment has been required for abdominal pain due to faecal impaction secondary to chronic self-neglect. He has a history of alcohol abuse, periodic violence, indecent exposure, and paranoid behaviour (he repeatedly asks to be rehoused because his neighbours are harming him with noise and 'rays' which affect his legs). He has been on a guardianship order but is not at present. He sleeps badly and has lost weight. He has consistently declined a trial of antipsychotic medication.

Dilemma Should Tom's refusal of medical treatment be respected or should his clinicians go ahead against his wishes?

Main topics Danger of underuse of concept of mental disorder; refusal of physical treatment in learning disabled person.

Other topics Balance of autonomy and beneficence; protection of others; rationality; distributive justice; diagnosis as the mobilizer of resources; values in psychiatric diagnosis; children's consent (case of R); consent and mental health law; gender bias in attributions of mental illness; normalization.

Tom Benbow, who is 53, suffers from moderate learning disability: his IQ falls between 35 and 50. The immediate difficulty confronting his clinicians concerns his unwillingness to consent to manual removal of faeces. Two days ago he presented at the local general hospital trust with abdominal pain, caused, as it turned out on examination, by severe constipation. As with several previous hospital admissions, he required manual evacuation of faeces under general anaesthetic. But he became fearful when this was explained to him, muttering that it might make his 'legs worse'. He left the casualty department without agreeing to the procedure.

The next day he returned, still anxious and in pain. This time he was persuaded to sign the consent form, but withdrew his consent in the anaesthetic room. The clinicians did not feel that it was possible to use the Mental Health Act in these circumstances. Instead, the hospital's consultant liaison psychiatrist called in Claire Gerrard, consultant psychiatrist for learning disability, who in turn brought in Tom's community worker from the learning disability team, Tony Bettio. Tom finally consented to the operation after a long discussion with Claire and Tony, and had three to four kilograms of faeces removed. Although he made a good recovery this time, the clinicians are concerned that repeated episodes like this (this was the fifth similar incident in four years) will harm Tom's already poor health.

In addition to his learning disability, Tom exhibits ideas which could be classified as delusional, and sometimes his behaviour is violent. He has several convictions for indecent exposure, usually following unusually heavy drinking. After the first such episode, dating back to his adolescence, he was placed on a restriction order of the Mental Health Act 1959. In the past ten years he has been moved, at his request, a total of nine times, always after threatening his neighbours with physical violence and banging on their doors at all hours of the night. His version of events is that his neighbours have their televisions too loud and are persecuting him, in a way that he finds difficult to describe. If Social Services staff resist his requests for rehousing, he often becomes violent: he threw a glass ashtray at the wall during one such discussion, and punched his social worker on the jaw in another.

The physical complaint — self-neglect resulting in impacted faeces — has been tackled successfully, in the past, with a guardianship order. Tom was put under an obligation to attend for medical treatment when asked, but he could still refuse consent to an enema or manual evacuation after assessment in hospital. He had three manual evacuations under general anaesthetic under this arrangement, but it was eventually felt that he was well enough for the order to be terminated. During the time he was on the guardianship order, however, his troubles with his neighbours escalated: there seems to be no relation between his constipation and his social difficulties.

Relief care for two days every fortnight was tried recently, to help him with his personal hygiene and to make sure that he was not neglecting his health. When Claire Gerrard assessed him on an in-patient basis, he talked of noise and 'rays' being sent by his neighbours to harm him, causing pain in his legs. He found it difficult to describe this further, and it was not clear whether it was some form of manipulation to make Social Services rehouse him, as he desired. He only talks about the 'rays' and their effect on his legs when he is trying to petition a member of the Social Services learning disability team for another change of address. He never gives the same story twice, and it is not at all clear whether he holds these beliefs with delusional intensity. There is no clear formal thought disorder: he is well orientated and his memory is reasonable. He seems to have some insight into his behaviour: when asked why he is neglecting himself, he says it is because he is trying to put pressure on the people involved in his care to get him a change of accommodation.

Tom is quite withdrawn. He has no contact with his numerous family, although they all live locally. He tends to interpret attempts to help as 'picking on me', although he accepts visits from the community learning disability team. He sleeps badly and has lost weight. He consistently declines antipsychotic medication on a therapeutic trial.

Tom Benbow's case, like most others in this book, could be discussed under any of several headings from medical ethics. The usual approach would be in terms of the principles of autonomy and beneficence (Beauchamp and Childress 1994; Gillon 1985) — is it right to override Tom's autonomy (his right to refuse treatment) in favour of beneficence (of improving his physical health)? Perhaps this discussion would also include the question of harm to others, not just to Tom — is the present pattern of management sufficient to protect others from Tom's verbal abuse and occasional physical violence?

An alternative approach might be in terms of rationality. Despite Tom's learning disability and the possibility of delusional fixation, there seems to be good evidence that his behaviour is intentional and his delusions less than robust. In terms of intentionally directing his actions towards a particular end — getting himself rehoused — he acts with a fair degree of success, although the underlying end may be less rational. Voltaire declared in his *Philosophical Dictionary* that madness meant 'to have erroneous perceptions and to reason correctly from them'. On that reading, Tom's behaviour looks at first to be irrational. Behaviour is termed rational when the starting point is appropriate to the situation and the beliefs are well founded; it is irrational when the underlying elements cannot be justified. The inference — the links from either sort of belief to action — may, however, be just the same (Wilkes 1988). With his fears about 'rays' affecting his legs, and his self-neglect so severe as to require manual evacuation of faeces, how can it be said that Tom's beliefs are appropriate to his situation?

Both informed consent and rationality are important issues in Tom's case, and we will discuss them, but not in the usual principlist manner. In addition, implicit throughout our discussion is another ethical topic, distributive justice — a topic too rarely considered in the progression from symptoms into diagnosis and classification. Is diagnosis evenly and fairly 'distributed' among patient groups? Or are some people more likely to attract a psychiatric diagnosis than others? Whether that is a benefit or a burden is another question.

Distributive justice in diagnosis is important because decisions about diagnosis precede and underpin those about management.

> It is the prerogative to diagnose that enables the psychiatrist to commit patients, against their wills, to psychiatric hospitals, that delineates the populations subjected to his care, and that sets in motion the methods he will use for treatment. And it is this prerogative that, therefore, should provoke perhaps the most fundamental — and the most serious — ethical examination. (Reich 1991, p. 102)

On the other hand, the power to diagnose and label mental illness is also the power to mobilize resources for the sufferer (Brody 1992). In Tom's case, are the clinicians doing enough to mobilize help? Tom seems to think not. He has taken it upon himself to get the help he thinks he needs — rehousing — by threatening his neighbours and deliberately neglecting his own health. We want to suggest, by comparison with a case involving a 15-year-old girl adjudged psychotic and treated compulsorily on the grounds of her 'violence' towards her father, that there are ethical issues about discrimination and fairness in the diagnostic judgements employed in Tom's case.

The risks of misuse of a positive psychiatric diagnosis are now familiar[1], thanks to the work of patients' rights organizations such as MIND and the National Schizophrenia Fellowship, the campaigns of the antipsychiatry movement, and the publicity given to abuses in Nazi Germany, the former USSR, and Japan (Müller–Hill 1991; Bloch 1991; Harding 1991). Perhaps because psychiatrists are increasingly aware of their possibly corrupting powers, the diagnostic process in some areas of psychiatry tends to result in a 'finding' of mental health rather than mental illness (Reich 1991, p. 104; Scheff 1966). In other areas — for example, in old age psychiatry — there appears to be a presumption in favour of a diagnosis of mental illness. Because psychiatric illness is commoner in old age, clinicians tend to play safe by over-diagnosing mental illness in the elderly (Oppenheimer 1991, p. 367) — a circular self-fulfilling prophecy. In somatic medicine, as in old age psychiatry, it has been said that false positives are less feared than false negatives:

> Whereas the judiciary's concern about error is expressed in the statement that it is better that ten [guilty] people go free than that one innocent person be punished, [somatic] medicine's concern about error is expressed in the statement that it is better that ten people be hospitalized unnecessarily than that one person should not be hospitalized and should die. (Peele 1991, p. 301)

The point of comparing clinicians' reluctance to intervene in Tom's case, with ready diagnosis and forcible treatment in the case of the 15-year-old girl, is to raise issues about fairness in diagnosis. In addition to seeing Tom's case in terms of informed consent, we also therefore want to discuss it under the umbrella of justice as fairness (Rawls 1971). As one of us has written elsewhere:

> ...given that mental illness is more overtly evaluative than physical illness...we should expect to find that the criteria by which the symptoms of mental illness are evaluated are more variable from person to person and for a given person on different occasions — than the corresponding criteria for the symptoms of physical illness. And overall, this is what is found. For example, the criteria by which we evaluate anxiety, a typical symptom of mental illness, are more variable than the corresponding criteria for, say, physical pain. (Fulford 1991, p. 87)

If justice is defined in Aristotelian fashion as treating equals equally, this variability makes justice particularly problematic in psychiatric diagnosis. The more evaluative nature of psychiatric diagnosis means that unintentional discrimination is an ever-present possibility. Comparing Tom's case with that of the 15-year-old girl, known simply as 'R', illustrates the danger (Devereux *et al.* 1993).

R had voluntarily entered the care of the local authority after a family conflict in which she damaged property, attacked her father, and threatened suicide. She had been known to Social Services for 12 years as a possible victim of emotional abuse and had previously been placed on the at-risk register. In therapy she was 'extremely argumentative, hostile and accusative'. After referral from a hospital psychiatric unit to a specialist adolescent care unit, she refused antipsychotic drugs on the grounds of their side-effects. The local authority initially gave permission for the medication but withdrew their consent after discussion with R, who, the authority thought, was competent to express her own wishes. She behaved calmly and rationally in discussion with her mental health social worker and with the consultant child psychiatrist, who judged that 'she is of sufficient maturity and understanding to comprehend the treatment being recommended, and is currently rational'. Nevertheless, the adolescent unit declared that it required freedom to administer treatment without R's consent if necessary. Without antipsychotic medication, the clinical team thought that R would be a victim of the 'revolving door' cycle for much of her adult life.

In the Court of Appeal judgement (1991) Lord Donaldson, Master of the Rolls, and Lord Justice Farquharson (Lord Justice Staughton expressing no opinion) held that a child with fluctuating mental capacity could never be competent to refuse treatment. R, it was held, probably did not understand the implications of refusing treatment, although it was generally agreed that she had a competent understanding of the side-effects of accepting antipsychotic medication. Although R was not found to be competent to refuse, Lord Donaldson went further. Notwithstanding the contrary opinion of Lord Scarman in the Gillick case (1985), even a competent child would only have the right to consent to treatment, not to refuse it — so long as someone with parental authority gave their consent. Lord Donaldson did not distinguish mental disability from mental disturbance. In this respect the case of R prompts thought about the instance of someone with learning disability.

What is the wider relevance of R's case to Tom Benbow? First, it focuses our attention on the grounds for compulsory treatment as a means of lessening the risk of violence to others. We want to suggest that the clinical team in Tom's case needs to focus not only on his harm to himself through self-neglect, but also on his violence to others — exposing himself, punching a social worker, throwing a glass ashtray, abusing and threatening his neighbours. Yet Tom is allowed to refuse antipsychotic medication which might lessen the risk of harm to others from his uncontrolled violence, whereas R is not, although her violence is limited to her father, less generalized, and perhaps a reaction to his abuse. Being 'extremely argumentative, hostile and accusative' seems to be enough to deny R her right to refuse. If she is being treated with antipsychotic drugs for defiance, she has a lot more to be defiant about now. This illustrates the second aspect of R's case which we want to highlight — the existence of distributive injustice in diagnosis. It seems plausible that young people, perhaps especially girls who break the conventional feminine mould by abandoning their home lives and dabbling in violence, are more likely to attract a diagnosis of mental illness or to be treated without their informed consent than are adult men with learning disability.

What is really being looked at in cases involving young people's consent to treatment is rationality, often an assessment of mental and emotional age as contrasted with chronological age. It needs to be stressed that we are not comparing Tom or R with an imaginary super-rational patient, but with the average patient who does not attract a diagnosis of mental illness. Patients of unquestioned competence to give informed consent to treatment have been found to have quite low levels of understanding. In one study, 20 men with a previous history of hospitalization for heart disease were informed in a taped interview before cardiac surgery of risks during the procedure, possible complications, likely benefits, probability of overall success, and alternative treatments. When interviewed again after the operation, only 25 per cent remembered that the possibility of death during surgery had ever been mentioned; 90 per cent had forgotten that less serious complications had also been discussed. Patients were best able to remember the benefits which had been predicted from a successful operation — indicating contamination by wishful thinking and hindsight. One patient stoutly maintained that he had been given no information at all: 'All he [the physician] did was lift up my shirt, put a stethoscope on my heart, and that was it'. This patient had been given half an hour of the surgeon's time (Robinson and Merar 1983).

Tom Benbow is actually being quite rational in terms of his own agenda — getting Social Services to rehouse him. There is nothing inherently irrational about this objective, although Tom does not recognize that moving will not solve his problems with his neighbours — but many people move house for no better reason. His methods, including violence, possibly manipulative reference to 'rays' affecting his legs, and self-neglect, appear less rational, but we need to be careful that we do not confuse our inherent revulsion at his methods with a diagnosis of mental illness. Tom might actually be using our revulsion to get what he wants. When asked why he doesn't improve his hygiene, avoiding further manual evacuations, he says that it is because he wants to be moved. He understands his own motivations to a considerable extent and seems well orientated.

Disparity in diagnosing mental health or mental illness is generally not purposeful or wilful, so it may seem odd to suggest that it could be unethical. But unintentional bias can be unfair, even discriminatory, in its results. We argue — controversially — that Tom's gender and perhaps even his learning disability are biasing clinicians towards a finding of (comparative) mental health, in the face of his violence and possible delusions. This may mean that he is not getting all the resources he needs, including psychotropic drugs for his violence, although on the face of it he might appear to have 'benefited' from the reaction against treating sexual offences, like his exhibitionism, as biologically determined and curable with drugs or surgery.

We suggest, then, that a wholesome awareness of the temptation to classify socially aberrant behaviour as mental illness has its 'down' side. More speculatively, it also seems possible that Tom's clinicians are working too hard to overcome their natural feelings of repulsion at the consequences of his self-neglect, the need for manual evacuation of faeces. Bending over backwards not to let their own 'irrational' feelings of repulsion contaminate their clinical judgement, they may be ignoring the influence of values on (what they take to be) the factual process of diagnosis (Fulford 1991).

Practitioner commentary (CASE 3.2)

Dr John Morgan Consultant Psychiatrist, Oxfordshire Learning Disability NHS Trust

The case of Tom Benbow illustrates some common dilemmas facing health and social workers. The historical changes to service models, often driven by institutional scandals, policies, and theoretical frameworks such as 'normalization' (Wolfensberger 1972) and 'social role valorization' (Wolfensberger 1983) have rightly ensured that independence, autonomy, and community presence are at the forefront of clinicians' considerations.

The theoretical framework of normalization and its subsequent development into social role valorization have had a particular influence on services to people with learning disabilities. The theory stresses that services should pursue models that reinforce positive social roles for those with disabilities. There is danger that this may foster a reluctance to assign diagnoses to individuals as this could be construed as unhelpful labelling, but some services may require classification of the individual as a means of accessing them. The training and experience gained by the professional mould their practice. One of the consequences is that some professions are more comfortable than others in categorizing individuals with disabilities. Such differing perspectives can have a powerful effect on multidisciplinary teams. The positive effects include the encouragement of differing viewpoints providing a richer source of material and interpretations. However, on the down side, such differences can create interprofessional tensions.

When faced with difficult situations as in Tom's case, the individual worker or team has to consider a number of factors, some of which may be in conflict. Working with people like Tom, who have chronic disabilities and fluctuating mental illnesses, is a long-term endeavour. Practitioners may well have to balance the provision of optimum care with that of maintaining a therapeutic relationship: for example, admitting him into a psychiatric hospital under a section of the Mental Health Act will allow him to obtain optimum management of his psychotic symptoms; but this risks damaging the long-term therapeutic relationship, with the result that he may be less likely to let anyone into his house in the future to monitor his mental state. Is it preferable, then, that he has less than optimal management of his psychosis in the community or that the therapeutic relationship remains intact? Of course in practice other risk factors, such as risk to himself or the public would be taken into account, but the example serves to illustrate that such decisions are judgements. The multidisciplinary team is important in providing a forum where such discussions can take place, but it is essential that the views of the person concerned, their carers, and advocates be taken into account.

Tom also presents dilemmas to practitioners because of his cognitive disabilities and the question to what extent he is able or willing to give consent. In practice, the issue of Tom's capacity to consent would usually be resolved by the appropriate member/s of the team assessing him with reference to a particular decision. The criteria for assessing this have been described elsewhere (see BMA and Law Society 1995, for example). One important thing to bear in mind is the complexity of the decision and the need to spend sufficient time with the individual to help them understand the relevant information — this may take several interviews using different types of information, such as pictures and symbols.

If it becomes apparent that the individual is unable to consent, the team can take action, provided it is necessary and in the person's best interest, under the legal concept of necessity. This of course raises the question of what is in Tom's best interest — an uncomfortable but vital question faced by many practitioners. In practice, the professionals would consult with the relevant carers, family, and other involved parties before making this judgement. One useful approach is to consider what are the consequences of taking action and of not doing so, enabling the practitioner to weigh up the options. Again, judgements made on the basis of inputs from all those concerned, including the multidisciplinary team, may be helpful here.

References (CASE 3.2)

Beauchamp, T.L. and Childress, J.F. (1994) *Principles of Biomedical Ethics* (4th edn). New York, Oxford University Press.

Bloch, S. (1991) The political misuse of psychiatry in the Soviet Union. In *Psychiatric Ethics* (2nd edn) (ed. Bloch, S. and Chodoff, P.), pp. 493–515. Oxford, Oxford University Press.

BMA and the Law Society (1995) *Assessment of Mental Capacity. Guidance for Doctors and Lawyers*. London, BMA.

Brody, H. (1992) *The Healer's Power*. New Haven, Yale University Press.

Devereux, J.A., Jones, D.P.H., and Dickenson, D.L. (1993) Can children withhold consent to treatment? *BMJ*, **306**:1459–61.

Fulford, K.W.M. (1991) The concept of disease. In *Psychiatric Ethics* (2nd edn) (ed. Bloch, S. and Chodoff, P.), pp. 77–99. Oxford, Oxford University Press.

Gillick v West Norfolk and Wisbech Area Health Authority (1985) 3 All England Reports 402.

Gillon, R. (1985) *Philosophical Medical Ethics*. Chichester, John Wiley.

Harding, T. (1991) Ethical issues in the delivery of mental health services: abuses in Japan. In *Psychiatric Ethics* (2nd edn) (ed. Bloch, S. and Chodoff, P.), pp. 473–91. Oxford, Oxford University Press.

Müller–Hill, B. (1991) Psychiatry in the Nazi era. In *Psychiatric Ethics* (2nd edn) (ed. Bloch, S. and Chodoff, P.), pp. 461–71. Oxford, Oxford University Press.

Oppenheimer, C. (1991) Ethics and psychogeriatrics. In *Psychiatric Ethics* (2nd edn) (ed. Bloch, S. and Chodoff, P.), pp. 365–90. Oxford, Oxford University Press.

Peele, R. (1991) The ethics of deinstitutionalization. In *Psychiatric Ethics* (2nd edn) (ed. Bloch, S. and Chodoff, P.), pp. 291–311. Oxford, Oxford University Press.

Rawls, J. (1971) *A Theory of Justice*. Cambridge (Mass.), Harvard University Press.

Re R (1991) 3 Weekly Law Reports 592.

Reich, W. (1991) Psychiatric diagnosis as an ethical problem. In *Psychiatric Ethics* (2nd edn) (ed. Bloch, S. and Chodoff, P.), pp. 101–33. Oxford, Oxford University Press.

Robinson, G. and Merar, A. (1983) Informed consent: recall by patients tested post-operatively. In *Moral Problems in Medicine* (2nd edn) (ed. Gorovitz, S. *et al.*). Englewood Cliffs (New Jersey), Prentice–Hall.

Scheff, T. (1966) *Being Mentally Ill: A Sociological Theory*. Chicago, Aldine.

Wilkes, K.V. (1988) *Real People: Personal Identity Without Thought Experiments*. Oxford, Clarendon Press.

Wolfensberger, W. (1972) *The Principle of Normalisation in Human Services*. Toronto, National Institute on Mental Retardation (NIMR).

Wolfensberger, W. (1983) Social Role Valorization: a proposed new term for the principle of Normalization. *Mental Retardation*, **21**:234–9.

Reading Guide

This Reading Guide covers models of disorder, their significance in relation to abusive uses of psychiatry for political or other non-medical purposes, and their importance in current clinical practice. Further reading on the role of values in psychiatric diagnosis is given in Chapter 4.

Models of disorder

An early but still excellent overview of models of disorder in mental health is A. Clare's 'The disease concept in psychiatry', in *Essentials of Postgraduate Psychiatry* (1979), edited by P. Hill *et al*. Illustrative original articles are reproduced in *Concepts of Health and Disease, Interdisciplinary Perspectives* (1981), edited by A.L. Caplan *et al*. Fulford has brought these reviews up to date in 'Modern conceptions of health and illness', in *Coping with Sickness: Perspectives on Healthcare Past and Present* (1996), edited by J. Woodward and R. Jütte, and in a long entry on 'Mental illness' for *The Encyclopaedia of Applied Ethics* (1998), edited by R. Chadwick.

A user-friendly introduction to the main models important in clinical work in psychiatry is *Models for Mental Disorder: Conceptual Models in Psychiatry* (1993, 2nd edn) by P. Tyrer and D. Steinberg. The different perspectives (biological, psychological, and social) important in psychiatry are carefully set out by McHugh and Slaveney (1983) in *The Perspectives of Psychiatry*. The medical model in psychiatry is well reviewed by Macklin in 'The medical model in psychoanalysis and psychotherapy' (1973).

Abusive uses of psychiatry

The debate between psychiatry and antipsychiatry was at its height in the 1960s and 1970s. The central claim of the antipsychiatrists in this debate was that all psychiatry is abusive in effect if not in intent, essentially because psychiatric disorders are moral not medical problems. Clear presentations of the antipsychiatry and pro-psychiatry extremes in the debate are, respectively, Szasz's *Insanity: the Idea and its Consequences* (1987) and Kendell's 'The concept of disease and its implications for psychiatry' (1975). Roth and Kroll's *The Reality of Mental Illness* (1986) is a direct reply to Szasz's arguments. An analysis of the assumptions common to anti- and pro-psychiatry theories, and hence a reconciliation of their positions, is developed by Fulford in Chapter 1 of his *Moral Theory and Medical Practice* (1989). The role of models in the abuse of psychiatry in the USSR is examined in Fulford *et al*. (1993).

Paul Chodoff's Chapter 4 in the third edition of *Psychiatric Ethics* (1999), edited by Bloch *et al.*, reviews a number of high-profile abuses of psychiatry in Nazi Germany, Japan, and the USSR. More detailed accounts of each of these are to be found in Chapter 22 (by Benno Müller–Hill), Chapter 23 (by Timothy Harding), and Chapter 24 (by Sidney Bloch) of the second edition (1991). Legal ramifications of the abuse of psychiatry are explored in Alan Stone's *Law, Psychiatry, and Morality* (1984). That psychiatry remains vulnerable to abusive manipulation is graphically illustrated by the American psychiatrists Alfred Freedman and Abraham Halpern's (1999) description of the growing involvement of psychiatrists in executions in some parts of the USA.

Models of disorder and current practice
Although the debate about models of mental disorder is less intense than it was in the 1960s and 1970s, the issues have certainly not gone away. Indications of the practical importance of models of disorder, especially in the new circum- stances of community care, are to be found in: 1) a large literature from patients and patient groups (for example, P. Campbell's 'What we want from crisis services' in *Speaking our Minds* (1996), edited by J. Read and J. Reynolds, 2) more systematic studies (for example, *Experiencing Psychiatry: Users' Views of Services* by Rogers *et al.* (1993), 3) official reports (for example, the 1995 *Report of the Clinical Standards Advisory Group on Schizophrenia*, Volume 1, which showed that an over-reliance on a consumer-led model could lead to seriously ill patients being neglected, and 4) in the ethical and clinical prob- lems posed by community care (see, for example, Rachel Perkins and Julie Repper's *Dilemmas in Community Mental Health Practice*, 1998). Anthony Colombo's *Understanding Mentally Disordered Offenders: a Multi-Agency Perspective* (1997) describes an empirical study of the role of different models of disorder in structuring practice. This includes operationalized definitions of each of the key models.

The *Declaration of Madrid*, the first code to spell out the importance of the 'user' voice in clinical decision making, was published in 1996 by the World Psychiatric Association.

Reading Guide: references

Campbell, P. (1996) What we want from crisis services. In *On Speaking Our Minds: Anthology* (ed. Read, J. and Reynolds, J.), pp. 180–4. London, MacMillan Press Ltd. (for The Open University).

Caplan, A. L., Engelhardt, T., and McCartney, J. (ed.) (1981) *Concepts of Health and Disease, Interdisciplinary Perspectives*. Addison–Wesley Publishing Company.

Chodoff, P. (1999) Misuse and abuse of psychiatry: an overview. In *Psychiatric Ethics* (3rd edn) (ed. Bloch, S., Chodoff, P., and Green, S.), Chapter 4. Oxford, Oxford University Press.

Clare, A. (1979) The disease concept in psychiatry. In *Essentials of Postgraduate Psychiatry* (ed. Hill, P., Murray, R., and Thorley, A.) New York, Academic Press, Grune and Stratton.

Colombo, A. (1997) *Understanding Mentally Disordered Offenders: a Multi-Agency Perspective*. Aldershot (England), Ashgate.

CSAG (1995) *Report of the Clinical Standards Advisory Group on Schizophrenia* (Volume 1). London, HMSO.

Freedman, A.M. and Halpern, A.L. (1999) The psychiatrist's dilemma: a conflict of roles in executions. *Australian and New Zealand Journal of Psychiatry*, 33:629–35.

Fulford, K.W.M. (1989, reprinted 1995; 2nd edn forthcoming) *Moral Theory and Medical Practice*. Cambridge, Cambridge University Press.

Fulford, K.W.M. (1996) Modern conceptions of health and illness. In *Coping with Sickness: Perspectives on Healthcare Past and Present* (ed. Woodward, J. and Jütte, R.). Sheffield, European Association for History of Medicine and Health Publications

Fulford, K.W.M. (1998) Mental illness. In *Encyclopaedia of Applied Ethics* (ed. Chadwick, R.). San Diego, Academic Press.

Fulford, K.W.M., Smirnoff, A.Y.U., and E. Snow. (1993) Concepts of disease and the abuse of psychiatry in the USSR. *British Journal of Psychiatry*, 162:801–10. Reprinted in 1996 in *Medical Ethics* (ed. Downie, R.S.), volume in *The International Research Library of Philosophy* series (series ed. J. Skorupski). Aldershot (England), Dartmouth.

Harding, T. (1991) Ethical issues in the delivery of mental health services: abuses in Japan. In *Psychiatric Ethics* (2nd edn) (ed. Bloch, S. and Chodoff, P.), pp. 473–91. Oxford, Oxford University Press.

Kendell, R.E. (1975) The concept of disease and its implications for psychiatry. *British Journal of Psychiatry*, 127:305–15.

Macklin, R. (1973) The medical model in psychoanalysis and psychotherapy. *Comprehensive Psychiatry*, 14:49–69.

McHugh, P.R. and Slaveney, P.R. (1983) *The Perspectives of Psychiatry*. Baltimore (USA), The Johns Hopkins University Press.

Müller–Hill, B. (1991) Psychiatry in the Nazi era. In *Psychiatric Ethics* (2nd edn) (ed. Bloch, S. and Chodoff, P.), Chapter 22. Oxford, Oxford University Press.

Perkins, R. and Repper, J. (1998) *Dilemmas in Community Mental Health Practice: Choice or Control*. Aberdeen (England), Radcliffe Medical Press.

Rogers, A., Pilgrim, D., and Lacey, R. (1993) *Experiencing Psychiatry: Users' Views of Services*. London, The MacMillan Press.

Roth, M. and Kroll, J. (1986) *The Reality of Mental Illness*. Cambridge, Cambridge University Press.

Stone, A. (1984) *Law, Psychiatry, and Morality*. Washington, American Psychiatric Press.

Szasz, T.S. (1987) *Insanity: The Idea and Its Consequences*. Chichester (England), John Wiley & Sons.

Tyrer, P. and **Steinberg, D.** (1993) *Models for Mental Disorder: Conceptual Models in Psychiatry* (2nd edn). Chichester (England), John Wiley & Sons.

World Psychiatric Association, Geneva (1996) Declaration of Madrid. (Reproduced with a brief commentary in 1999 in *Psychiatric Ethics* (3rd edn) (Bloch, S., Chodoff P., and Green S.A.), Appendix — Codes of Ethics, pp. 511–31. Oxford, Oxford University Press.)

Diagnosis: rationality, responsibility, and values in psychiatric classification

Ethical and scientific considerations cannot be fully disentangled in psychiatric classification and diagnosis

In the last chapter we were concerned with the overall concept of mental disorder. We found that mental disorder is understood in a number of different ways in the context of everyday practice, and that among these different 'models', it is important to strike a balance between medical and moral conceptions. In this chapter we move from the general to the specific, from the broad concept of mental disorder to three particular aspects of it which are ethically significant in psychiatric diagnosis: rationality (in Case 4.1, Martin McKendrick); responsibility (in Case 4.2, Delia Jarrett); and descriptive psychopathology (in Case 4.3, Simon Greer).

At first sight these three aspects of the concept of mental disorder make odd bedfellows. Rationality and responsibility, we can see in a general way, both bridge ethics and psychiatric diagnosis: both concepts are, on the one hand, the concern of law and moral philosophy, and, on the other, closely connected with our conceptions of madness. But why psychopathology? After all, for many psychiatrists, descriptive psychopathology is the very basis of the scientific account of mental disorder by which they take their subject to be marked out as a genuine branch of medicine.

In fact, it is precisely the *dis*junction between moral concepts, such as rationality and responsibility, and the medical concepts of psychopathology, which brings them together in this chapter. The difficulties that psychiatrists, lawyers, and others have found in defining mental disorder have led them to concentrate on what each regards as more tractable aspects of the concept. Lawyers and ethicists, understandably enough, have focused on the overtly moral aspects of mental disorder. The definition of mental disorder, they have in effect said, may be hard to pin down, but it is the irrationality and/or the loss of responsibility involved in mental disorder with which we are concerned.

Rationality and responsibility are concepts we understand, so let us concentrate on these.

Psychiatrists, by contrast, have had greater success with the *scientific* endeavour of defining the symptoms of mental disorder — of developing a *descriptive* psychopathology. Consistently then, with the medical model, there has been a move to confine psychiatric diagnostic assessments to these symptoms. Here the psychiatrist, like any other medical specialist, can offer expertise as, in the old-fashioned but still current legal phrase, a 'man of science'. It is recognized that a diagnosis of mental disorder carries ethical and legal implications. But these implications are for experts of other kinds — lawyers and moral philosophers in the case of rationality, a lay jury in the case of 'folk' concepts like responsibility.

The Butler Committee, set up by the UK Government to review the treatment of mentally disordered offenders prior to the introduction of the Mental Health Act 1983, took this line explicitly (Butler 1975). As we noted in Chapter 2, it reviewed the connections between psychopathological concepts and the loss of responsibility which justifies the status of mental disorder as a legal excuse. It argued that it is only with a *psychotic* disorder that a person has traditionally been regarded as not responsible for their actions; but, it continued, since there is no accepted definition of 'psychosis', the law should be framed in terms of a number of particular psychotic symptoms, specifically, certain kinds of delusion, hallucination, and disturbances of cognitive functioning. Psychiatrists, the Butler Committee concluded, could then be asked to give expert evidence only as to the presence of these specific symptoms, leaving questions of responsibility to the judge and jury.

As things turned out, this was one of the Butler recommendations which did not make it into the Mental Health Act 1983. In the UK, and indeed in most countries around the world (Fulford and Hope 1996), mental health law is cast in terms of the broad notion of 'mental disorder'. As we noted in Chapter 2, even countries such as Denmark, which start out by limiting involuntary treatment to psychotic disorders, go on to add a rider to the effect that it may be extended to other relevantly similar conditions. But the attempt to disentangle descriptive psychopathology from moral and ethical concepts remains one to which psychiatrists are inclined. The DSM, for example, includes a disclaimer against its use in ethical and legal contexts — a paragraph in DSM–III (APA 1987) which is expanded into a full page in DSM–IV (APA 1994). Disentangling is also the approach of many lawyers and ethicists. We had an example of this in Chapter 2 with the work of the American bioethicists, Tom Beauchamp and James Childress, on the justification of involuntary treatment. You will recall that in a valuable review of different theories of responsibility relevant to psychiatry, they argued that judgements of responsibility involve

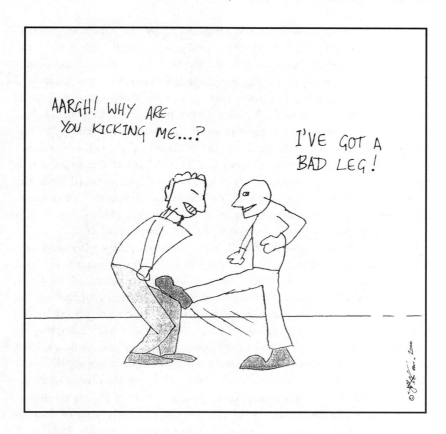

judgements of value. But this disentangling diagnosis from ethics, has the consequence that judgements of responsibility involve '*moral not* medical considerations [our emphasis]' (Beauchamp and Childress 1989, p. 84).

We will see in a moment that there are dangers in this strategy of disentangling. We should note first, though, that as a strategy it is in itself perfectly sound. It has indeed good scientific precedents. The theory of relativity, no less, was a product in part of Einstein's strategy of disentangling a tractable aspect of the concept of time, viz. its measurement with clocks. We may not be able to define 'time' but, so this approach implies, at least we can measure it. Forget about defining 'time' then; specifying the procedures or 'operations' that we go through to measure time is enough. Such 'operational criteria' are sufficient for our use of the concept of time in practical science. In the case of relativity, they were sufficient to generate a whole new class of physical theory.

'Operational criteria' is the buzz word, too, in modern psychiatric diagnostic classifications. The use of specific inclusion and exclusion criteria to

define categories of mental disorder, introduced by the American psychiatrist Robert Spitzer in DSM–III (APA 1987), was directly inspired by the
success of the operational approach in physics. Indeed, behind the operational criteria of modern psychiatric diagnostic classifications, there is a
classic story of scientific progress. This starts with careful descriptions of
the phenomena of interest (the descriptive psychopathology of Jaspers,
Kraepelin, and others in the early years of the twentieth century); premature aetiological theories are then rejected in favour of a classification based
on symptoms and symptom clusters (in ICD–8, WHO 1967); and the reliability of psychiatric diagnosis takes a quantum leap forward with the
development of formal procedures for eliciting these symptoms (for example,
the Present State Examination, Wing *et al.* 1974) and carefully designed field
trials (for example, the US-UK Diagnostic Project, Cooper *et al.* 1972).

So where's the ethics in all this? Well, in the first place philosophers and soci-
ologists have shown that the 'classic' story of science misrepresents progress
even in physics. The crucial switch from aetiology to symptoms in ICD–8 was
recommended to the WHO by the British psychiatrist, Irwin Stengel, on the
basis of a paper on the classic account of scientific classifications by the
philosopher of science Karl Hempel (1961). But Hempel was one of the last
philosophers of science to believe in the classic account. There are now known
to be a whole series of points at which meaning and significance are built into
the development of scientific theory. Thus all scientific theories, as the
American philosopher of science, W.V.O. Quine, famously put it, are under-
determined by the data (Quine 1948). In other words, for any set of data, an
open-ended family of theories is possible. We select from possible theories, of
course, but we select according to principles of economy (Occam's famous
razor), elegance, and so forth. More radically though, the very 'data' on which
our theories are based are, necessarily, selected. If you doubt this, try giving a
complete (*complete*, mind) description of an everyday object like a chair. You
will find that the process is essentially open-ended — there is no *definitive*
description; you *have* to select — and, again, you select according to criteria of
significance, relevance, and so forth.

What you observe about a chair is, of course, except in some very extreme
philosophical theories, not unconnected with the real chair! The point is that
even with everyday physical objects like chairs, our observations reflect a good
deal of ourselves. If this is true of objects like chairs, how much more so will it
be the case with the 'observations' of human experience and behaviour on
which psychopathology is built. Karl Jaspers, to whom above all we owe modern descriptive psychopathology, repeatedly emphasized the importance of
meanings as well as causes in psychopathology, of understanding as well as
explanation (Jaspers 1913). Recent work in the philosophy of psychiatry has

shown the continuing importance of values in shaping our diagnostic concepts (see, for example, Fulford 1994 and Sadler 1996).

In psychiatric diagnosis then, concerned as it is with human experience and behaviour, we should not be surprised to find that questions of meaning and significance cannot be wholly disentangled from the 'objective' observations on which a scientific model of diagnosis has traditionally been based. This is the point of departure for the three cases examined in this chapter. The difficulties encountered with the concept of mental disorder have led to attempts to focus on aspects of the concept which have seemed more tractable. These attempts have gone in two equal and opposite directions — either assimilation to (supposedly) higher-level concepts (rationality and responsibility) or restriction to (supposedly) lower-level concepts (the specific symptoms of mental disorder and the syndromes defined by clusters of these symptoms which make up psychopathology). The danger, though, is that the very success of this disentangling approach may lead us to lose sight of the original problem or, worse still, to suppose that we have resolved the original problem by resolving one of its component parts.

The cases we discuss in this chapter illustrate the strengths but also the limitations of the disentangling approach. We focus in each of them on one of the three particular aspects of psychiatric diagnostic concepts with which we are concerned in this chapter — rationality (Case 4.1), responsibility (Case 4.2), and psychopathology (Case 4.3), respectively. This allows us to explore the ethical significance of each of these in some detail in the context of everyday clinical practice. But in each case, we argue, the ethical significance of the concept in question is integral to, and cannot be disentangled from, psychiatric diagnostic assessment. In the first case, Martin McKendrick, judgements of rationality are at the *heart* of the clinical problem of how to respond to his request for euthanasia. In the second case, Delia Jarrett, attributions of responsibility go *hand in hand* with fluctuating views about her diagnosis of 'marginal personality disorder'. In the third case, Simon Greer, the *crucial* differential diagnosis, between delusion and religious experience, actually turns not on the facts about his experiences and behaviour but on a series of value judgements.

It is significant that the aspects of psychiatric diagnosis around which the issues raised by these cases revolve — rationality, responsibility, and values respectively — have at best a low profile in psychiatric education. This is a further reflection of the narrowly medical model of psychiatry outlined in Chapter 1. Yet all three aspects of psychiatric diagnosis are current 'hot topics' in practice. Thus, rationality is very much back on psychiatry's agenda; it is at the heart of requests for 'psychiatric euthanasia' (as in our first case in this chapter: see also Burgess and Hawton 1998). Judgements of rationality are important, too, in a range of issues about advance directives and mental disorders (Savulescu and Dickenson 1998). They are also the key to our understanding of children's consent (Dickenson and Jones 1995). Responsibility, similarly, has swung into prominence, notably in connection with risk and the disputed concept of personality disorder. The current review of mental health legislation in the UK looks set, on the one hand, to extend psychiatry's powers of compulsion (thus reducing the responsibility of users), and, on the other, to make psychiatrists responsible for the actions not only of those with recognized psychiatric illnesses but of those with personality disorders. Difficulties of attributing responsibility, let alone of human rights and justice, are at risk of being subordinated to political contingencies in this process.

So far as values are concerned, they are not merely back on psychiatry's agenda, but at the top of its agenda — in the very criteria on which modern scientific classifications of disorder are based. As we will see in the diagnosis in the case of Simon Greer, in the third case in this chapter, the key distinction between spiritual experience and a schizophrenic illness turns essentially on a series of value judgements. These value judgements, moreover, are not merely implicit in the diagnostic distinction but explicit in the DSM's own 'Criterion B' for schizophrenia. Such value judgements are not widely recognized for what they are, but once they are, they are evident not only throughout psychiatric classification (Fulford 1994) but also in the processes by which diagnostic categories are defined (Sadler 1996). Those for whom the validity of psychiatry as a science is taken to depend on a value-free classification of psychiatric disorders will be concerned by this; as we noted in Chapter 1 (and again in the Reading Guide to Chapter 2), there is continuing debate about the relationship between fact and value generally, not just in psychiatric diagnosis. But at a practical level, there is a growing recognition of the de facto importance of values in diagnosis, for example, in cross-cultural psychiatry (Fulford 1999) and in connection with the user's voice being heard in how their problems are understood (Campbell 1996).

The practical and theoretical problems surrounding rationality, responsibility, and values in psychiatry, have been compounded by recent case law, notably the case of 'C', in which it was held that delusions *per se* do not invalidate autonomous choice. 'C' was an elderly man in Broadmoor who chose not to have a potentially life-saving amputation of a gangrenous leg; he based his decision on the delusional belief that he was an experienced surgeon. The court, however, upheld his decision on the basis of expert testimony to the effect that this was the kind of decision that would be reasonable for people like Mr C to make (Re C 1994). The court was in effect identifying with Mr C's values (that he would rather be dead with his leg than alive without it), however delusional (and hence irrational) their justification.

Legal argument in *Re C*, it should be said, was not explicitly in terms of values. Rather it reflected a growing trend, at least in the law in England and Wales, to replace diagnostic criteria for involuntary treatment (like 'mental disorder' or 'delusion') with criteria of incapacity. The nub of the decision in *Re C* was that the rationality of a person's choice is to be judged by common criteria for the delusional and the non-delusional cases. Those criteria, following a major review by the Law Commission (1995), a Government Green Paper (Lord Chancellor's Department 1997), statements from professional bodies such as the BMA (1995), and so forth, are, broadly, that the person concerned can:

1 understand and retain the treatment information;

2 believe the information;

3 weigh up the information in a balanced way;

4 come to a decision based on that information.

These criteria currently apply only to treatment for a physical disorder: had *Re C* been concerned with treatment for a mental disorder, then the Mental Health Act 1983, with its diagnostic criterion of 'mental disorder', would have been pertinent. But there is a strong move to abolish specific mental health legislation, like the Mental Health Act 1983, altogether, and to replace it with a generic 'incapacity act' (Szmukler and Holloway 1998, with replies by Fulford 1998 and Sayce 1998).

The replacement of diagnostic criteria with generic incapacity criteria for involuntary psychiatric treatment could have a number of advantages; it might reduce stigma, for example, as George Szmukler and Frank Holloway (1998) argue. But it could be highly abusive in effect if it failed to acknowledge the particular difficulties of judgements of rationality in mental disorder. This is especially so with the ethically central case of delusion. As we saw in Chapter 2, delusion is the central case of mental illness as an excuse in law (and correspondingly the form of psychopathology most commonly involved in involuntary psychiatric treatment). Bioethicists, such as Beauchamp and Childress, as well as psychiatrists, have assumed that this is because those who are deluded lack the capacities required for autonomous choice, and hence that delusion can be assimilated to cases such as dementia and unconsciousness. Yet it is far from clear what capacities are disturbed in the case of delusion. In dementia and unconsciousness there is disturbance of cognitive capacities; but no disturbance of cognitive functioning uniquely characteristic of delusion has yet been identified (Garety and Freeman 1999).

So far as the proposed legal criteria are concerned, as *Re C* shows, those who are deluded may well be deemed competent. Of course, the decision of the patient, in the case of involuntary psychiatric treatment, is by definition different from that to which everyone else has come; this is why the treatment is involuntary. In order for the proposed generic criteria of incapacity to cover the case of delusion, therefore, we have to make value judgements of the *quality* of the decision to which the patient has come: in a word, is their decision a good or a bad decision? This is why the expert testimony in R*e C* — that people like C often choose to refuse amputation — was crucial. It showed that C's choice was a good one as measured by his peers. But this is also the second level at which generic incapacity legislation may be abusive in effect. For as we have seen, in psychiatry, as against physical medicine, the relevant values are particularly *diverse*. Hence criteria which depend on *shared* values, like the proposed generic criteria of incapacity, are a recipe for the values of the majority being imposed on the minority. And, as the abuse of psychiatry in the former USSR showed (Fulford *et al.* 1993), the risks here will be especially large if the value judgements concerned are not recognized for what they are — if the generic incapacity criteria are thought to be objective scientific criteria and a matter solely for expert witnesses to determine.

All the dangers of the disentangling approach — of focusing on the parts and neglecting the whole — are thus inherent in this proposal. Generic incapacity legislation seems attractive (in part) because (we believe) we know how to define incapacity. In some circumstances this is right. As we noted in Chapter 2, Beauchamp and Childress successfully redefined judgements of rationality in terms of specific capacities for the case of physical disorders and for certain mental disorders, notably dementia. But in the absence of criteria for delusion — the ethically central case of irrationality in mental disorder — we are at risk of wrongly assimilating judgements of delusional irrationality to other, more tractable, but quite different, cases. The mismatch between the criteria for incapacity appropriate for, say, dementia, and the diagnostic criteria for delusion, means that people will be judged irrational when they are rational, and vice versa! As we saw in Chapter 3, either alternative can be equally abusive.

All of which is not to say that definition is a pointless exercise. As we have several times noted, much useful work has been done in law and ethics through attempts to define the criteria for rationality, responsibility, capacity, and so forth, more precisely. In psychiatry, similar attempts have clarified the criteria for the wide variety of different kinds of psychopathology with which we are concerned. But appreciating the role of definition needs to be balanced by two considerations, one negative and one positive. The negative consideration is that there is a limit to the practical utility of explicit definitions of the concepts like mental disorder. This is the bottom line of the cases described in this chapter. Teasing out the problems raised by Martin McKendrick, Delia Jarrett, and Simon Greer — in terms of rationality, responsibility, and descriptive psychopathology, respectively — helps to clarify the issues involved. But here, as with other mental disorders, rationality and responsibility cannot be *wholly* disentangled from psychopathology, and psychopathology cannot be *wholly* disentangled from rationality and responsibility.

The positive consideration is that if criteria are not sufficient, we should look as well to the *processes* by which such concepts are applied in practice. The rationale for this is that we are often better at *using* concepts (that is, the process) than at *defining* them. We return to the distinction between use and definition, and to the importance of process, in Chapter 8 in connection with the user's voice and the role of the multidisciplinary team.

References

American Psychiatric Association (3rd edn, revised, 1987; 4th edn 1994) *Diagnostic and Statistical Manual of Mental Disorders*. Washington DC, American Psychiatric Association.

Beauchamp, T.L. and **Childress, J.F.** (1989) *Principles of Biomedical Ethics* (3rd edn). Oxford, Oxford University Press.

BMA and the Law Society (1995) *Assessment of Mental Capacity: Guidance for Doctors and Lawyers*. London, BMA.

Burgess, S. and **Hawton, K.** (1998) Suicide, euthanasia, and the psychiatrist. *Philosophy, Psychiatry, and Psychology*, **5/2**:113–26.

Butler, the Rt. Hon., Lord. (1975) *Report of the Committee on Mentally Abnormal Offenders, Cmnd., 6244*. London, HMSO.

Campbell, P. (1996) What we want from crisis services. In *On Speaking Our Minds: Anthology* (ed. Read, J. and Reynolds, J.), pp. 180–4. London, MacMillan Press Ltd. (for The Open University).

Cooper, J.E., Kendell, R.E., Gurland, B.J., Sharpe, L., Copeland, J.R.M., and **Simon, R.** (1972) *Psychiatric Diagnosis in New York and London*. London, Oxford University Press.

Dickenson, D. and **Jones, D.** (1995) True wishes: the philosophy and developmental psychology of children's informed consent. *Philosophy, Psychiatry, and Psychology*, **2/4**:287–304.

Fulford, K.W.M. (1994) Closet logics: hidden conceptual elements in the DSM and ICD classifications of mental disorders. In *Philosophical Perspectives on Psychiatric Diagnostic Classification* (ed. Sadler, J.Z., Wiggins, O.P., and Schwartz, M.A.), Chapter 9. Baltimore, Johns Hopkins University Press.

Fulford, K.W.M. (1998) Replacing the Mental Health Act 1983? How to change the game without losing the baby with the bathwater or shooting ourselves in the foot. Invited commentary on Szmukler, G. and Holloway, F. Mental health legislation is now a harmful anachronism. *Psychiatric Bulletin*, **22**:666–8.

Fulford, K.W.M. (1999) Philosophy and cross-cultural psychiatry. In *Mental Health Service Provision for a Multi-Cultural Society* (ed. Bhui, K. and Olajide, D), Chapter 2. London, W.B. Saunders, Ltd.

Fulford, K.W.M. and Hope, T. (1996) Informed consent in psychiatry: comparative assessment of Section 5 of the National Reports — Report for Biomed 1 project (published as Control and Practical Experience).In *Informed Consent in Psychiatry: European Perspectives on Ethics, Law and Clinical Practice* (ed. Koch, H.-G., Reiter–Theil, S., and Helmchen, H.), pp. 349–77. Baden–Baden, Nomos Verlagsgesellschaft.

Fulford, K.W.M., Smirnoff, A.Y.U., and Snow. E. (1993) Concepts of disease and the abuse of psychiatry in the USSR. *British Journal of Psychiatry,* **162**:801–10. Reprinted in 1996 in *Medical Ethics* (ed. Downie, R.S.), volume in *The International Research Library of Philosophy* series (series ed. J. Skorupski). Aldershot (England), Dartmouth.

Garety, P. A. and Freeman, D. (1999) Cognitive approaches to delusions: a critical review of theories and evidence. *British Journal of Clinical Psychology,* **38**:113–54.

Hempel, C.G. (1961) Introduction to problems of taxonomy. In *Field Studies in the Mental Disorders* (ed. Zubin, J.), pp. 3–22. New York, Grune and Stratton. Reproduced in 1994 in *Philosophical Perspectives on Psychiatric Diagnostic Classification* (ed. Sadler, J.Z., Wiggins, O.P., and Schwartz, M.A.), pp. 315–31. Baltimore, The Johns Hopkins University Press.

Jaspers, K. (1913) *Allgemeine Psychopathologie.* Berlin, Springer. In translation in 1963 as *General Psychopathology* (translated by Hoenig, J. and Hamilton, M.W.). Manchester, Manchester University Press. New edition in 1997, with a new foreword by McHugh, Paul R. Baltimore, The Johns Hopkins University Press.

Law Commission (1995) *Mental Incapacity.* London, HMSO.

Lord Chancellor's Department (1997) *Who Decides? Making Decisions on Behalf of Mentally Incapacitated Adults. CM 3803.* London, The Stationery Office Ltd.

Quine, W. (1948) On what there is. *Review of Metaphysics,* **2**. Reprinted in 1953 in *From a Logical Point of View* (Quine, W.). Cambridge (Mass.), Harvard University Press.

Re C (adult: refusal of medical treatment) (1994) 1 All ER 819.

Sadler J.Z. (1996) Epistemic value commitments in the debate over categorical vs. dimensional personality diagnosis. *Philosophy, Psychiatry, and Psychology,* **3**:203–22.

Savulescu, J. and Dickenson, D. (1998) The time frame of preferences, dispositions, and the validity of advance directives for the mentally ill. *Philosophy, Psychiatry, and Psychology,* **5/3**:225–46.

Sayce, L. (1998) Mental health legislation is now a harmful anachronism. *Psychiatric Bulletin,* **22**: 669–70.

Szmukler, G. and Holloway, F. (1998) Mental health legislation is now a harmful anachronism. *Psychiatric Bulletin,* **22**:662–5.

Wing, J.K., Cooper, J.E., and Sartorius, N. (1974) *Measurement and Classification of Psychiatric Symptoms.* Cambridge, Cambridge University Press.

World Health Organisation (1967) *Manual of the International Statistical Classification of Diseases, Injuries and Causes of Death (ICD–8).* Geneva, WHO.

World Health Organisation (1973) *The International Pilot Study of Schizophrenia. Volume 1.* Geneva, WHO.

CASE 4.1
Martin McKendrick — rational and irrational suicide

Synopsis A 42-year-old man, with a history of repeated suicide attempts, says that he has nothing to live for and wants to die. He has auditory hallucinations and persecutory delusions. Trials of various medications and periods of detention under the Mental Health Act have proved ineffective. He has no social contacts.

Key dilemma Is his wish to die rational?

Main topic Judgements of rationality.

Other topics Suicide; Suicide Act 1961; Chabot case; Dutch law on assisted suicide; action and rationality; euthanasia; identity; medical model of psychiatry; paternalism; Kant; Re C; best interests.

Like Delia Jarrett, Martin McKendrick has a long history of involvement with psychiatric services, dating back to adolescence, when he made the first of many suicide attempts. His mother died when he was twelve, and he was largely brought up by an older sister; his father had abandoned the family when Martin was a little boy. Martin, now forty-two, lives alone and has lost contact with his sister. But he continually hears her voice, he says, telling him that he is evil and that he ought to kill himself. He also believes that his sister is poisoning his food.

Martin has taken repeated overdoses, usually of paracetamol, requiring medical intervention in several cases. Twice he also slashed his wrists. He eats little but smokes and drinks heavily. His sister appears to have been anorexic, and his own weight is below eight stone.

Although Martin seeks help, he has always been poorly compliant with medication and follow-up. Often he has presented asking for admission, only to self-discharge after a few day, ignoring follow-up arrangements. He has been detained under the Mental Health Act several times, but finds compulsory admission very distressing; his eating patterns worsen and his self-harm behaviour escalates. Therapeutic trials of several different medications, including antidepressants, were used while Martin was under section, but with only minimal improvement; the hallucinations and suicidal thoughts remain. ECT has also been tried; his delusions become less fixed, but his desire to die does not alter.

Martin's experience of compulsory admission leads him to the despairing conclusion that psychiatrists can do nothing for his constant suffering. The only thing the doctors could do for him, he says, would be to help him end his life. When at home he has no daily contacts, apart from psychiatric services. He spends his days with the curtains drawn, afraid to venture outside or even look through the window. He has no activities, despite repeated offers and suggestions. Martin gets no enjoyment from life, he says, and he sees no better prospects for the future.

In contrast to the case of Elizabeth Orton, there appears little doubt in this case that the patient, Martin McKendrick, has some form of mental illness: one that is also chronic and unamenable to treatment. Martin's case raises the issue of whether a person with a mental illness can make a rational request. Our next case (Delia Jarrett) will raise the question of whether a person with mental illness can still be responsible for her own behaviour. In neither case can we simply assume that the presence of mental illness rules out rationality and responsibility, and with them, rights. Martin's case also requires us to consider the even harder question — whether a request to die should be granted, even if it is rational. But can a request to die be rational?

The first point to make is that we cannot simply assume that Martin is mentally ill because he wants to die. There are other indicators here of mental illness, but the wish to die is not itself automatically one of them. In Martin's case, is his misery so deep that his wish to die is reasonable? Or is his suicidal impulse the manifestation of his mental illness? At one pole of the argument, one might view Martin's mental state as an exaggerated version of the modern identity, not as an aberration or illness at all. With the decline in the West of fixed, unchallengeable moral systems, particularly those centred on religious dictates, and the expectation that individuals should instead forge their own values, a sense of emptiness and the absence of a moral 'horizon' are increasingly common. Perhaps this is even linked in psychopathology to the decline in hysterias, phobias, and fixations (as the stuff of Freud's clinical life) and the upsurge in depression and suicidal tendencies (Taylor 1989, p. 19).

The opposite way of looking at Martin's suffering would be represented by the medicalized model of suicide. We sometimes hear reference to 'the disease of suicide': for example, in health promotion, where reducing the level of suicide is talked of in the same breath as encouraging people to improve their diet in the interests of minimizing coronary artery disease. In our society, suicide is often linked with mental illness, and with a medical model of psychiatric disorder; but in other societies it is regarded as a virtuous or rational act (the suicide of Seneca, for example). So why does the idea of rational suicide seem paradoxical to us?

Heyd and Bloch (1991) argue that it is next to impossible for clinicians to view suicide as rational, because intentional self-harm represents such a grave affront to the psychiatrist's own value system. Whereas other psychiatric conditions present a problem to be solved, drawing on the clinician's professional skills, deliberate self-harm represents a slap in the face:

> ...most medical and psychiatric problems are concerned with the adjustment of the right means to a given end that is basically shared by doctor and patient; suicide however focuses on the end itself, about which the two parties may hold polarly opposite views. Suicide is not only a functional problem to which therapeutic techniques are applied but also an existential one — in both the literal and the philosophical senses of the word. The question is not how to achieve a better, more fruitful life, but whether to live at all. (Heyd and Bloch 1991, p. 243)

In addition, the number of people who successfully attempt suicide while receiving psychiatric care shows up the uncomfortable limits of the psychiatrist's powers. In Martin's case, those limits are particularly clear: drug treatment and ECT have largely failed. When, if ever, should clinicians write off further treatment as futile? Is there really nothing the clinicians can do for Martin except help him to die?

This was the argument made to the Dutch psychiatrist, Dr Boudewin Chabot. Dr Chabot's patient, Mrs B, a physically fit woman in middle age, had lost her first son to suicide and her second son to cancer. Divorced from an alcoholic and violent husband, she had no further desire to live, and asked Dr Chabot, who was treating her for depression, to help her die.

Martin's clinicians are bound by Section 2 of the Suicide Act 1961, making it an imprisonable crime if one person 'aids, abets, counsels or procures the suicide of another, or an attempt by another to commit suicide'. In contrast, Dutch physicians are able to meet requests for assisted suicide and euthanasia so long as they adhere to legally prescribed guidelines and a statutory reporting procedure, even though euthanasia formally remains a criminal offence under Articles 293 and 294 of the penal code. Dutch law on assisted suicide (in which the patient takes the fatal dose) and euthanasia (in which the doctor gives a lethal injection) does allow intractable mental suffering to be considered on the same plane as unpalliatable physical pain, when a request for euthanasia is made.

In passing judgment on the Chabot case in June 1994, the Dutch Supreme Court found Mrs B competent to request assisted suicide, despite expert testimony that she was clinically depressed. It acquitted Dr Chabot, explicitly rejecting the prosecutor's contention that 'help in assistance with suicide to a patient where there is no physical suffering and who is not dying can never be justified'. In this sense the court accepted a medical model of mental illness. But should it have done so? 'The particular problem that is raised by "psychiatric euthanasia" ' — strictly speaking in this case, psychiatric assisted suicide — 'is the dubious boundary between psychiatric illness and understandable unhappiness' (Ogilvie and Potts 1994, p. 492).

Like Mrs B — although over a longer period of time — Martin has experienced a series of losses: father, mother, sister. Unlike Martin, Mrs B had not simply failed to respond to antidepressants: she had refused to take them. But Dr Chabot felt that this was part of her right to refuse treatment. The question, however, is whether her refusal of treatment, and her request for suicide, were actually caused by her depression. The same can be asked about Martin. If so, then granting a depressive's wish for assisted suicide would be no more justifiable than giving emetics to a bulimic at their request. Accepting a medical model of mental illness could just as well have led to intervention aimed at preventing rather than abetting her suicide. Indeed, this is the more likely form of reasoning.

Testifying against Dr Chabot, along these lines, at the Dutch Medical Council hearing which followed Chabot's acquittal by the Supreme Court, Dr van den Hoofdakker (a psychiatrist specializing in the treatment of depression) put forward a cleft stick argument. Either Mrs B was Dr Chabot's patient, in which case it was his professional duty to cure her rather than help her die, or he was acting as her friend, in which case he should have had no access to the drugs which he administered to bring about her death. (Mrs B, together with several other patients, had actually been living in Dr Chabot's house.) The Dutch Medical Council did decide to censure Dr Chabot, despite his acquittal by the judicial system.

Let us recapitulate. We have implicitly assumed a syllogism something like this in our discussion so far:

1 Requests made by rational patients ought to be honoured.

2 Martin and Mrs B have made requests to die.

3 These requests ought to be honoured if Martin and Mrs B are seen as rational, but if their depressive states are so powerful as to undermine rationality, the requests ought to be disallowed.

Thus our discussion has centred on the question of the patient's rationality. But there is an argument for focusing instead on the rationality of the action, as distinct from that of the patient. Considerations from both practice and law would support this second course.

One Dutch critic of assisted suicide and euthanasia has written: '...the request of the patient is not in practice the basis on which physicians decide to perform euthanasia, but rather they base such decisions on the condition of the patient' (Jochemsen 1994, p. 212–13). This may seem perfectly right and proper: doctors should not automatically honour patients' requests. But it does mean that doctors rather than patients usually decide whether life is worth living, and that can lead not only to paternalism but to more worrying consequences. On the one hand, in 1990, euthanasia or aid in suicide was given in 2700 cases out of 9000 requests; on the other, 1000 lives were terminated without a specific request from the patient (Remmelink Commission 1991). Although this worrying figure includes many patients in a comatose state and near the end of life, about one quarter were competent to some extent and had a life expectancy of several more weeks. In addition, pain relief in dosages almost certain to cause death was given without the patient's request in about 60 per cent of such cases (Van der Maas *et al.* 1992, Chapter 8.3.1).

Practically speaking, then, doctors who focus on the rationality of the patient rather than the action may be too readily tempted into paternalism. The argument in favour of focusing on rationality of actions rather than patients also gains support from English law. In Re C (1994), as we saw earlier in this chapter, a 68-year-old schizophrenic patient detained in a secure hospital refused amputation of a gangrenous leg under the influence of his delusion that the doctors were torturers, whereas he himself was a world-famous surgeon. His refusal of consent was upheld, however, partly on expert testimony that other people of his age and condition frequently refused amputations in vascular disease — either preferring to die intact, or fearing that the first amputation might just be one of several. In other words, the action of refusing amputation was perfectly normal or rational in Mr C's circumstances, despite his own evident irrationality. Another way of putting this is to say that Mr C's irrationality was not all-pervasive: he was deemed to understand the nature and purpose of the treatment, as well as the consequences of refusal. By concentrating on the treatment action being considered, rather than on his general mental state, what was rational in his mind was highlighted.

The direction in which our argument has been tending seems to be that Martin's deliberate self-harm should not necessarily be judged as an irrational action. There is an argument against that — the Kantian claim that suicide is inherently contradictory and therefore irrational in a logical sense. A similar critique would be this: no matter how great Martin's suffering, he cannot improve his condition by killing himself, because there will be no one's condition to be improved after he is dead. It cannot be in someone's best interest to die, because we are appealing to the interests of an entity which will not exist.

Even if suicide were considered as a rational action, however, that would not mean that the psychiatric team is morally bound to aid and abet Martin's suicidal impulses. (We have already seen that they are legally obliged not to, regardless of his mental state; neither a mentally healthy nor a mentally disordered person is competent to request what the law forbids.) Martin's clinicians should resist what may be construed as his attempts to make them feel guilty for their inability to work any real improvements in his condition, and to play on that guilt by asking them to help him end his life. They may well regret their inability to cure his condition, but that is no reason for them to help him kill himself. Failure to prevent suicide — incidentally, the leading cause of malpractice suits against US psychiatrists — is different from actively assisting it.

Opponents of euthanasia and assisted suicide have always predicted that legalization of physician-assisted death would put the most vulnerable most at risk — the elderly, people with learning disability, the depressed (Hendin and Klerman 1994). If we see Mrs B as the victim of an evil fate rather than an active agent performing an autonomous act, it looks as if she was doubly victimized: first by the deaths of her sons; secondly, and ironically, by Dr Chabot's undoubtedly sincere sympathy. Even if the action of suicide may be rational, and even if the disease model does not apply, there are good reasons why clinicians should resist assisting it.

This is a purely negative conclusion. The more troubling question, in practice, might be whether Martin's clinicians should continue trying to prevent him from killing himself, even if he sincerely believes there is no meaning or value in his life. If self-harm is not a disease, perhaps there is no requirement to prevent it — still less to 'cure' it. Health care practitioners' responsibilities are of course not limited to people who are ill (preventive medicine being a case in point). But a duty of care to those who are *not* suffering from a disease is certainly not implied by the health care practitioner's duty of care to those who *are* suffering from a disease. The focus of this case, then, has been on the medicalization of self-harm versus the possible rationality of suicide, as symbolic of the entire question about what counts as mental illness.

Practitioner commentary (CASE 4.1)

Sally Burgess Senior Psychiatric Registrar, Oxfordshire

In approaching Martin's case from a clinician's viewpoint, I considered two other questions to be of even greater importance than whether or not his suicidal wishes were rational. These questions were: Does Martin really wish to die? And if so, is this wish enduring? Martin's behaviour shows considerable ambivalence both to suicide and to psychiatric treatment. Cases such as this are not uncommon (Burgess and Hawton 1998). There may be many reasons why Martin repeatedly harms himself other than a true enduring wish to end his life. His suicidal expressions and behaviours may be a metaphor for his distress, his frustration, and his anger with the failures of treatment.

There is a difference here between Martin's case and that of Dr Chabot's patient. Mrs B approached Dr Chabot as someone whom she believed might well assist her in killing herself. She was aware Dr Chabot had volunteered himself to the Dutch Voluntary Euthanasia Society. Thus, Dr Chabot could have greater confidence, increased by his subsequent close contact with her, that Mrs B was seriously committed to the idea of suicide. Martin, on the other hand, presents to psychiatrists whom he knows from past experience are bound to be using all means possible to prevent his suicide. Thus it seems less likely that he has a clear, consistent desire to end his life. A consideration of the motivation behind Martin's suicidal behaviours is important in understanding and treating his illness. It is vital if there were any question of 'psychiatric euthanasia'.

The case also raises issues regarding a clinician's duty towards patients like Martin. Dickenson and Fulford put forward (but reject) the suggestion that further treatment should be written off as futile, and that there may be nothing that can be done for Martin except in helping him to die. I feel a distinction needs to be drawn here between treatment and cure. As doctors, we may not be able to cure Martin, but we can certainly continue to treat him. Such treatment could focus on minimizing his symptoms and caring for him through his suffering. In practical terms, this might involve using medication to reduce psychotic symptoms, supportive psychotherapy, and admission to hospital when he requests it. It may also involve a decision to avoid future detention and involuntary treatment, which in the past appears to have served to increase Martin's distress. The primary aim of treatment is thus changed from prevention of suicide to maximization of Martin's quality of life.

This approach is akin to treatment of other incurable (and possibly fatal) diseases. The fact that cancer, ischaemic heart disease, and dementia may not be cured does not lead to doctors refusing to treat patients with these conditions. If these patients die despite treatment, it is not generally seen as a failure on the part of their doctors. Martin's illness could be seen in these terms — as a chronic and incurable condition that, despite treatment, may in the end be fatal. Dickenson and Fulford note that there should not be a requirement to 'cure' self-harm. As Thomas Szasz wrote, to do this one must be able to exercise complete control over a patient, reducing him to a social state below that of a slave (Szasz 1986). Perhaps our management of such cases should avoid these two extremes — of colluding with a patient's belief that the only escape is death, or forcing him to go on living, no matter what his life is reduced to in the process.

References (for CASE 4.1)

Burgess, S. and Hawton, K. (1998) Suicide, euthanasia, and the psychiatrist. *Philosophy, Psychiatry and Psychology*, **5/2**:113–26.

Hendin, H. and Klerman, G. (1994) Comment: 'Physician-assisted suicide: the dangers of legalization'. *American Journal of Psychiatry*, **150/1**:143–5.

Heyd, D. and Bloch, S. (1991) The ethics of suicide'. In *Psychiatric Ethics* (2nd edn) (ed. Bloch, S. and Chodoff, P.), pp. 242–64. Oxford, Oxford University Press.

Jochemsen, H. (1994) Euthanasia in Holland: an ethical critique of the new law. *Journal of Medical Ethics*, **20/4**:212–17.

Ogilvie, A.D. and Potts, S.G. (1994) Assisted suicide for depression: the slippery slope in action? Learning from the Dutch experience. *BMJ*, **309**:492–3.

Re C (1994) 1 All ER 819 (FD).

Remmelink Commissie onderzoek medische praktijk inszke euthanasie (1991) *Rapport Medische Besslissingen rond het Levenseinde* (Report on Euthanasia and Other Medical Decisions concerning the End of Life). Den Haag,SDU-Uitgeverij.

Szasz, T. (1986). The case against suicide prevention. *American Psychologist*, **41**:806–12.

Taylor, C. (1989) *Sources of the Self: The Making of the Modern Identity*. Cambridge, Cambridge University Press.

Van der Maas, P.J., Van Delden J.J.M., and Pijnenborg, I., (1992) Euthanasia and other medical decisions concerning the end of life. *Health Policy*, **22(1/2)**:1–262.

CASE 4.2

Delia Jarrett — is the patient responsible for her behaviour?

Synopsis A 35-year-old woman with a history of repeated hospital admissions, delinquency, and marginal psychotic symptoms is the subject of a complaint of neglect by MIND against the mental health team.

Key dilemmas Is she capable of taking responsibility for her actions? Or should the mental health team take responsibility for her?

Main topics Attributions of responsibility (legal and ethical); akrasia.

Other topics Social control; voluntary action; rationality; *mens rea* (capacity to form a criminal intention); capacity; character; personality disorder; Kant; Hurley; Re C; criminal law; intention; rationality; Plato.

Delia Jarrett is a 35-year-old woman with an extensive psychiatric history dating back to the age of 16. Diagnoses of her condition have been many and various including personality disorder, substance abuse, bipolar affective disorder, schizo-affective disorder, schizophrenia, and various combinations of these.

She and her older brother, Thomas, were raised by an elderly aunt and uncle in Barbados, after their parents' death in a traffic accident during Delia's early childhood. When Delia was twelve, the family emigrated to Britain, and she attended a local comprehensive school, where her behaviour was normal for some time. At fifteen, however, she began to play truant, to shoplift, and to abuse drugs. The next year she gave birth to a full-term baby which was subsequently adopted.

Her first contact with psychiatric services came shortly afterwards, when she was found wandering down an airport runway while a plane was trying to land. She told the airport authorities that she was chasing the pretty lights of the plane, but informed police that she was trying to get a lift to see some friends. Delia was admitted informally but then detained under a section of the Mental Health Act. During her stay, which lasted approximately one month, she was diagnosed as manic and treated with Haloperidol, up to 90 mg per day. As on many subsequent admissions, however, the issue of drug abuse just prior to contact with psychiatric services could not be ruled out, although she claimed not to be using drugs at the time. Following discharge, which was hasty and unplanned, she rapidly dropped out of contact with psychiatric services, despite clinicians' efforts to stay in touch.

By the time Delia was eighteen, her aunt and uncle had died, and she came into a small inheritance from them, which she spent on a holiday in Africa for herself and a boyfriend. During the holiday she was admitted on a compulsory basis to a psychiatric hospital, and her boyfriend abandoned her. Her brother Thomas had to fly out and bring her back home. This became a pattern: throughout her life Delia has repeatedly returned to Thomas for help, promising not to lead such a disorganized life. Her brother has complained to psychiatric services that Delia is completely irresponsible — she cannot feed or clothe herself reliably, cannot manage money, is often aggressive and sometimes violent, abuses drugs, and once tried to set fire to his house. Although Thomas helped her financially many times, he has now taken out an interdict against her coming back to his home. But she has taken to breaking in and causing damage when he and his wife are not there.

Delia's subsequent admissions have often followed incidents in which she has been picked up by police. In one case, she stole a car but was placed on probation for a year after the responsible psychiatrist stated that her mental state would have affected her actions and her capacity to form the intention to commit a crime. In another instance, she was arrested after wandering around in the middle of the city streets, jumping in front of passing cars. On admission, her thought was disordered, and she appeared to be visually hallucinated. She insisted that she had killed a baby, and also that she was pregnant. Her urine showed the presence of amphetamines. Again she was detained under a section of the Mental Health Act, remaining in hospital for ten weeks with a diagnosis of hypomania and probable personality disorder. She required high doses of neuroleptics, which seemed to control acute episodes of mental illness but had little effect on her behavioural problems. And again there was doubt as to whether she was really mentally ill, had a personality disorder, was abusing illicit substances — or possibly a combination of all three.

Discharged to a therapeutic community, Delia deliberately sabotaged her placement, as she admitted later, by smearing faeces and splashing urine in the toilet. She then dropped out of regular contact with psychiatric services and returned to a drug-dealing boyfriend, who was known to be violent to her. A complaint was made by the local branch of MIND about gross inadequacies in provision of care, accusing the hospital of turning a blind eye. Delia was now roaming the streets barefoot, talking to imaginary companions, and wandering in and out of traffic. The consultant concerned, Samantha George, replied that compulsory admissions and drug therapies had shown no long-term improvements in Delia's condition. She added that she was not sure that Delia had ever been mentally ill, and that she wondered if past admissions had been due to intoxication or other drug abuse.

Meanwhile, Delia has just been arrested again — after throwing a brick through the window of a police car, stationary at traffic lights, barely missing the driver. She told the locum senior registrar that she was hearing voices telling her to go to prison. When asked whether she realized that she could have killed somebody, she replied, 'As long as it's a policeman, that's all right'.

There is considerable doubt among the clinical team about whether Delia has ever been frankly psychotic, but her reasoning is often so bizarre that mental disorder must be suspected. Although medication seems to help in the short term, it does result in severe side-effects, worsening her restlessness. The clinicians have persisted pragmatically with a low-dose depot regime, but she often defaults from her appointments. To complicate the picture yet further, her behaviour does seem to improve while she is in hospital if staff impose strict guidelines, stating clearly what is acceptable and unacceptable. It is unclear therefore how much of her behaviour is under her own control.

This case makes an interesting companion to Case 3.1, Elizabeth Orton: in both, the patient first comes into psychiatric care through referral from the statutory services (the police in Delia Jarrett's case, Social Services in the case of

Elizabeth Orton). Both examples raise troubling issues of personal responsibility and social control. And for different reasons, both question the meaning of a psychiatric diagnosis. Although Delia is far more clearly disturbed than Elizabeth, it is not at all certain that either of them is mentally ill, or that mental health services can effect a 'cure'. If the patient is not mentally ill, it would probably be presumed that she is responsible for her own behaviour. But even if she is mentally ill, to what extent are her actions under her own control?

There are two general conditions, very roughly speaking, which must be fulfilled before attributing responsibility for an action (Flew 1979, p. 284):

1 The agent knows what he or she is doing.

2 The agent's desires and /or intentions influence the action.

Are these conditions met in Delia's case? We might have considerable doubts about the first condition. On the one hand, Delia's behaviour does improve if staff set strict guidelines. This seems to indicate that she knows what she is doing and knows that it is unacceptable. Conversely, depot medication does not improve her behaviour greatly, once she is out of the controlled hospital environment in which staff can set guidelines for her. So again, her behaviour seems to be under her conscious control and not simply determined by psychopharmacology.

But what would it mean to say that Delia freely chooses how she acts? Isn't this much too hard on her? There is a strong element of disabling compulsion in her behaviour — the opposite of free choice. This view (meaning that she is not really responsible for her actions) predominated in the testimony of the psychiatrist at Delia's trial for car theft. Her mental state, in his opinion, affected her capacity to form an intention, in this case a criminal intention.

Let us clarify one point before proceeding any further. The discussion in this case is primarily about ethics, and only secondarily about the criminal law. Courts in the United Kingdom (although not so much in the USA) are jealous of their ultimate prerogative to decide whether the defendant possesses *mens rea* (the capacity to form and implement a criminal intention). The psychiatrist's role in court, strictly speaking, is merely to testify on whether a mental abnormality might affect that capacity — not to state whether or not the defendant could be held responsible for the crime (Mason and McCall Smith 1991, p. 409). Particularly in extraordinary cases, this is an important caveat. In the trial of the 'Yorkshire Ripper', Peter Sutcliffe, the jury, by returning a guilty verdict, deliberately rejected psychiatric evidence that Sutcliffe was mentally disordered in such a way that he was not responsible for his actions. But in terms of everyday ethical dilemmas, clinicians can and must decide the question of whether or not the patient is responsible for his or her actions; whether a mental illness lessens or negates that moral responsibility.

However, even a diagnosis of mental illness does not itself establish, in either ethics or law, that a person is definitely not responsible for their actions. That would be to accept full-fledged determinism — to argue that a mentally ill person's actions are wholly determined by their mental illness. But there always remains the question of whether he or she could have acted other than as they did.

On the Kantian principle of 'ought implies can', we should only hold people responsible for what they can do or control. In this sense, the legal and ethical approaches to personal responsibility do coincide. A diagnosis of mental illness only tells us something about the person's ability to control their actions in general; it does not tell us that, in this particular case, Delia could not have done otherwise. At most, there is a statistical relationship — for example, the probabilistic tendency of certain psychiatric conditions to be associated with criminal conduct, such as shoplifting with depression (Mason and McCall Smith 1991, p. 411).

Put another way, Delia's case is not just a clinical or technical question about diagnosis — mental illness, personality disorder, or substance abuse? — but an ethical dilemma about whether even if she is mentally ill, she could still be held responsible for her conduct. We cannot assume a simple causal relationship between mental illness and criminal actions (Duff 1990, p. 39). There are at least two reasons why not. First, even in the case of those who are mentally healthy, there is no simple causal relationship between mental state and action. A sane person could also be tempted to steal a car, but if she does not act on that temptation, we do not just attribute her law-abidingness to her good mental health; we distinguish between good mental health and good moral character. Second, and conversely, mental abnormality does not necessarily indicate moral 'abnormality'. Just as even a person with diagnosed mental illness may still be capable of autonomous judgements, such as refusal of consent to treatment (Re C 1994), so they may still be able to make considered moral choices and avoid illegal behaviour.

This brings us into the territory of the second condition (the effect of the agent's desires and intentions upon the action) and also introduces another concept from moral philosophy — akrasia, or weakness of will. On the one hand, we want to resist the easy conclusion that mentally ill and mentally healthy people ought always to be treated differently in terms of attributing responsibility. It is consistent, on the other hand, to try to understand the actions of someone who may have mental illness, like Delia, in terms which are more conventionally applied to agents whose capacity is not in doubt but who may not always act according to their better judgements or good intentions.

Why should weakness of will — an all too familiar phenomenon to most of us — be considered problematic in philosophy? Akrasia has troubled philosophers since classical times because of its implications for intentionality and rationality. Although most fully discussed in Aristotle, the concept first arises in Socrates' claim that no one knowingly and willingly seeks the greater of two evils or the lesser of two goods (Protagoras 352b). We usually assume that a rational agent intentionally performs X rather than Y because he wants to do X more than Y; so if he really wants to do Y, what can make him do X?

In the present case, we could magic the problem away simply by saying that Delia is not rational. Akratic action is usually defined as uncompelled, intentional action conflicting with an individual's better judgement. (Mele 1995, p.59). Does Delia have a better judgement? But first of all, we are not certain that Delia has a mental illness, rather than a personality disorder or a problem of substance abuse.

Secondly, even if Delia is mentally ill, we cannot automatically equate mental illness with irrationality, since the mentally ill may be able to demonstrate rationality in some spheres. In the case of C, a schizophrenic detained in a secure hospital was judged competent to refuse consent to a surgical procedure because his ability to deal with personal finances, for example, demonstrated a level of rationality which enabled him to understand the consequences of refusal. The philosopher Susan Hurley advises, 'The general rule is: Attribute irrationality with restraint; be as charitable as possible' (Hurley 1989, p. 159). In support of her maxim she cites a warning which psychiatrists are likely to find particularly apt: 'To see too much unreason on the part of others is simply to undermine our ability to understand what it is they are so unreasonable about.' (Davidson 1984, p. 153).

Third, we have argued against treating mental illness as so aberrant that the conventional concepts of moral philosophy simply do not apply — notions such as personal responsibility or, now, akrasia. Such an approach would be both disempowering and patronizing, as well as logically confused. But by treating Delia's actions as akratic rather than necessarily irrational, we accord her a 'privilege' also given to the mentally well. Attributions of akrasia are similar in some ways to attributions of irrationality (Hurley 1989, p. 159), but not so wholesale. We allow that the mentally well can be weak-willed or inconsistent, too, at certain times. This is less of a blanket judgement than simply calling Delia irrational, and it seems to fit the facts of her case better. We can delineate particular circumstances in which she is particularly weak-willed (with her abusive boyfriend or after drug use) and when she seems to have some control over her actions (in a hospital environment where staff set firm boundaries). Perhaps her latest episode actually shows some self-awareness and rationality: she knows herself well enough to realize that she has most control over her actions in a secure environment. The 'voices' telling her to get herself arrested so that she can go to prison or, more likely, back into hospital, are speaking a certain truth. Perhaps she recognizes that she is so frequently weak-willed that this is the best, most rational alternative for her.

We might even say that Delia displays a perverse strength of will in holding to the course that will get her what she wants (a secure environment) and in defending her action in throwing the brick. Similarly, she deliberately sabotages her placement in a less secure environment, overcoming natural revulsion at smearing urine and faeces on the wall in another display of strong will. Whether an action is weak-willed or strong-willed does not depend on its moral content. I can act akratically in not performing a wicked or irrational deed that I had already determined to do (Mele 1995, p. 61). Hence Lady Macbeth's reprimand to her husband, 'Infirm of purpose!' (Macbeth, II, ii , 52) Akratic action may have a virtuous motive but still be akratic, and seen as such by the agent. Even though Macbeth's hesitations about murdering Banquo are virtuous, rooted in clan loyalty and the duties of a host, he begs to be relieved of them:

> ...Come, seeling night,
> Scarf up the tender eye of pitiful day,
> And with thy bloody and invisible hand
> Cancel and tear to pieces that great bond
> Which keeps me pale!
>
> (III, ii, 45–9)

On the other hand, an agent can also exercise self-control in resisting an immoral action. This commonsense truth leads into such difficulties with the concept of akrasia that it might seem better to abandon it altogether. If akrasia can be demonstrated both in resisting and in following one's 'better judgement', what use is the concept? In common parlance we get around the problem of akrasia by saying 'I acted against my better judgement'; but this still implies the use of some other form of judgement, and only introduces further problems about what kind of judgement this could be. There is a risk of infinite regress here.

Perhaps the best course, and the one which best describes Delia's case, involves distinguishing weakness of will from weakness of character (Mele 1995, p. 63). In deciding on a course of action which conflicts with one's better judgement or good intentions, but sticking with it, it is the latter that is exhibited, not the former. Weakness of character fits Delia's continual failure to make good her promises to Thomas about leading a less disorganized life. It also describes her inability to act according to her better judgement except when made to do so by staff. (Again, neither weakness of character nor weakness of will is necessarily the same as weakness of reason: better judgements may be supported by appetites, emotions, and all sorts of motives — not just intellect.)

What does this suggest in the clinical context? If it is weakness of character which leads Delia to miss many of her appointments for receiving depot medication, a psychopharmacological solution is not likely. Nor is it really appropriate if Delia is not mentally ill or if her illness is not improved long-term by medication, as seems to be the case. Giving Delia the benefit of the doubt about mental illness — following Hurley's advice to ascribe irrationality sparingly — may also encourage clinicians to make her act more responsibly.

Practitioner commentary (CASE 4.2)

David Osborn MRC Clinical Research Fellow and Hon. Specialist Registrar in Adult Psychiatry, Department of Psychiatry and Behavioural Sciences, Royal Free and University College Medical School, London

Delia's case will resonate with all mental health practitioners. Psychiatric clinics and in-patient units grapple with clinical pictures similar to hers on a daily basis. The uncertainty of her symptoms and behaviour generates a multitude of possible diagnoses and treatment options. In part, this is because few patients fit into perfect textbook categories. The manic patient with no co-morbid diagnosis (such as alcohol-related problems, drugs, or a hint of a personality disorder) is the exception rather than the rule. Equally uncommon is the personality-disordered patient without occasional or prolonged affective or psychotic symptoms. For Delia, the quest for a golden, all-encompassing diagnosis has been associated with the treatment extremes of very high-dose antipsychotic medication and referral to a therapeutic community — the most intensive form of non-biological psychiatric treatment. Neither has proved helpful in the long term.

The challenge to the clinical team is that the prevailing problem, and therefore diagnosis and treatment, may change hour to hour and day to day as well as year to year. The team's diagnostic flavour of the week will depend on the clinical symptoms of the week. When Delia is aroused and hallucinated she must be considered psychotic. If illicit drugs are discovered, then the diagnosis will relate to those. But the picture a month later, when she is free from drugs, may generate yet another diagnostic theory perhaps relating to her early losses and adolescent antisocial behaviour. None of these are wrong, and none are mutually exclusive. In addition, none of these diagnoses or theories automatically determines whether Delia is responsible for her actions. Her ability to control her actions may vary as frequently as her behaviour. The dilemma for clinicians is being able to hold these differing pictures together as one coherent overview. The further challenge is to tread the line between being over-paternalistic on the one hand or neglectful on the other hand (as alleged by MIND in the case).

Patients' degree of responsibility and practical decision-making ability will always vary from time to time, depending on matters as diverse as what symptoms they are currently suffering from, what life stresses they are experiencing, and what drugs (illicit or prescribed) they are taking. Their responsibility and capacity to make decisions depend on multiple factors which are time-, place-, and task-specific (Osborn 1999). It is only rarely that given levels of responsibility and capacity can be applied to a patient across the board, at all times, in all situations. There are times when Delia has been totally coherent and in control of her actions. This has led the team to question whether she has ever been psychotic. At these times it would be extremely controlling to deny her the freedom to make her own decisions — where to live, whom to see, and what drugs to take. The team can only advise her what they think would constitute sensible planning. It is unfortunately at these 'rational' times that she defaults from services. But that is her choice, and not necessarily irrational. At other times she presents in crisis, and at this point things have changed. Her management plan must therefore adapt itself accordingly. After careful assessment, this may involve medication, detention under the Mental Health Act, psychotherapy, or a combination of all three.

After overseeing a catalogue of fruitless treatment strategies with patients such as Delia, the temptation is to make sweeping generalizations about them. An example is the (not infrequent) assertion that further in-patient treatment is not indicated on the basis that previous attempts have been unhelpful (as alluded to by Dr George in Delia's case). The opposite extreme would be prolonged detention or the imposition of enforced monitoring such as that embodied by the UK supervision order. Rules (sometimes written in clinical notes) such as 'she never benefits from admission' or 'she must always be held accountable for her behaviour' can become attractive to weary clinicians when they review an extensive, unproductive psychiatric history. Such rules may occasionally guide junior doctors who are unfamiliar with the patient, as when they assess a patient late at night. But in general, they are rules simply in danger of being broken or of being wrong; they discount how widely a patient's presentation and competence may vary over time and place.

Psychiatric predictions, as the title of this book reminds us, are based on probability and likelihood, rather than certainty. The very chaos of Delia's career, so far, makes any future predictions precarious. They may be right seven times out of ten, but on three occasions they will be wrong. There is probably no single clinical answer or truth regarding her diagnosis or her treatment, and her care package must relate to the problems that present at any one time, each time she presents. Equally her responsibility for her actions must be carefully assessed and viewed as time- and action-specific. Her responsibility for the diet she chooses is a different ability from her responsibility for setting a fire or launching an aggressive assault on a police car. Only careful assessment of Delia at the time of any incident can shed light on her *current* ability to take responsibility for her actions. Even then, it should not be simply by reference to a psychiatric diagnosis (or lack of one) that she is taken to be responsible or not responsible for her actions. Recent work has shown that many people with mental disorders, including schizophrenia, are perfectly capable of making rational decisions in a whole range of domains, irrespective of their symptoms (see, for example, Grisso and Applebaum 1995; Kitamura *et al.* 1998; Wirshing *et al.* 1998; and Wong *et al.*, forthcoming). Equally, many people without formal psychiatric diagnoses are at times compromised in this ability.

So is there a case for accusing the team of neglect? This claim places a requirement on the team to police Delia, even though they can find no current reason to force her to comply with their treatment, never mind to accept their wider advice. Although Delia's picture fluctuates, she has arguably had no prolonged period of unequivocal mental illness. Psychiatrists in the UK face the possibility of being made responsible for dangerousness *per se*, regardless of whether it is associated with mental disorder. But it would in my view be paternalistic to treat Delia further against her will when she is not in crisis. That is not to say that any reports of concern should be ignored. Each time she arouses concern, her care will need reviewing. Delia's mental health and her needs may be ever-changing.

The concern of MIND seems to be that Delia has gone back to an abusive boyfriend. Whilst this appears undesirable, it seems far from the remit of her mental health team. Many women (and men) live in abusive, destructive, counterproductive relationships. Some have mental health problems and others do not. Only rarely will the mental health problem be the determinant of why the person stays in that relationship. Decisions to stay or leave will be influenced by multiple social and psychological factors. Even if Delia is mentally ill, this does not automatically render her unable to make decisions about relationships. To believe that it does is to stigmatize mental illness further. Whilst a clinical team should show their concern and support for a patient, it is not within their jurisdiction to determine what relationship anyone, including Delia, chooses. We care about our patients and would prefer not to see them in harmful relationships, but in the absence of mental disorder, our role does not extend to a social one which allows us to sanction chosen partners.

Delia's future will inevitably include further clinical and social dilemmas. Responsibility for forensic actions may play a further part in her assessment; each action will require separate assessment. In the same way that

Delia may be responsible enough to decide whom she has relationships with, there may be times when her criminal actions are deemed within her control. She will then be required to face the penalty for those actions. But it is important that the mental health team always remain robust and willing to reassess and consider her predicament as it develops. Even if she has not been mentally ill so far, she may develop a mental illness in the future; she certainly has a life loaded with the risk factors for such an illness. Reluctance to be involved with her treads dangerously close to repeating the patterns of rejection and loss that have characterized her childhood and young adult life. At the very least, there may well be new treatment options available in the future. Neuroleptics have at least shown some efficacy for Delia, if only in the short term. With the new armoury of more gentle antipsychotics, unpleasant side-effects are far more avoidable. This in itself might open a new chapter in treatment adherence for Delia. At all events, the clinical team will need to remain cohesive and responsive for the sake of both Delia and themselves.

References (CASE 4.2)

Davidson, D. (1984) Belief and the basis of meaning. In *Inquiries into Truth and Interpretation* (ed. Donaldson, D.) Oxford, Clarendon Press.

Duff, R.A. (1990) *Intention, Agency and Criminal Liability*. Oxford, Blackwell.

Flew, A. (1979). *A Dictionary of Philosophy*. London, Pan Books.

Grisso, T. and Appelbaum, P.S. (1995) The MacArthur Treatment Competence Study: III. Abilities of patients to consent to medical and psychiatric treatments. *Law and Human Behaviour*, **19**:149–74.

Hurley, S.L. (1989) *Natural Reasons: Personality and Polity*. Oxford, Oxford University Press.

Kitamura, F., Tomoda, A., Tsukuda, K., Tanaka, M., Kawakami, I., and Mishima, S. (1998) Method for assessment of competency to consent in the mentally ill. *International Journal of Law and Psychiatry*, **21**:223–44.

Mason, J.K. and McCall Smith, R.A. (1991) *Law and Medical Ethics*. London, Butterworths.

Mele, A.R. (1995) *Autonomous Agents: From Self-Control to Autonomy*. Oxford, Oxford University Press.

Osborn, D.P.J. (1999) Research and ethics: leaving exclusion behind. *Current Opinion in Psychiatry*, **12**:601–4.

Protagoras. In *The Collected Dialogues of Plato*. (1961) (ed. Hamilton, E. and Huntington, C.). New York, Pantheon Books.

Re C (1994) 1 All ER 819 (FD).

Wirshing, D., Wirshing, W., Marder, S., Liberman, R.P., and Mintz, J. (1998) Informed consent; assessment of comprehension. *American Journal of Psychiatry*, 155:1503–11.

Wong, J.G., Clare, I.C.H., Holland, A.J., Watson, P.C., and Gunn, M. (forthcoming) The capacity of people with a 'mental disability' to make a health carer decision. *Psychological Medicine.*

CASE 4.3

Simon Greer[1] — schizophrenia or religious experience?

Synopsis A middle-aged African-American lawyer reacted to a racially inspired threat of legal action from his colleagues by suddenly becoming convinced that he was 'the living son of David' with a special mission from God. He based this on random wax marks ('seals') outlining words and phrases in his Bible. Although he came from a Baptist background, he had not previously been particularly religious, and his 'seals' carried no significance for anyone else, including members of his own cultural group.

Key dilemma Is Simon suffering from a psychotic illness (such as schizophrenia) or is this a religious experience? (And what has all this to do with ethics?)

Main topics Value judgements and psychiatric diagnosis; delusion and religious experience

Other topics Delusional perception; thought insertion; ICD–10 and DSM–IV; Criterion B for schizophrenia; concept of mental disorder; cross-cultural psychiatry; abuse of psychiatry; user perspective; relativism.

Simon, 40 years old, was a senior African-American professional, from a middle-class Baptist family. Although not particularly religious in outlook, he had had occasional, relatively unremarkable, psychic experiences at various times in his life. These had led him to seek the guidance of a professional 'seer', whom he occasionally consulted on major life events and decisions.

His story was that his hitherto successful career was now threatened by legal action from his colleagues. Although he claimed to be innocent, mounting a defence would be expensive and hazardous. He had responded to this crisis by praying at a small altar which he set up in his front room. After an emotional evening's outpouring, he discovered that the candle wax had left a 'seal' or 'sun' on several consecutive pages of his Bible, covering certain letters and words. He described his experiences thus: 'I got up and I saw the seal that was in my father's Bible and I called X and I said, you know,

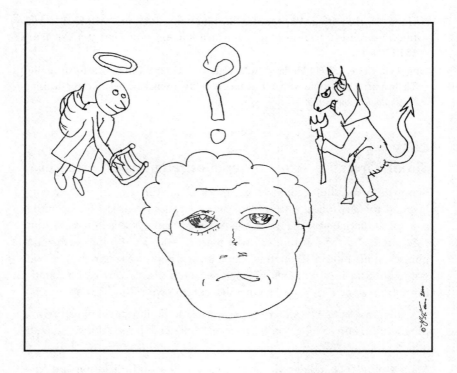

"Something remarkable is going on over here". I think the beauty of it was the specificity by which the sun burned through. It was…in my mind, a clever play on words.' Although the marked words and letters had no explicit meaning, Simon interpreted this event as a direct communication from God, which signified that he had a special purpose or mission.

After this first episode, Simon received a complex series of 'revelations', largely conveyed through the images left in melted candle wax. He carried photos of these, which most observers found unimpressive, but which were, for him, clearly representations of biblical symbols, particularly from the book of Revelations (the bull, the 24 elders, the arc of the covenant, and so on). He interpreted them as signifying that 'I am the living son of David…and I'm also a relative of Ishmael, and…of Joseph'. He was also the 'captain of the guard of Israel'. He found this role carried awesome responsibilities: 'Sometimes I'm saying — O my God, why did you choose me, and there's no answer to that'. His special status had the effect of 'increasing my own inward sense, wisdom, understanding, and endurance' which would 'allow me to do whatever is required in terms of bringing whatever message it is that God wants me to bring'.

His beliefs were highly systematized, in that he interpreted much of his ongoing experience in terms of them. His colleagues were agents of Satan, trying to thwart him, and his career successes were evidence of God's special favour. Relatively trivial obstacles which he encountered in daily life — such as having a cold at the time of the interview — were satanically motivated trials of purpose. In the course of these experiences, Simon had both heard God's voice and seen 'prophetic' visions. He expressed these beliefs with full conviction 'The truths that are up in that room are the truths that have been spoken of for 4000 years'. When confronted with scepticism, he commented: 'I don't get upset, because I know within myself, what I know'.

He also described experiences of his thoughts being 'short-circuited'. 'If you're sitting and watching television, and then somebody turns on the vacuum cleaner, and the TV goes on the fritz, it's like that'; and again, 'the things that come are not the things that I have been thinking about...they kind of short-circuit the brain, and bring their message'.

Simon had no insight in the sense (defined in the PSE, symptom 104) that he considered his mental processes to be completely normal. He had told various friends and ministers about them, and believed that 'no-one really thought I was crazy because...they've known me all my life...and I think God would not permit it, to be honest with you'. However, he was careful to conceal what was happening from his colleagues, as he recognized that they would perceive it as suspect. Moreover, while his beliefs were clearly subculturally influenced, other members of his cultural group regarded them as abnormal. Indeed, he was puzzled by the way in which certain of the ministers he had consulted drew attention to their messianic overtones. He had 'stopped talking to some of the ministers' and he commented that 'people want to take it away from me, and say "I'm glad that you don't see it as something especially for you"...they'll try and dismiss me out of the equation, which I find fascinating'.

Most psychiatrists presented with Simon's case history respond to it as a 'technical' problem in differential diagnosis rather than as an 'ethics' case. There is a duty of care involved, of course, as in all differential diagnosis. But this is assumed to be limited to a responsibility for, first, carefully eliciting the facts of Simon's case history and mental state, and, second, matching these against the full range of relevant diagnostic possibilities. One of us (Bill Fulford) has presented Simon's case history in a variety of teaching contexts. On the question of diagnosis, reactions vary. But among psychiatrists (whether trainees or seniors) and other mental health professionals, Simon is generally assumed to be suffering from some form of psychotic illness, probably either schizophrenia or schizo-affective disorder. Other possibilities commonly noted include hypomania, organic psychosis (drug induced?), stress-induced psychosis, brief psychotic episode, and hysterical psychosis.

In putting forward this differential diagnosis, the presence of 'first rank' symptoms is emphasized. Simon's reaction to the wax seals has the form of a delusional perception — a primary delusion which is 'based on sensory experiences' and involves the subject 'suddenly becoming convinced that a particular set of events (have) a special meaning' (PSE symptom 82). Similarly, though less clear-cut, his description of thoughts coming into his head suggests thought insertion (PSE symptom 55) — they 'are not the things I have been thinking about…They kind of short-circuit the brain, and bring their message'. These symptoms, combined with his complete lack of insight, suggest a diagnosis of schizophrenia, although the grandiose element in Simon's thinking raises the possibility of hypomania or of the hybrid schizo-affective disorder.

To resolve these and other diagnostic possibilities, most groups point out that we need more information about the course of Simon's condition: the International Classification of Diseases (ICD–10, WHO 1992) requires any one first-rank symptom to be clearly present for four weeks or more for a diagnosis of schizophrenia; with hypomania, the mood change and grandiose delusions will come to dominate the picture; organic psychoses (other than drug-related disorders) are likely to show deterioration in cognitive functioning (memory, level of consciousness, and so on); brief psychotic episodes and stress-induced psychoses should both, by definition, have resolved within two or three months; and hysterical psychoses (like all hysterical disorders) may be the prodroma of other more serious underlying pathology, organic or functional.

So, how did Simon's story evolve?

The case continues:

A year after the initial interview, he made contact again. He reported that in the interval his career had flourished and that he had used some of the money he had made to set up a new charitably oriented institution. His revelations had continued, indeed they had increased in frequency and scope, but they had been entirely beneficial in his life. They had given him the conviction to contest and win the law suit against him, and more generally to succeed as a high-achieving black person in a predominantly white, racist context. He had high self-esteem, firm moral convictions, and a strong sense of purpose in life. He confided that his mission involved unifying 'true Christianity' (a 'return to the ancient ways of the worship of the Lord') and 'true Islam'. He had plans to announce himself live on TV but was waiting for the right signs.

The good outcome of Simon's story comes as a surprise to most psychiatrists. They have generally assumed, with this story, that Simon must be ill, or at any rate that he has been referred (or possibly referred himself) to a psychiatrist. Hence the problem is taken to be one of differential diagnosis — of what kind of illness Simon is suffering from, rather than whether he is ill at all. In fact, Simon had been nowhere near a psychiatrist. His story came to light, in Mike Jackson's original study, through an organization in Oxford called The Alister Hardy Centre, which records people's experiences of spiritual and paranormal phenomena.

When this further background is filled in, psychiatrists, and indeed others, react in two quite different ways. For some, it confirms the diagnosis of schizophrenia (because Simon's symptoms have persisted) albeit with, as a participant in one seminar put it, a 'remarkably benign course'. For others, the 'benign course' precludes pathology of any kind, requiring a complete revision of the original diagnosis, a reappraisal of Simon's experiences not as a form of psychotic illness but rather as a religious or spiritual experience. This split vote shifts the diagnostic problem into a more overtly ethical frame. The ethical issue (and it is an issue about which at this stage discussion tends to become ethically heated) is the need to avoid the equally abusive outcomes of, on the one hand, treating 'saints as psychotics' (Storr 1997) — the spiritual counterpart of the treatment in the former USSR of political dissidents as schizophrenics (see Introduction to Chapter 3) — and, on the other, denying treatment to those who are really ill (recall John Wing's comment in Chapter 2 that denying involuntary treatment to someone who is suicidally depressed is 'morally repellent' (Wing 1978, p. 244).)

But can the issue, albeit ethically laden, not be resolved by the methods of traditional scientific psychopathology? After all, it has been recognized for many years that some forms of religious experience may be phenomenologically similar to madness: both show, for example, synchronicity, time distortion, loss of self–object boundaries, synethesias, and so forth. Indeed, William James described paranoia as 'a sort of religious mysticism turned upside down' (James 1902, p. 426). Careful observations of the details of the experiences concerned, however, in the work of foundational figures such as Jaspers, Bleuler, and Kraepelin, led to the recognition of discrete psychopathological syndromes based on specific symptoms including, in the case of schizophrenia, the first-rank symptoms. Moreover, the power of this approach of careful and systematic observation has been further vindicated in recent psychiatry through the successes of such studies as the US–UK Diagnostic Project (Cooper *et al.*, 1972) and the International Pilot Study of Schizophrenia (WHO 1973) in establishing internationally acceptable diagnostic criteria. This, is turn, has been the basis of the recent explosive growth of neuroscientific advances in understanding the brain bases of psychiatric disorders and the development of new and more specific drug treatments.

Defining mental disorders descriptively, then, has an excellent pedigree. Applying this approach to Simon's case seems initially to support the first of the two reactions to his good outcome — that he has schizophrenia. Simon has at least one, and possibly two, first-rank symptoms which, persisting as they have done for more than six weeks, satisfy the ICD–10 criteria for schizophrenia. His good outcome thus has to be understood as an exception which proves the rule. True, he does not *appear* ill, let alone seem to be suffering a severe illness of the kind schizophrenia generally turns out to be. But the rule (marking out those forms of madness which are medical disorders by descriptively defined symptoms) is sufficiently important that we should retain it even in the face of an occasional self-contradiction (Simon has a disorder but is not disordered).

There is a twist, though, to the 'defining mental disorders descriptively' story, which supports the *other* main initial reaction to Simon's story — the reaction that he was not ill at all. The twist comes if we move from the World Health Organisation's ICD–10 to the American Psychiatric Association's DSM–IV (APA 1994). For the DSM has added an additional criterion for the diagnosis of schizophrenia, criterion B, that the person concerned shows 'social/occupational dysfunction'. This means, in an adult, that 'for a significant portion of the time since the onset of the disturbance, one or more major areas of functioning such as work, interpersonal relations, or self-care are markedly below the level achieved prior to the onset' (APA 1994, p. 285).

According to DSM, therefore, Simon does *not* have schizophrenia or any other psychotic disorder. He could possibly have persistent delusional disorder, by DSM criteria, except that this diagnosis is limited to those who have never met the criteria for schizophrenia (APA 1994, p. 301). So far so good. The DSM, by introducing this additional criterion B, makes a lot more sense clinically of cases like Simon's than the ICD. The twist, though, is a double twist. For the DSM, like the ICD, aims to provide a scientific (and hence value-free) basis for the diagnosis of mental disorders: in its introduction, for example, it says of itself that it was the product of 'a formal evidence-based process' (p. xv), that it drew on 'the widest pool of information' (p. xv), and that in arriving at final decisions, the Task Force 'reviewed all of the extensive empirical evidence' (p. xvi). Indeed, the DSM authors considered that 'the major innovation of DSM IV lies not in any of its specific content changes but rather in the systematic and explicit process by which it was constructed' and that 'more than any other nomenclature of mental disorders, DSM IV is grounded in empirical evidence' (p. xvi).

Perhaps because of the strongly scientific self-image of DSM and ICD, clinicians tend not to recognize that criterion B depends on a series of *value judgements*. Thus, it requires, not merely a change in social/occupational functioning but a change for the *worse:* there must be '*dys*function' (that is, functioning '*below* the level previously achieved'). Indeed, DSM–III, in which criterion B first appeared, actually described it in overtly evaluative terms as involving a *deterioration* in social or occupational functioning (APA 1980, p. 189).

The value judgements involved in applying criterion B show that the diagnostic problem in Simon's case (and by extension, in the diagnosis of all psychotic disorders) is, in the sense of the term used in this book, inescapably ethical in nature. That is to say, the diagnosis of such disorders, as defined by DSM itself, although clearly involving matters of fact, also and inescapably involves value judgements. There are of course more conventional ethical aspects to diagnosis as well. There is a general duty of care, for example, as we have already noted. In Simon's case, moreover, the good outcome of his story takes us into the ethics of balancing moral (spiritual) and medical (schizophrenic) interpretations, and hence of avoiding abusive misdiagnosis (either way). But the crucial point here is that the diagnosis actually turns, at least in the DSM, on a series of value judgements. The DSM, it should be said, in a section considering the definition of mental disorder (APA 1994, p. xl1–xl2), emphasizes that psychopathological interpretations of human experience and behaviour should never be based *solely* on deviation from social norms. But this implies, consistently with the inclusion in DSM of criterion B, that a value judgement is at least *necessary*.

Is there any way of escaping from the necessity for making value judgements in the diagnosis of schizophrenia? As we noted in Chapter 2 (and again in the introduction to this section), the apparent conflict between these value judgements and psychiatry's self-image as a scientific medical discipline has led to exploration of a number of possible escape routes. One such escape route is simply to avoid the problem. This comes in two forms — denial, and what might be called 'peaceful coexistence'.

Taking the denial escape route first, this involves collapsing the categories of religious experience and psychosis. As with the wider debate between moral and medical models of mental disorder, this has been attempted in both directions: for some, all madness is a form of religious (or at any rate, spiritual) experience (R.D. Laing, although not denying the reality of mental illness, considered it to be a form of spiritual quest — Laing 1967); for others, all religious experience is madness (the Group for the Advancement of Psychiatry argued in 1976 that all spiritual experience is psychopathology of one kind or another). The 'peaceful coexistence' escape route, on the other hand, draws on the fact (widely recognized particularly by theologians, historians, anthropologists, and others familiar with the heterogeneity of human experience and behaviour) that spiritual experience and madness are not mutually exclusive categories. The psychiatrist and anthropologist Roland Littlewood has described no less than five ways in which experiences which would be regarded as psychopathological by medical psychiatry may become transformed through social processes into meaningful cognitions and actions; his case study of the transformation of delusions into a new religion in Trinidad has become an important classic (Littlewood 1993 and 1997).

Neither of these approaches is effective in avoiding the problem here. Merely collapsing one category into the other fails to account for the prima facie distinction between them. This is the basis of a general argument against either polarized extreme in the psychiatry/antipsychiatry debate: a theory which seeks to collapse mental disorder *either* into moral *or* into medical categories must explain why, if the moral and medical categories are not distinct, they *appear* to be so (see Fulford 1989, Chapter 1, for a full account of the constraints on theory in this area). In the absence of such an account, therefore, either kind of collapse is potentially abusive, treating saints as psychotics or denying treatment to those who most clearly need it. The 'peaceful coexistence' approach, by contrast, although avoiding these abusive consequences, and also enormously fruitful in charting the richness of human experience in this area, begs the question. This is clear from the two-way table (see Table 4.1) by which Littlewood illustrates his argument. The claim that both psychosis and religious experience may be either present or absent in a given case presupposes the distinction between them; this surely remains true whether the categories are understood in realist, or as Littlewood prefers, conventionalist terms (Littlewood 1997, p. 68).

If the problem of value judgements appearing in psychiatric diagnosis cannot be avoided, can the value judgements concerned at least be circumscribed or ring-fenced to preserve a value-free core of medical theory? A number of authors have attempted this second kind of escape route (see Reading Guide to this chapter, section on values). Among these, the distinction drawn by Christopher Boorse (1975) between disease and illness might seem attractive in Simon's case: disease is dysfunction, he argues, while illness is a disease which is serious enough to be incapacitating. Hence, rather as Boorse concludes that homosexuality is a disease but not an illness (Boorse 1976), so Simon could be said to be suffering from a disease but not to be ill. As noted in Chapter 2, there are a number of general conceptual difficulties inherent in this position (Fulford 1989, Chapters 3 and 6). But even if these could be overcome, it would seem hardly less abusive to be told that one's deepest spiritual experience, let alone one's sexual orientation, is a disease than an illness.

A recent variant on this approach is Jerome Wakefield's analysis of disorder as a harmful dysfunction, where dysfunction is defined scientifically by reference to an evolutionarily established species-typical design (Wakefield

Table 4.1 Littlewood's two-way table of the co-occurrence of religious experience and psychosis

Religious experience	Psychosis	
	Present	Absent
Present	A	B
Absent	C	D

Littlewood argues on anthropological grounds that religious experience and psychotic illness are not mutually exclusive. He defines these categories, respectively, as 'something close to psychiatry's recognition of major mental illness' (psychosis) and, as 'something like an anthropological notion of religious or spiritual experience' (Littlewood 1997). Hence, Simon would fall into Group A if we accept his experiences as first-rank symptoms of schizophrenia which, nonetheless, carry enlightenment; if we do not accept his experiences as first-rank symptoms he would fall into Group B. Corresponding allocations for Groups C and D follow if we deny that his experiences are religious at all. Littlewood's approach, therefore, far from resolving the diagnostic problem of the distinction between religious experience and psychosis, recreates it in even more difficult form. And it becomes even more complex if we follow his further suggestion of a 16-way table reflecting the different perspectives of 'professionals' and of the individual concerned.

1995). This is close to the spirit of DSM. Criterion B was apparently introduced not to distinguish psychotic illness from its non-pathological counterparts, but to distinguish the severe illness of schizophrenia from the less severe schizophreniform disorder (which although a disorder, in DSM terms, does not involve deterioration in life functioning; see APA 1994, p. 289). Simon, it should be said straightaway, could not be diagnosed as suffering from a personality disorder of any kind, because his experiences represent a marked change for him. (Personality disorders differ from diseases in being essentially stable patterns of maladaptive experience or behaviour present from late adolescence onwards.) Wakefield's distinction, though, could be applied to Simon's case roughly along the lines that his first-rank 'symptoms' represent a departure from the species-typical design (hence he has a dysfunction); but since this is not in his case harmful, he does not have a disorder.

Wakefield's analysis, like Boorse's, has the (to many) abusive consequence of labelling atypical spiritual experiences, like atypical sexual orientations, as dysfunctions. In Wakefield's case though, the need to preserve a value-free definition of pathology seems even more transparently unacceptable (Fulford, 2000). Wakefield's analysis requires that *any* departure from a species-typical norm, whether or not disadvantageous, is a dysfunction. This is doubtful, evolutionarily — natural selection, after all, being driven by departures from species-typical norms in the form of mutations and other sources of variation. But taken literally, it makes *improved* function (as in Simon's case) a species of *dys*-function! Good may come out of evil: a paralysis, for example, may lead to a life which is more focused. As one of the founders of modern psychiatry said specifically of madness and religious experience, 'What right have we to believe God under any obligation to do his work by means of complete minds only?' (Maudsley 1886, p. 257; quoted in Littlewood 1997). But in Simon's case, it is his experiences, *in and of themselves,* which are good. And as one of us has shown elsewhere, the effects even of recognized brain pathology, such as a brain tumour, are not in themselves necessarily pathological (Fulford, 2000*b*). What right have we therefore, in such cases, to assume an 'incomplete mind'? Simon's mind could have been *more* complete; to the extent that his experiences were empowering, it *was* more complete.

Wakefield's version of the conceptual escape route leads inevitably, therefore, like Boorse's, to the potentially abusive construal of Simon's spiritual experiences as pathology. To call Simon's experience a disease but not an illness (with Boorse), or a dysfunction but not a disease (with Wakefield), is to deny the deep spiritual importance to Simon of his experiences. This is not abusive in intent, but it is abusive in effect. Mike Jackson, the psychologist from whose work Simon's story is derived, showed in a wider epidemiological survey the extent of user dissatisfaction with the failure of psychiatrists to recognize the significance of people's spiritual and religious experiences (Jackson, 1997). Such failure is a consequence of our wider failure to recognize the diversity of human values in the areas with which psychiatry is concerned. As we noted in Chapter 1, values are present in diagnosis in all areas of medicine, but they become diagnostically important where, as in psychiatry, medicine is concerned with areas of human experience and behaviour in which people's values differ.

A third escape route that we need to consider avoids the abusive consequence of labelling spiritual experience as pathology, but only at the expense of admitting values back into the diagnostic process. This escape route is clinical. It comes in three forms — phenomenological, cross-cultural, and aetiological. We will deal with the phenomenological and cross-cultural escape routes here and return to the aetiological in the next chapter.

The phenomenological escape route is illustrated by Andrew Sims' work as a psychopathologist on religious experience and psychosis. Criticizing Jackson and Fulford's account of Simon and similar cases (1997), Sims (1997, p. 80) argued that the required distinction depends on 'detailed psychopathological examination'. This involves exploring empathically the 'meaning' of the subject's account to establish 'the precise subjective state and nature of (their) experiences'. Sims then described a useful check-list of points of differentiation between religious experience and psychotic illness (derived from a fuller treatment in Sims 1988). Many of these points of differentiation are practically rel-evant, but, like Littlewood's proposal already described, they presuppose the distinction: thus, Sims refers to the diagnostic importance of a course 'consis-tent with the natural history of mental disorder' and 'symptoms of known psy-chiatric illness' (p. 80). But the 'crucial difference', Sims concludes, is that in the case of religious experience 'not only do the subjects themselves regard their experiences as being basically good and life-enriching, but so does any reason-able external observer' (Sims 1997, p. 81).

In Sims' account, then, it is the value judgements 'basically good and life-enriching' which turn out to be diagnostically crucial. Essentially, the same surfacing of values is evident in the second empirical approach, that of the contribution of cross-cultural psychiatry to psychiatric diagnosis. As with other important aspects of psychiatric diagnosis, DSM has been particularly forward in incorporating cross-cultural factors into psychiatric diagnosis: DSM–IV includes a whole appendix on cultural formulation (APA 1994, pp. 843–9); and its V Codes (which cover conditions that may come to the attention of clinicians but are explicitly *not* pathological) includes a category of 'Religious or Spiritual Problem' (APA 1994, p. 685). Simon avoids the lat-ter category because his experience is not 'distressing' and hence is not a 'problem' in DSM's terms. The value judgements involved in this diagnosis are self-evident. But can a 'cultural formulation' distinguish Simon's experi-ences from schizophrenia or other psychotic illness without introducing value judgements?

Cultural formulations of Simon's and other similar cases are discussed by Francis Lu, David Lukoff, and Robert Turner (1997) in another com-mentary on Jackson and Fulford's account. These three authors have been at the forefront of the development of culture-sensitive uses of the DSM. Like Sims, they emphasize that traditionally defined symptoms (as in the PSE) have to be assessed contextually. Here, though, the relevant context is said to be the individual's cultural norms. Turning to DSM itself, we find that it is with respect to these cultural norms that 'the meaning and perceived severity of the patient's symptoms' (APA 1994, p. 844) should be assessed. Simon's experiences, Lu *et al.* argue, are 'probably consistent with his African-American background'. They say 'probably' because Simon had not previously been particularly religious, the meanings he read into the wax seals were not evident to others, and at least some of the ministers (of religion) he consulted were concerned at the messianic overtones of his experiences. Even so, Lu *et al.* continue, 'his lack of impairment and positive outcome' help us substantiate the conclusion that his experiences are not psychopathological. Note, therefore, the signifi-cance of the two value judgements — lack of impairment and positive outcome — introduced here. In relation to a further case, Sean, reported in the same paper (Jackson and Fulford 1997), these value judgements turn out to be diagnostically central. Sean's experiences were *wholly* outside his cultural context. Nonetheless, Lu *et al.* argue, they were not pathological because they had 'a profoundly *positive* [authors' emphasis] effect on his life' (Lu *et al.* 1997, p. 76).

Again, then, if we press the traditional, supposedly exclusively science-based approach to diagnosis in relation to Simon's case, value judgements emerge as diagnostically crucial. To recognize this, as we stressed in Chapter 1, is not to diminish the importance of science in psychiatry. It is rather to emphasize that values, as well as facts, may be important diagnostically. In many areas of physical medicine, as we noted in Chapter 1, the values relevant to diagnosis can be ignored because they are shared and hence unproblematic. But the danger of extrapolating from such areas to psychiatry is that in psychiatry the relevant values are often *not* shared and hence *cannot* be ignored. Denial of values was an important factor in the abusive uses of psychiatry in the former USSR (Fulford *et al.* 1993). As the experience of Soviet psychiatry showed, a failure to recognize the evaluative element in psychiatric diagnosis is a recipe for imposing one person's or one group's values on another behind a mask, and with the authority, of objective science.

The practical corollaries of recognizing the importance of values in making a diagnosis in Simon's case are, straightforwardly:

1 that we should take the patient's values as seriously as the professional's in considering how their experiences and behaviour should be understood (thus extending traditional bioethics' principle of autonomy from treatment to diagnosis);

2 that where there are *differences* of values, we should seek to come to a balanced perspective.

Just how we do this is a matter of good practice skills. It requires, first, a knowledge of people's likely needs and wishes in a given clinical situation (as we have several times noted, professionals, just because they *are* professionals, are particularly likely to misunderstand their patients' values —see especially, Chapter 2, p. 23). A balanced perspective also requires good skills of ethical reasoning. As we noted in Chapter 2, principles reasoning and casuistry may both be complementary to perspectives in this respect. But a balanced perspective requires, above all, good communication: for exploring the patient's values in a given case and for effective sharing of perspectives between members of the multidisciplinary team. This indeed gives multidisciplinary teams a new and important role; in the traditional medical model, it provides only a variety of treatment skills. In a 'fact + value' model, the different perspectives of different team members may be crucial to the balance of values on which diagnostic assessment, in a case like Simon's, may critically depend.

These corollaries (to which we return in Chapter 8) may seem obvious, but the dominance of the traditional medical model in psychiatry has meant that we have been late in recognizing their importance. The 'skilled psychopathologist' to whom Sims refers — empathically exploring the 'meaning' of an individual's experience, feeling their way into 'the situation of the other person' until they have 'understood the respondent's subjective experience' — is an ideal of good communication skills which the experiences of those concerned show is all too rarely met. In Mike Jackson's larger study (already noted), he found that many of those who had tried to talk to psychiatrists about their spiritual experiences felt that they were immediately labelled as 'mad', and that most people with such experiences avoid contact with psychiatrists altogether! It is only recently, and then only because of the efforts of such pioneers as Sims in the UK, and Lu, Lutcoff, and Turner in the USA, that psychiatrists have begun talking to people about their religious beliefs (Cox, 1996).

Similar comments apply to cultural formulation. The cultural formulation outlined by DSM reminds us that in coming to a balance of values, the perspective of the individual's own culture (and indeed of their age and gender) is centrally important. But even today we still talk of 'culture-bound syndromes' as though there could be such a thing as a culture-free psychiatry (Fulford 1998); many outside the 'white Western' culture of origin of psychiatry regard our practice as still highly culture-*in*sensitive (see, for example, several chapters in Bhui and Olajide 1999).

Simon's case history, therefore, although initially appearing to pose only technical problems of differential diagnosis, has turned out to be ethically laden in a number of key respects. Besides a general duty of care (to carry out the diagnostic assessment thoroughly), there was a critical need to avoid the equally abusive misdiagnoses either of spiritual experience as psychotic illness, or of psychotic illness as spiritual experience. Distinguishing spiritual experience and psychosis turned, again critically, on a series of value judgements embodied (though not always recognized for what they are) in criterion B for schizophrenia as specified in the DSM. Attempts to escape the required value judgements, either by avoidance or by prescriptive redefinition aimed at preserving a value-free 'core' to medicine, turned out to be abusive in effect (though not of course in intent). The cross-cultural escape route, although conceived as being within traditional empirical diagnostic methods, led back to the central diagnostic importance of values — those of the patient (in the case of phenomenology) and those of society (in the case of cultural formulation).

The danger perceived by those committed to an exclusively scientific view of psychiatric diagnosis in acknowledging values is relativism — of 'anything goes'. As one of us has argued elsewhere (Fulford, 1998), this is not a danger in practice so long as human values are more or less coherent. Law and aesthetics, for example, are both value-based; but in neither discipline is it true that 'anything goes'. And in diagnosis, anyway, the point is not that values should replace facts but that we need to recognize the importance of values alongside facts. So in the 'fact + value' model of medicine advocated here, even if human values were totally at odds, diagnosis would still be constrained by facts.

The opposite, and far less well-recognized danger (Fulford 1998*b*), though, is of *consensus*. If 'coming to a balanced perspective' means the tyranny of the many over the one, then, to quote Anthony Storr again, we really are at risk of 'condemning saints as psychotics' (Storr 1997). The abusive consequences of consensus were tragically demonstrated in the former USSR, in which the dominant Soviet ethic, masked behind a strongly medical (that is, exclusively fact-based) model of mental disorder, led to political deviance being diagnosed as psychotic illness (Fulford *et al.* 1993). In principle, there is a cleft stick here between relativism (everyone's values count equally) and consensus (the majority values prevail). In practice, professionals are obligated to pay particular (though not exclusive) regard to the values of their particular patients. Where these seem directly to conflict with those of society there may be a need to act against the wishes of the patient. This is of course often true, by definition, in forensic psychiatry. It is important, though, to note that in many of the tragedies involving psychiatric patients harming others, the patients themselves, far from refusing treatment, have been most vocal in asking for help.

In such cases, then, it has been *denial* of the patient's values which has been the operative factor. In a majority of cases the issue is not, of course, as stark as this; it is far from clear whether the experiences of the person concerned are good or bad, rational or irrational, incapacitating or empowering. Good practice in such cases, therefore, is in part about becoming more aware of the values involved. This requires, in Sims' (1997) terms, a careful and empathic exploration of the subject's experience, starting from and building on their values and beliefs. This in turn requires not an ethics of anything goes but a tolerance of diversity and a recognition, contrary to the objectivist view of psychiatry, that so long as psychiatry is concerned with real people, there will be no privileged perspective from which psychiatric diagnoses can be made determinate (Fulford 1998).

Practitioner commentary (CASE 4.3)

Dr Mike Jackson Clinical Psychologist, University of Wales, Bangor

The central point of this discussion is that in terms of the facts of Simon's case — the content and form of the experiences he describes — his experiences cannot be distinguished from a psychotic episode. Instead, as the authors make crystal clear, our clinical inclination not to call it mental illness turns on a judgement about values. This raises two further issues beyond the process of diagnosis. The first concerns the implications of this for biological theories which involve concepts of organic dysfunction in the brain. The second concerns the design of research studies which aim to identify psychopathological factors in the psychoses.

Something is clearly distinctive about the way that Simon's brain is processing information. The fact that the 'output' is psychotic in form and content would suggest that if we could understand the neural processes involved, they would be closely similar to, or indistinguishable from, those of psychotic patients whom we are more comfortable in viewing as mentally ill. In Simon's case, however, we cannot justify applying the concept of an organic dysfunction, because he is not ill or dysfunctional. Indeed, if we could specify the differences in brain function between psychotic patients and 'normals', such cases would suggest that we need to be able to explain how these differences may also lead to enhanced function for some individuals.

This conclusion follows more forcefully if we consider a broader range of cases of benign spiritual experience, in which psychotic phenomenology, such as vivid hallucination, are associated with enhanced life functioning, such as recovery from depression and the development or renewal of a sense of meaning and purpose in life. Given that a conservative estimate of the incidence of spiritual experience is around 30 per cent in the general population (Hay 1987), we might argue that the psychological processes involved in generating such experiences are 'normal', and normally adaptive. I have suggested elsewhere (Jackson 1991 and 1997) that such experiences might be viewed as special cases of a more general, adaptive, problem-solving process, which is also described in the process of artistic and scientific creativity (Batson and Ventis 1982; Grof and Grof 1986; Kris 1952) and in the assimilation model of therapeutic change (Stiles *et al.* 1992).

This raises the question of what determines the outcome for a given individual, or why, in William James' (1902) terms, some find 'seraphs' and others, 'snakes'. Rather than searching for the core of psychopathology in the mechanisms which support hallucination and delusion formation, then, it may make more sense to ask the question: why is it that in some individuals, these schizotypal processes become dysfunctional? For the purposes of research, this suggests that in order to isolate the critical variables which can inform us about psychopathology, the ideal comparison group in aetiological studies of psychosis would be 'healthy schizotypes' like Simon, who have the psychotic phenomenology without the psychopathology.

In the meantime, there is a need for further research into the 'grey area' between benign spiritual experience and psychosis, to clarify some of the questions raised by cases such as Simon. Another study in this series (Lewis and Jackson, in preparation) has used more formal and quantitative measures of psychotic symptoms to assess the degree of overlap between spiritual experiences reported by respondents to a questionnaire survey and ratings of acutely psychotic in-patients. To briefly summarize the findings, in the spiritual experience group, substantial symptom ratings were found for auditory and visual hallucinations, religious delusions, depression, ideas and delusions of reference, thought insertion and withdrawal, delusions of being controlled, and delusions of mind-reading. For some of these measures (for example, religious delusions and delusions of control), their scores were higher than for the acute in-patients. On other measures such as anxiety, persecutory delusions, thought broadcasting, and social functioning, the spiritual experience group were more like control subjects.

A further study in progress is examining the claim that spiritual experience is indeed benign in its pragmatic effects. The testimony of individuals reporting such experiences is clearly subjective (and arguably, rather biased) in this respect, and it is not unusual for unambiguously psychotic individuals to also feel that their experience is useful to them. As a first step in going beyond first-person accounts, we are in the process of examining the perspective of friends and family on the spiritual experiences of a set of volunteers.

References (CASE 4.3)

American Psychiatric Association (3rd edn, revised, 1987; 4th edn 1994) *Diagnostic and Statistical Manual of Mental Disorders*. Washington DC, American Psychiatric Association.

Batson, C.P. and Ventis, L.W. (1982). *The Religious Experience*. Oxford, Oxford University Press.

Bhui, K. and Olajide, D. (ed.) (1999) *Mental Health Service Provision for a Multi-Cultural Society*. London, W.B. Saunders Ltd.

Boorse, C. (1975) On the distinction between disease and illness. *Philosophy and Public Affairs*, **5**: 49–68.

Boorse, C. (1976) What a theory of mental health should be. *Journal of Theory Social Behaviour*, **6**:61–84.

Cooper, J.E., Kendell, R.E., Gurland, B.J., Sharpe, L., Copeland, J.R.M., and Simon, R. (1972) *Psychiatric Diagnosis in New York and London*. London, Oxford University Press.

Cox, J.L. (1999) Psychiatry and religion: a general psychiatrist's perspective. In *Religion and Psychiatry* (ed. Bhugra, D.), Chapter 11. London, Routledge.

Fulford, K.W.M. (1989, reprinted 1995; 2nd edn forthcoming) *Moral Theory and Medical Practice*. Cambridge, Cambridge University Press.

Fulford, K.W.M. (1998*b*) *Dissent and dissensus: the limits of consensus formation in psychiatry*. In *Consensus Formation in Health Care Ethics*, pps 175–192 eds, H.A.M.J. ten Have, and H.M. Saas. Kluwer: Philosophy and Medicine Series.

Fulford, K.W.M. (1999) Philosophy and cross-cultural psychiatry. In *Mental Health Service Provision for a Multi-Cultural Society (ed. Bhui, K. and Olajide, D.),* Chapter 2. London, W.B. Saunders, Ltd.

Fulford, K.W.M. (2000) Teleology without Tears: Naturalism, Neo-Naturalism and Evaluationism in the Analysis of Function Statements in Biology (and a Bet on the Twenty-first Century). *Philosophy, Psychiatry and Psychology*, **7/1**:77–94.

Fulford, K.W.M. (2000*a*) Philosophy meets psychiatry in the twentieth century— Four looks back and a brief loof forward. In Louhiala, P., Stenman, S. (eds.): *Philosophy Meets Medicine*. Helsinki: Helsinki University Press; p. 116–34.

Fulford, K.W.M. (2000*b*) Disordered minds, diseased brains and real people in *Philosophy, Psychiatry and Psychopathy: Personal identity in mental disorder*. (ed. Heginbotham, C.), Chapter 4 Avebury Series in Philosophy in association with The Society for Applied Philosophy. Aldershot (England): Ashgate Publishing Ltd.

Fulford, K.W.M., Smirnoff, A.Y.U., and Snow. E. (1993) Concepts of disease and the abuse of psychiatry in the USSR. *British Journal of Psychiatry*, **162**:801–10. Reprinted in 1996 in *Medical Ethics* (ed. Downie, R.S.), volume in *The International Research Library of Philosophy* series (series ed. J. Skorupski). Aldershot (England), Dartmouth.

Grof, S. and Grof, C. (1986) Spiritual emergency: the understanding and treatment of transpersonal crises. *Re-vision*, **8**:7–20.

Group for the Advancement of Psychiatry (1976) *Mysticism: Spiritual Quest or Psychic Disorder?* New York, G.A.P. Publications.

Hay, D. (1987) *Exploring Inner Space* (2nd edn). Harmondsworth, Penguin Books.

Jackson, M.C. (1991) A study of the relationship between spiritual and psychotic experience. Unpublished D.Phil thesis, Oxford University.

Jackson, M.C. (1997) Benign schizotypy? The case of spiritual experience. In *Schizotypy. Relations to Illness and Health* (ed. Claridge, G.S.). Oxford, Oxford University Press.

Jackson, M. and Fulford, K.W.M. (1997) Spiritual experience and psychopathology. *Philosophy, Psychiatry, and Psychology,* 4:41–66. Commentaries by Littlewood, R.; Lu, F.G. *et al.*; Sims, A.; and Storr, A.; and response by authors, pp. 67–90.

James, W. (1902) *The Varieties of Religious Experience.* New York, Longmans.

Kris, E. (1952) *Psychoanalytic Explorations in Art.* New York, International Universities Press.

Laing, R.D. (1967) *The Politics of Experience.* Harmondsworth, Penguin Books.

Lewis, H.W. and Jackson, M.C. (in preparation) *Spiritual and psychotic experiences: phenomenological similarities and differences.*

Littlewood, R. (1993) *Pathology and Identity: The Work of Mother Earth in Trinidad.* Cambridge, Cambridge University Press.

Littlewood, R. (1997) Commentary on Jackson and Fulford's 'Spiritual experience and psychopathology'. *Philosophy, Psychiatry, and Psychology,* 4/1:67–74.

Lu, F.G., Lukoff, D., and Turner, R.P. (1997) Commentary on 'Spiritual experience and psychopathology'. *Philosophy, Psychiatry, and Psychology,* 4/1:75–8.

Persinger, M.A. (1983). Religious and mystical experiences as artefacts of temporal lobe function: A general hypothesis. *Perception and Motor Skills,* 57, 1255–1262.

Sims, A. (1988) *Symptoms in the Mind: An Introduction to Descriptive Psychopathology.* London, Baillière Tindall.

Sims, A. (1997) Commentaries on 'Spiritual experience and psychopathology'. *Philosophy, Psychiatry, and Psychology,* 4/1:79–82.

Stiles, W.B., Meshot, C.M., Anderson, T.M., and Sloan, W.W. (1992). Assimilation of problematic experiences: the case of John Jones. *Psychotherapy Research,* 2:81–101.

Storr, A. (1997) Commentary on Jackson and Fulford's 'Spiritual experience and psychopathology'. *Philosophy, Psychiatry, and Psychology,* 4/1:83–6.

Wakefield, J.C. (1995) Dysfunction as a value-free concept: a reply to Sadler and Agich. *Philosophy, Psychiatry, and Psychology,* 2:233–46.

Wing, J.K. (1978) *Reasoning about Madness.* Oxford, Oxford University Press.

Wing, J.K., Cooper, J.E., and Sartorius, N. (1974) *Measurement and classification of psychiatric symptoms.* Cambridge, Cambridge University Press.

World Health Organisation (1973) *The International Pilot Study of Schizophrenia. Volume 1.* Geneva, WHO.World Psychiatric Association, Geneva (1996) Declaration of Madrid. (Reproduced with a brief commentary in 1999 in *Psychiatric Ethics* (3rd edn) (Bloch, S., Chodoff P., and Green S.A.), Appendix — Codes of Ethics, pp. 511–31. Oxford, Oxford University Press.)

World Health Organisation (1992) *The ICD–10 Classification of Mental and Behavioural Disorders: Clinical Descriptions and Diagnostic Guidelines.* Geneva, WHO.

Reading Guide

The cases in this chapter, reflecting the pivotal role of diagnosis in psychiatric ethics, have covered a wide range of issues. In this Reading Guide we focus on the three topics in its title — responsibility, rationality, and the role of values in shaping psychiatric classifications and diagnostic concepts.

Responsibility

The role of mental illness as an excuse in law (that is, as a condition which renders the accused not responsible for their actions) has been widely debated, particularly in relation to the 'insanity defence' and related legal pleas. Classic treatments include Nigel Walker's *Crime and Insanity in England and Wales* (1967) and the philosopher Anthony Flew's *Crime or Disease?* (1973). The first chapter of R.A. Duff's *Trials and Punishments* (1986) offers a careful philosophical treatment of the grounds for exempting mentally disordered people from criminal responsibility. More recently, Lawrie Reznek's *Evil or Ill?* (1998) includes a valuable review of the issues and Dan Robinson's *Wild Beasts and Idle Humours* (1996) provides a scholarly historical *tour de force*. There is a considerable sociological literature on the status of illness generally as a condition which excuses from responsibility (going back to Talcot Parson's *The Social System*, 1951).

A helpful introduction to the philosophical deep waters of determinism and responsibility is Mary Warnock's 'Freedom, responsibility and determinism' (Chapter 5 in her *An Intelligent Person's Guide to Ethics*, 1998). A more extended treatment is John Lucas' *Responsibility* (1993). Other philosophical texts include Jonathan Glover's *Responsibility* (1970) and Chapter 6, 'Risk, responsibility, rationality and consent' in Donna Dickenson's *Moral Luck in Medical Ethics and Practical Politics* (1991). John Harris' *Violence and Responsibility* (1980) offers a thought-provoking treatment.

A clear introduction to legal responsibility from the perspective of philosophy of law is H.L.A. Hart's *Punishment and Responsibility* (1968). A valuable recent addition to legal work on responsibility is Nigel Eastman and Jill Peay, *Law without Enforcement: Integrating Mental Health and Justice* (1999).

Rationality

Although there is a large philosophical literature on rationality and irrationality, the rich variety of different forms of irrationality represented by psychopathology has been largely ignored. An important exception is Gardner's *Irrationality and the Philosophy of Psychoanalysis* (1993). A detailed analysis of rationality linked to competencies is given in Chapter 3 of Beauchamp and Childress' *Principles of Biomedical Ethics* (4th edn, 1994). This is one of the few bioethical accounts to take seriously the problem of judgements of rationality in psychiatry.

Fulford and Hope, in 'Psychiatric ethics: a bioethical ugly duckling?' (1993), have argued that the competencies approach works well for organic conditions like dementia but fails to account for the kind of irrationality exhibited by the functional disorders. A more detailed treatment of the failure of traditional accounts of rationality to explain the ethical and legal status of delusion and other psychotic symptoms is given in Chapter 10 of Fulford's *Moral Theory and Medical Practice* (1989); this is developed further in his 'Value, action, mental illness, and the law' (1993) and 'Responsibility, mental illness and psychiatric experts' (1996). An amusing compilation of fallacies and illicit mental short-cuts can be found in Stuart Sutherland's *Irrationality: The Enemy Within* (1992).

Rationality and its gendered interpretation is well elucidated in Genevieve Lloyd's *The Man of Reason: 'Male' and 'Female' in Western Philosophy* (1993). A feminist reconstruction of rationality, which tries to apply the traditional philosophical link between agency and rationality to women's position, can be found in the section 'Rationality and its discontents' in Donna Dickenson's *Property, Women and Politics: Subjects or Objects?* (1997).

Many aspects of the rationality (or otherwise) of suicide are explored in a thematic issue of *Philosophy, Psychiatry and Psychology* on 'Suicide and psychiatric euthanasia' (Volume 5/2; 1998). This issue includes a series of case studies by Sally Burgess and Keith Hawton (1998) together with commentaries and supporting articles by philosophers, lawyers, and practitioners. Henry Tam's *Punishment, Excuses and Moral Development* (1996) is a useful edited collection covering issues of responsibility from a number of perspectives — legal, bioethical, sociological, and so on. Jonathan Glover's *Causing Death and Saving Lives* (2nd edn, 1992) remains a readable and thought-provoking pioneering work, written from a utilitarian viewpoint.

Values in psychiatric classification and diagnosis

Chapters 9 (by Bill Fulford) and 10 (by Walter Reich) in *Psychiatric Ethics* (1999), edited by Bloch *et al.*, are concerned with ethical aspects of psychiatric diagnosis. A valuable edited collection covering most of the key conceptual issues in psychiatric diagnosis and classification is *Philosophical Perspectives on Psychiatric Diagnostic Classification* (1994), edited by Sadler *et al.* This book was published to coincide with the appearance of DSM–IV; it has a foreword by Allen Frances, the Chair of the DSM–IV Task Force.

Chapters 3, 4, and 5 of Fulford's *Moral Theory and Medical Practice* (1989) show that, while values help to define diagnostic concepts in all areas of medicine, they are especially important practically in psychiatry because of the diversity of human values in the areas of experience and behaviour with which psychiatry is concerned. (See also Chapter 1 of this book.) An edited collection, including canonical, first-hand, and original materials, and structured around the stages of the clinical process, is Fulford *et al.*'s *Healthcare Ethics and Human Values* (forthcoming).

A further useful collection is an issue of *The Journal of Medicine and Philosophy*, edited by L. Kopelman, on 'Philosophical issues concerning psychiatric diagnosis' (1992). The *Philosophy and Medicine* book series has included a number of volumes on philosophical and ethical aspects of classification and diagnosis, in particular *The Ethics of Diagnosis* (1992), edited by José Luis Reset and Diego Gracia, which covers historical, anthropological, and sociological perspectives. Volume 15 of the *Episteme* book series on *Diagnosis: Philosophical and Medical Perspectives* (1990), by Laor and Agassi, includes a number of relevant chapters, in particular Chapter 4, 'Ethics of diagnostic systems', which examines the issues from the novel perspective of systems analysis.

Simon, the person whose story is described in Case 4.3, was first reported at length, together with other similar cases, in Jackson and Fulford's 'Spiritual experience and psychopathology' (1997). The study from which these cases were drawn was reported in full in Mike Jackson's 'Benign schizotypy? The case of spiritual experience' (1997), in *Schizotypy: Relations to Illness and Health*, edited by G.S. Claridge. This included an epidemiological study showing the extent to which psychiatrists are insensitive to religious and spiritual beliefs and experiences. The significance of Simon's case for our understanding of the role of values in diagnosis, particularly in cross-cultural psychiatry, is explored in Fulford's article 'From culturally sensitive to culturally competent mental health care: a seminar in philosophy and practice skills' (1999). For a valuable edited collection on the relationship between psychiatry and religion, see D. Bhugra's *Psychiatry and Religion* (1996).

Articles on the importance of values in all areas of psychopathology appear regularly in the international journal, *PPP— Philosophy, Psychiatry and Psychology*. Besides Jackson and Fulford (already mentioned), examples include L.M. Kopelman's 'Normal grief: good or bad? Health or disease?' (1994); Moore *et al.*'s 'Mild mania and well-being' (1994); J.Z. Sadler's (1996) 'Epistemic value commitments in the debate over categorical vs. dimensional personality diagnosis' (1996); and Sadler and Agich's 'Dysfunction as a value-free concept' (1995).

Reading Guide: references

Beauchamp, T.L. and **Childress, J.F.** (1994) *Principles of Biomedical Ethics* (4th edn). Oxford, Oxford University Press.

Bhugra, D. (1996) *Psychiatry and Religion.* Context, Consensus and Controversies. London and New York: Routledge.

Burgess, S. and **Hawton, K.** (1998) Suicide, euthanasia, and the psychiatrist. *Philosophy, Psychiatry, and Psychology*, 5/2:113–26.

Dickenson, D. (1991) *Moral Luck in Medical Ethics and Practical Politics.* Aldershot, Avebury Press.

Dickenson, D. (1997) *Property, Women and Politics: Subjects or Objects?* Cambridge, Polity Press.

Duff, R.A. (1986) *Trials and Punishments.* Cambridge: Cambridge University Press.

Eastman, N. and Peay, J. (1999) *Law Without Enforcement: Integrating Mental Health and Justice.* Oxford and Portland (Oregon), Hart Publishing.

Flew, A. (1973) *Crime or Disease?* New York, Barnes and Noble.

Fulford, K.W.M. (1989, reprinted 1995; 2nd edn forthcoming) *Moral Theory and Medical Practice.* Cambridge, Cambridge University Press.

Fulford, K.W.M. (1993) Value, action, mental illness and the law. In *Action and Value in Criminal Law* (ed. Shute, S., Gardner, J., and Horder, J.), pp. 279–310. Oxford, Oxford University Press.

Fulford, K.W.M. (1996) Responsibility, mental illness and psychiatric experts. In *Punishment, Excuses and Moral Development* (ed. H. Tam). Aldershot (England), Avebury Press.

Fulford, K.W.M. (1999) Chapter 9 in *Psychiatric Ethics* (3rd edn) (ed. Bloch, S., Chodoff, P., and Green, S.A.). Oxford, Oxford University Press.

Fulford, K.W.M. (1999) Philosophy and cross-cultural psychiatry. In *Mental Health Service Provision for a Multi-Cultural Society* (ed. Bhui, K. and Olajide, D.), Chapter 2. London, W.B. Saunders Ltd.

Fulford, K.W.M. and Hope, R.A. (1993) Psychiatric ethics: a bioethical ugly duckling? In *Principles of Health Care Ethics* (ed. Gillon, R. and Lloyd, A.), Chapter 58. Chichester (England), John Wiley and Sons.

Fulford, K.W.M., Dickenson, D. and Murray, T.H. (eds) (forthcoming) *Healthcare Ethics and Human Values.* Oxford, Blackwells.

Gardner, S. (1993) *Irrationality and the Philosophy of Psychoanalysis.* Cambridge, Cambridge University Press.

Glover, J. (1970) *Responsibility.* London, Routledge and Kegan Paul.

Glover, J. (1997) *Causing Death and Saving Lives.* Harmondsworth, Penguin Books, 2nd edn.

Harris, J. (1980) *Violence and Responsibility.* London, Routledge and Kegan Paul.

Hart, H.L.A. (1968) *Punishment and Responsibility: Essays in the Philosophy of Law.* Oxford, Oxford University Press.

Jackson, M.C. (1997) Benign schizotypy? The case of spiritual experience. In *Schizotypy. Relations to Illness and Health* (ed. Claridge, G.S.). Oxford, Oxford University Press.

Jackson, M. and Fulford, K.W.M. (1997) Spiritual experience and psychopathology. *Philosophy, Psychiatry, and Psychology,* 4:41–66. (Commentaries by Littlewood, R.; Lu, F.G. *et al.*; Sims, A.; and Storr, A.; and response by authors, 67–90.)

Kopelman, L.M. (ed.) (1992) Philosophical issues concerning psychiatric diagnosis. *The Journal of Medicine and Philosophy*, **17**/2.

Kopelman, L.M. (1994) Normal grief: good or bad? Health or disease? *Philosophy, Psychiatry and Psychology*, **1**:209–20 (with commentaries by Dominian, J. and Wise, T.N. 221–4; response by Kopelman, 226–7)

Laor and Agassi (1990) *Diagnosis: Philosophical and Medical Perspectives.* Volume 15 of the *Episteme* book series. The Netherlands, Kluwer.

Lloyd, G. (1993) *The Man of Reason: 'Male' and 'Female' in Western Philosophy.* University of Minnesota Press.

Lucas, F.R. (1993) *Responsibility.* Oxford, Clarendon Press.

Moore, A., Hope, T., and Fulford, K.W.M. (1994) Mild mania and well-being. *Philosophy, Psychiatry and Psychology*, **1**:165–92 (with commentaries by Nordenfelt, L. and Seedhouse, D.)

Parsons, T. (1951) *The Social System.* Glencoe (Illinois), Free Press.

Reich, W. (1999). Chapter 10 in *Psychiatric Ethics* (3rd edn) (ed. Bloch, S., Chodoff, P., and Green, S.A.). Oxford, Oxford University Press.

Reset, J.L. and Gracia, D. (1992) *The Ethics of Diagnosis.* Volume 40 in *Philosophy and Medicine* series (series ed. Engelhardt, T. and Spicker, S.). The Netherlands, Kluwer.

Reznek, L. (1998) *Evil or Ill?*

Robinson D. (1996) *Wild Beasts and Idle Humours.* Cambridge (Mass.), Harvard University Press.

Sadler, J.Z. (1996) Epistemic value commitments in the debate over categorical vs. dimensional personality diagnosis. *Philosophy, Psychiatry, and Psychology*, **3**:203–22. (Commentaries by Livesley W.J. and Luntley M., 223–30)

Sadler, J.Z. and Agich, G.J. (1995) Dysfunction as a value-free concept: a reply to Sadler and Agich. *Philosophy, Psychiatry, and Psychology*, **2**:233–46.Sadler, J.Z., Wiggins, O.P., and Schwartz, M.A. (ed.) (1994) *Philosophical Perspectives on Psychiatry Diagnostic Classification.* Baltimore, Johns Hopkins University Press.

Sutherland, S. (1992) *Irrationality: The Enemy Within.* Harmondsworth, Penguin Books.

Tam, H. (1996) *Punishment, Excuses and Moral Development.* Aldershot, Avebury Press.

Walker, N. (1967) *Crime and Insanity in England.* Edinburgh University Press.

Warnock, M. (1998) *An Intelligent Person's Guide to Ethics.* London, Duckworth.

CHAPTER 5

Aetiology: causal and meaningful connections

Understanding meanings is no less important than explaining causes in mental health practice and research

There is a widespread belief that the problems with psychiatric diagnosis we encountered in the last two chapters will be resolved once we have a better picture of the underlying causes of mental disorder in the brain. The cases described in this chapter all show, in different ways, that this belief — the belief that 'brain trumps mind' — is mistaken in principle and may be abusive in practice.

For many people, and not only in psychiatry, the very 'reality' of mental illness depends on the demonstration of a brain lesion. A recent newspaper report of the discovery of an abnormality in the temporal lobe of patients with anorexia nervosa described how this would relieve the guilt that parents felt. The doctor concerned would be able to say, 'There is a major biological factor happening in your daughter's brain...causing her to behave this way. It is not your fault.' (*Sunday Times*, 13 April 1997). Thomas Szasz (whose rejection of mental illness as a myth we noted in Chapter 3) said in an interview with Jonathan Miller on the BBC that he will believe schizophrenia is a genuine disease if and when it is shown to have a causal basis in brain pathology equivalent to the lesions underlying neurological disorders. Similarly the courts, faced with issues of attributing responsibility, are impressed by brain scans, EEGs, and so forth — the implication being that the accused's behaviour is a product of a brain lesion rather than of their own will. Philosophers committed to a medical model of disease have argued that advances in our knowledge of brain functioning will clarify the boundary between deviance and disorder (for example, Boorse 1975; Wakefield 1995).

In psychiatry, the belief that 'brain trumps mind' has its origins, or at any rate its justification, in the medical model. Building on the work of Karl Jaspers and others in the early years of the twentieth century, psychiatry has made important advances by clarifying the symptoms of mental disorder — by developing a descriptive psychopathology. Historically, this is the equivalent of the symptom-based classifications of bodily disorders produced in the eighteenth century by such foundational figures as Thomas Sydenham. It was on the basis of these classifications that advances in histology, bacteriology, and so on, in the nineteenth century, were to give us our present causally based classifications of diseases. Psychiatry, therefore, so this line of thinking goes, will follow a similar path. Jaspers' descriptive psychopathology is the basis on which advances in genetics and neuroscience will build to clarify the brain pathologies underlying mental disorders. These pathologies, like pathologies in any other part of the body, will be products of complex causal chains, including psychological and social factors. But as the final causal pathway, brain pathologies will allow us to resolve our present difficulties about whether someone is or is not mentally ill, as readily as we can nowadays resolve questions about whether someone is or is not physically ill.

Exploring the metaphysical assumptions lying behind the belief that brain trumps mind would take us into many of the deepest areas of general philosophy. We noted some of these earlier —freedom and determinism, the nature of free choice, volition, the will, not to mention the mother of all philosophical problems, the relationship between mind and brain! And even without diving into these deep philosophical waters, the issue of the relationship between meanings and causes goes back at least as far as the nineteenth-century debate about the relationship between the natural and the human sciences (the so-called *Methodenstreit*). Karl Jaspers, influenced by this debate, believed that, important as the causes of mental disorder may be, in psychiatry we cannot avoid being concerned also with meanings (Jaspers 1913). Sigmund Freud thought much the same. But whereas Freud, at least in his early work, believed that psychology would eventually be reduced to neuroscience, Jaspers believed that the barriers to such a reduction might never be overcome — that brain would never trump mind.

Modern philosophy remains divided on this question. Many philosophers, though, subscribe to some form of a position called 'non-reductive monism'. This is the view that the mind is part of the natural world — that there is no separate 'mind stuff' as René Descartes famously claimed (hence 'monism' rather than 'dualism'); but that, all the same, the mind cannot be reduced to the brain, at least not in the way that, say, much of chemistry can be reduced to physics (hence 'non-reductive'). The inspiration for this is the computer. Software is not the same as hardware; you can run any given computer file on a number of different computers and knowing what file a computer is running can tell us nothing definite about the hardware. There is no software–hardware connection; and hence there is no 'reduction' from software to hardware, at least not in this sense of the term. As with computers, though, this does not imply that the mental is somehow other-worldly or non-physical. On the contrary, modern representational theories of mind locate the causal powers of mental states (that is, their ability to cause each other and to cause actions) precisely in their meaningful (that is, information-bearing) content (see Bolton and Hill, 1996, for a carefully worked out application of this approach to mental disorders[1]).

As the Reading Guide at the end of this chapter indicates, this is an area in which philosophy of mind and neuroscience research are rapidly coming together, not least in psychiatry. Deep though as the theoretical problems are, they are but the flip-side of problems with which psychiatrists, and indeed all those concerned with mental disorders, have to deal in their day-to-day clinical work. This is illustrated by the cases described in this chapter. Both cases show, in different ways, that, as Jaspers recognized, brain does not trump mind. Both thus raise, in principle, the deep metaphysical problems just noted. Given the depths of these problems, we will not be attempting to actually *resolve* them in this chapter! But we will be indicating the limitations of a framework which seeks to resolve them merely by limiting attention to causes. And we will be illustrating the rich resources from ethical and other aspects of philosophical theory which are available to us in taking the meanings of mental disorders as seriously as their causes.

Our first case, that of Jane Gillespie, examines the importance of meanings in a case of depression. Careful sociological research over the last twenty years or so has identified a number of social (as distinct from biological) risk factors for depression: for example, having lost your mother at an early age (see Brown and Harris 1978). Such factors might suggest that a biopsychosocial model of the causes of depression could be developed in a positivistic frame without regard to the meanings of these experiences for the individuals concerned. In fact, George Brown himself, one of the key figures in this field, has been at pains to emphasize that work in this area depends on judgements by skilled interviewers of the likely significance of an event for the person concerned (see, for example, Brown 1989).

Jane Gillespie's case provides a graphic illustration of the importance of this for ethical reasoning specifically in psychiatry. Her depression, which was precipitated by an assault, was linked to her having been abused as a child by her father. But the significance of the assault for *her* was that it undermined her carefully constructed sense of 'being in control' which she had built up as a defence against her experience of being abused. It was this that was at the heart of the ethical dilemma for the mental health team. They felt that she should be in hospital because she was at risk of suicide, but she was adamantly against being hospitalized; to have used a 'section' would have taken the last vestige of her crucial 'sense of control'. Dilemmas of this kind are a common feature of risk management in suicide (Burgess and Hawton 1998).

Our second case, that of Francesca Gindro, tackles meanings and causes in the heartland of psychopathology — delusions. Francesca Gindro developed a variant of erotomania in the course of psychotherapy. Erotomania proper is a monosymptomatic paranoid psychosis in which the patient develops a delusional belief that some particular person is in love with them. Francesca Gindro, who was in psychotherapy following her failure to have a baby, developed the delusional belief that her psychotherapist had agreed to donate his sperm and that this would allow her to have a successful pregnancy.

This is a complex and multilayered case. At its deepest theoretical level, it reopens long-running debates about the unconscious sources of experience and behaviour, one paradigm of which is psychoanalysis. Psychoanalytic explanations of psychotic experience, although frequently presented as causal theories (Freud's so-called 'hydrodynamics of the mind'), essentially involve meaningful relations. This is one reason why the scientific status of these theories has been so widely contested. But recent philosophy has generated a range of hermeneutic and other meaning-driven reconstructions of psychoanalytic theory (for example, Ricoeur 1970). We focus on a recent theory along these lines in Francesca Gindro's case — the philosopher Sebastian Gardner's account of self-deception and its relationship to irrationality (Gardner 1993). We are not therefore dependent on meaning-free (and in this sense, causal or scientific) psychoanalytic theory for a 'meaning-ful' account of the mind. And at least in Francesca Gindro's case, it is stretching credibility to believe that her delusions were not meaningfully related in *some* way to her disappointment in not being able to have a baby.

In descriptive psychopathology, we typically distinguish between *form* and *content*. Traditionally, the form of a symptom has been considered to be more significant diagnostically than its content. Form tells us what kind of symptoms we are dealing with, while content is context-dependent (a product of a particular patient's personal experiences and cultural background). Thus we distinguish obsessional from delusional beliefs by, among other things, the presence or absence of insight. Francesca Gindro is said to lack insight because she is unable to recognize that her beliefs about her therapist are irrational. Lack of insight, as a general defining characteristic of the *form* of delusions (whatever their *content* in a given case), crucially determines a range of management issues, from the choice of specific treatment through to the appropriateness or otherwise of the use of the Mental Health Act.

The form–content distinction, as employed in descriptive psychopathology, is a helpful heuristic. It allows us to characterize and organize the features of a patient's mental state in a way which is prima facie relevant to research and treatment. As with all heuristics though, it is at risk of being required to carry a greater theoretical burden than it can bear. We have already seen that form, as traditionally understood in psychopathology, is not sufficient to demarcate pathology from non-pathology. (Simon Greer's experiences (Chapter 4), although not pathological, had the form of first-rank schizophrenic symptoms.)

In the case of delusions, moreover, there are general grounds, connected with the form of delusions themselves, for believing that the distinction between delusional and non-delusional thinking lies in practical reasoning (the reasons people give for their actions) rather than in some (as yet to be identified) specific disturbance of cognitive functioning (Fulford 1989, Chapter 10). We develop this point in the discussion of Francesca Gindro's case. Its significance, as we will see, is that practical reasoning has traditionally been the concern of philosophers and lawyers rather than of neuroscientists and psychologists. Practical reasoning is where issues of responsibility, guilt, excuse, and so forth arise. This is not to say that science cannot or should not be concerned with practical reasoning. This is indeed one of the areas in which philosophy and neuroscience are converging. But it *is* to say that this is yet another situation in which a narrowly medical–scientific model, limited to a positivistic concern with the form of symptoms, may not be focused where the action really is.

An exclusive focus on form, narrowly conceived, is thus not sufficient for psychiatry's theoretical purposes. And, when it comes to the *practical* purposes

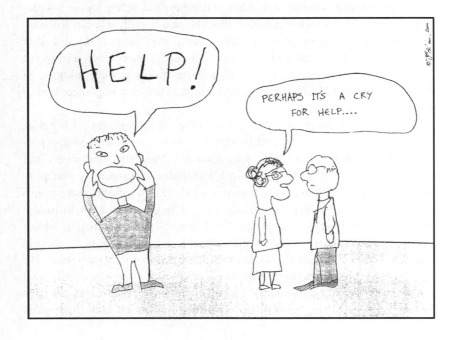

of psychiatry, this focus has been directly counter-productive. This is in part because the focus on form has led psychiatrists to neglect what is often most significant from the patient's point of view, the *content* of their symptoms. What really matters to Francesca Gindro is that her therapist is going to help her have a baby. Merely to write this off as delusional, to discount it, will therefore be, at the very least, abusive. It will also reduce the scope for co-operation in management, non-specifically in the case of drug treatments, but specifically in the case of cognitive–behavioural approaches, which start from and build on the patient's beliefs and values.

Good practice in psychiatry does require a careful account of the content of a particular patient's experiences as well as of their form (Sims 1997). But good practice, if we are to believe the reports of patients, is less widespread than psychiatrists are inclined to believe. There is all too often a gulf between the patient's values and beliefs and those of the doctor (or indeed of other professionals – see, for example, Campbell 1996). Important areas are avoided altogether: religious beliefs, for example, are taboo for most psychiatrists. Whether we like it or not, therefore, the emphasis on form has skewed our attention away from the meaningful content of symptoms.

Just how we concern ourselves with meanings as well as causes is another matter. As with our other cases, we offer no final resolution of the dilemmas presented by Jane Gillespie and Francesca Gindro. But if there is no final resolution of such cases, modern ethical theory offers a range of techniques for exploring meanings. We note a number of these in Jane Gillespie's case —narrative and other forms of hermeneutic ethics being especially relevant (Newton 1997; Lindemann Nelson 1997). Besides ethical theory, ethnography and other qualitative sociological methods, semiotics, discursive psychology, and recent developments in hermeneutics (building on the phenomenologies of Merleau–Ponty and Heidegger) may all illuminate the meaningful content of ethical issues in particular cases.

These developments in ethical theory are especially significant for the relationship between philosophy and psychiatry. For much of this century, philosophy has been split into two main schools — 'analytic' philosophy and so-called 'continental' philosophy (which includes hermeneutics and phenomenology). The difference in approach of these two schools corresponds broadly to the causes/meanings distinction. It is true that both include a wide variety of different disciplines, but broadly speaking, analytic philosophy has been concerned with logic and with the foundations of physical science, whereas continental philosophy has been concerned with subjective experience and the meanings of texts. There was no analytic–continental split at the start of the twentieth century when Jaspers was developing his key ideas; the split is now closing up again, with philosophers in many parts of the world increasingly drawing on both disciplines. This is a well-established trend in general philosophy, and one which comes to a natural focus in psychiatry in the need for both causal and meaningful accounts of mental disorder.

References

Bolton, D. and Hill, J. (1996) *Mind, Meaning and Mental Disorder: the Nature of Causal Explanation in Psychology and Psychiatry.* Oxford, Oxford University Press.

Boorse, C. (1975) On the distinction between disease and illness. *Philosophy and Public Affairs*, **5**: 49–68.

Brown, G.W. (1989) Life events and measurement. In *Life Events and Illness* (ed. Brown, G.W. and Harris, T.O.), pp. 49–94. New York, Guildford Press; London, Unwin and Hyman.

Brown, G.W. and Harris, T.O. (1978) *Social Origins of Depression: a Study of Psychiatric Disorders in Women.* London, Tavistock Publications, New York, Free Press.

Burgess, S. and Hawton, K. (1998) Suicide, euthanasia, and the psychiatrist. *Philosophy, Psychiatry, and Psychology*, **5**:113–26.

Campbell, P. (1996) What we want from crisis services. In *On Speaking Our Minds: Anthology* (ed. Read, J. and Reynolds, J.), pp. 180–4. London, MacMillan Press Ltd. (for The Open University).

Fulford, K.W.M. (1989, reprinted 1995; 2nd edn forthcoming) *Moral Theory and Medical Practice.* Cambridge, Cambridge University Press.

Gardner, S. (1993) *Irrationality and the Philosophy of Psychoanalysis.* Cambridge, Cambridge University Press.

Jaspers, K. (1913) Causal and meaningful connexions between life history and psychosis. Reprinted in 1974 in *Themes and Variations in European Psychiatry* (ed. Hirsch, S.R. and Shepherd, M.), Chapter 5. Bristol, John Wright and Sons Ltd.

Lindemann Nelson, H. (1997) *Stories and Their Limits: Narrative Approaches to Bioethics.* London, Routledge.

Newton, A.Z. (1997) *Narrative Ethics.* Cambridge (Mass.), Harvard University Press.

Ricoeur, P. (1970) *Freud and Philosophy* (trans. Savage, D.). London, Yale University Press.

Sims, A. (1997) Commentary on 'Spiritual experience and psychopathology'. *Philosophy, Psychiatry, and Psychology*, **4/1**:79–82.

Sunday Times (13 April 1997) 'Anorexia trigger found in the brain'.

Wakefield, J.C. (1995) Dysfunction as a value-free concept: a reply to Sadler and Agich. *Philosophy, Psychiatry, and Psychology*, **2**:233–46.

CASE 5.1
Jane Gillespie — agent and patient in depression

Synopsis A 42-year-old woman has become depressed and suicidal after being attacked by the father of a baby on a paediatric ward while she was the nurse in charge. She was abused physically by her father as a teenager. She has a supportive husband, three grown-up sons (all doing well), and a successful nursing career. But she has a continuing problem with a bullying manager at work. She refuses admission for fear of losing her job. To be admitted on an involuntary basis would further aggravate her sense of loss of control and hence of failure.

Key dilemma Whether to admit, aggravating her fear of loss of control, or risk suicide.

Main topic Autonomy and control in depression.

Other topics Meanings and causes in the aetiology of depression; suicide risk; nature of psychosis; ECT; feminist ethics; responsibility; psychiatric ethics (marginality); agency; freedom; determinism; intentionality; abuse (child).

Jane Gillespie, now forty-two, deliberately became pregnant when she was sixteen in order to get away from her father's physical abuse. Her other siblings, she says, never stood up to their father, and all his anger fell on her because she resisted his control. Her mother had died when she was eight. Although she had two young children by the time she was twenty, she managed to get her nursing qualification and helped to support the family by working night shifts. She and her husband now have three grown-up sons, one of whom still lives at home. Jane began studying for a paediatric intensive care nursing qualification when the youngest boy was ten, and she now has a ward managerial position at a large metropolitan hospital trust.

Three years ago, Jane was assaulted by a distressed relative in the paediatric intensive care unit. The father of a critically ill baby had become convinced that Jane was going to 'pull the plug' and let the child die. He barred the ward door when no other nurses were present and then hit her, causing a fractured jaw. Although Jane finally persuaded her attacker to let her go, the assault, together with overwork and what she describes as constant bullying by an unsympathetic line manager in the hospital, provoked a full-blown depression.

Jane was tormented by the feeling that she had lost control over her life, that she was worthless, that nothing she did was right. She was unable to complain to her line manager about the assault because she felt that it would call her competence into question: 'He already thinks I'm totally useless.' Meanwhile, she was being required to meet constantly tighter fiscal and efficiency targets for the intensive care unit, which was chronically understaffed. Her husband, George, became convinced that Jane was suicidal — not for the first time, he says — and urged her to see their GP. Jane agreed reluctantly, but did tell the GP that she had indeed been contemplating suicide for a long time, even before the assault.

Referred to an out-patient psychiatric clinic, Jane made little progress with 'talking cures': she was reserved and rather taciturn. Psychopharmacology was also problematic: although her mood lifted a little on a combination of antidepressants and lithium, she developed lithium tremors, which were noticed at work. Her sleep pattern became irregular and she started to wake earlier than usual. Her sense of failure and inadequacy worsened, and she decided to refuse treatment. To her mind, it was doing more harm than good. She thought more than ever about killing herself, she said, especially if she lost her job. But she resisted any efforts at liaison between psychiatric services and her line manager — he was not to know that she was receiving psychiatric treatment, she insisted.

By now Social Services had become involved in the case, and an application had been made to the magistrates' court for a Section 2 order under the Mental Health Act 1983. This gives the clinicians power to admit patients compulsorily for assessment over a 28-day period. Although this course had not been requested by Jane's principal clinician, specialist registrar Bella Tannenbaum, and although Jane's husband resisted it on the grounds that it would reinforce Jane's feelings of lacking control, the order was granted. During the period of compulsory admission, on the basis of her persistently low mood and distorted sleep pattern (she was continuing to wake early), Jane was formally diagnosed as suffering from endogenous depression by the consultant, Henry Walsingham. He recommended a course of ECT, which did seem to alleviate Jane's symptoms somewhat.

Since that time, however, Jane has only had brief periods of remission from her depression. She has had two more short compulsory admissions to hospital, this time under Section 3 of the Mental Health Act. Each time she has managed to hide the real nature of her illness from her line manager, but she feels that he is becoming increasingly suspicious. There is little change in her expressed desire to end her life, although she has never actually made a suicide attempt. Jane accepts ECT willingly, and even requests it, but Bella feels that this is at the expense of cognitive therapy, together with some form of counselling, which she would prefer to pursue.

Jane is now being treated on an out-patient basis again. She has made some progress with cognitive therapy. However, she relapsed after a counselling session in which she discussed her feelings about her father; she found this session particularly unpleasant, she said, because Christmas was coming, with its obligatory family reunion. The clinicians are reluctant to section her again: she is vehemently opposed, and certain that another bout in hospital would cost her her job. She insists that none of her patients is being put at risk and that if anything, she is particularly careful and scrupulous when she feels depression coming on. If she lost her job because her competence was put in doubt, she says, that would be the ultimate failure.

Bella is also left feeling very uncertain about how far to probe, and about whether Jane is using both the threat of suicide and the request for ECT as forms of control. As Bella puts it, 'If Jane's not 110 per cent in control, she feels like a failure. Sectioning takes away all her powers of control, and reinforces her sense of herself as a failure. But what happens if I don't section her, and she kills herself?'

This is a case in which 'technical' diagnostic decisions are deeply intertwined with ethical choices. In this respect it is of course no different from the cases described in the last two chapters. However, in those earlier cases, the diagnostic assessments were made at the level of symptoms, the level of the patient's experiences, and of their observed behaviour. In this case, by contrast, the diagnosis is made at the level of aetiology. The diagnostic label 'endogenous depression', traditionally contrasted with 'reactive depression', implies a process which wells up from within, a product of internal disturbances of functioning, as far beyond the control of the sufferer as a heart attack or appendicitis. 'Reactive depression', too, may imply loss of control to the extent that the sufferer is overwhelmed by events, but here, the label suggests, we retain some power of *re*action, of fighting against adversity, or at any rate of circumventing it. Endogenous depression, with its presumed origin in our genes and brain amines, offers no escape; as with the lesions underlying physical disorders, we are literally, patients — the passive objects of a disease process, rather than free agents.

It is with the practical consequences of the denial of agency implicit in the label 'endogenous' that we will be concerned in this discussion. Our aim will not be to set out the overtly ethical issues as such, still less to resolve them. The dilemma, as expressed by the specialist registrar, Bella Tannenbaum, is to do with suicide risk. Jane Gillespie needs to feel '110 per cent in control', as Bella puts it. She is tormented with feelings of worthlessness and guilt because she has failed in her responsibilities, abjured her self-image of someone who is competent in her highly responsible position. On this view of her situation, suicide may be, for Jane Gillespie, the last hope for control. But is her perspective merely a product of a depressive illness?

In essence, the dilemma is whether to admit Jane Gillespie on an involuntary basis or to respect her wishes. If she is ill, if her suicidal feelings are symptoms of a disease process, then admission to hospital may be justified; if on the other hand her suicidal feelings reflect 'true wishes', then whatever the risks, they should be respected.

The ethical issues here are thus, in many respects, similar to those considered in relation to Case 4.1, Martin McKendrick. But our aim in this chapter will be to explore and to make explicit some of the factors which lie behind Dr Tannenbaum's dilemma being so acute in this particular case. The key factor to emerge will be the extent to which the term 'endogenous' invites us to think of Jane Gillespie's situation in purely causal terms and thus to neglect the meanings which, we argue, are aetiologically (and hence also, in this case, ethically) crucial.

A preliminary point to consider is whether this is a non-issue, diagnostically speaking, given that notwithstanding the consultant psychiatrist Dr Walsingham's diagnosis, the categories of 'endogenous' and 'reactive' depression have been replaced in our official classifications by the categories 'major' and 'minor' depression. With this change of name, have we not changed the game? After all, the whole thrust of the development of modern classifications of mental disorders has been to abandon premature and ill-founded aetiological theories in favour of a descriptive (symptom-based) approach. In the case of depression, moreover, it has been known for some time that, contrary to the claims of earlier psychopathologists, there are no significant differences in symptoms between cases which appear to come 'out of the blue' (endogenous) and those which are meaningfully related to some life event (reactive).

There are, though, a number of reasons for believing that, in the case of depression at least, the game has not changed. In the first place, despite the official change in nomenclature, the diagnostic use of 'endogenous' is remarkably persistent. One explanation for this is that it reflects a continuing belief in a subcategory of depressions that are caused by diseases and are hence outside the scope of meaningful relations. In the second place, psychotic symptoms, which were closely associated with the category of endogenous depression (the two were sometimes used synonymously), remain a feature of major depression (they are included, for example, as a 'specifier' in DSM–IV; APA 1994, p. 376). And, as we saw in Chapter 2, it is with psychotic mental disorders that we take a patient's responsibility for their actions to be most deeply compromised. In such disorders, this seems to imply, what the person does is not meaningfully related to their beliefs and values but is 'caused by their disease'.

In the third place, and most decisively, major depression itself is defined, in large part, by the presence of what are known in psychiatry as 'biological symptoms' — early waking, weight loss, fixed diurnal variation of mood, and psychomotor retardation (slowing down of thought and behaviour). Such symptoms reflect disturbances in the 'deep' centres of the brain concerned with the control of vegetative functions. They signal, moreover, that the patient is likely to respond to 'physical' treatments such as antidepressant drugs and ECT. Hence, even where these symptoms occur in a depression which is clearly reactive to some life event (for example, grief), they suggest the presence of a causal process acting, somehow, in addition to, or in despite of, or outside the orbit of, the meaning of that event for the person concerned.

The game then, despite a change of name, really *is* the same. Major depression, like endogenous depression, though less overtly, still implies an underlying causal disease process[2]. Consistent with Henry Walsingham's diagnosis we can indeed discern at least one kind of clear causal story in Jane Gillespie's case — a social–causal story. Putting this story in terms of conventional psychiatric formulations of aetiology, there are at least two likely *predisposing factors* for Jane Gillespie's depression: childhood (physical) abuse and early loss of her mother. There is also a clear *precipitant,* at least for this episode of her depression, in the attack on her when she was in charge of the ward. And there are *maintaining factors,* notably the continuing pressures at work through lack of resources and her line manager's (perceived) bullying.

Factors of this kind have undergone an interesting evolution in psychiatric thinking in recent years. They have a 'commonsense' relationship to depression, in that we can all understand how any or all of them could make someone feel depressed. Yet not everyone who experiences such events becomes depressed. It took a large research programme, combining advanced clinical instruments (like the PSE) with sophisticated statistical and social science empirical methods, to bring a degree of clarity to whether and, if so, in precisely what ways, these factors are related to depression. George Brown and Tirrel Harris' book, *The Social Origins of Depression* (1978), which we noted in the introduction to this chapter, drew together the results of this programme of research in a sophisticated causal model of depression. The spirit of their book is positivistic: they avoid having to deal in individual meanings by limiting their variables to factors which most people would find distressing (their 'contextual scales', see their Chapter 5) and which, like loss of a parent, are capable of unambiguous identification. It is a reflection of the power of this approach that their model has largely survived the test of time. But they warn of the limitations of a meaning-free approach in their Chapter 5, on 'Meanings'; and as we noted, George Brown's continuing work in this area has emphasized the importance of judgements of the significance of events for individuals in this model of depression (see, for example, Brown 1989).

The relationship between meanings and causes in social science research, as

Brown and Harris are the first to point out in Chapter 5 of *The Social Origins of Depression*, is a matter of long-running philosophical debate. It has its origins in a discussion about method in the social sciences in the nineteenth century — the *Methodenstreit*. It continues today — and with renewed urgency as developments in artificial intelligence and the neurosciences come on stream — as a key question in the philosophy of mind (see Reading Guide). The *Methodenstreit*, as we note in the introduction to this chapter, was a crucial influence on Karl Jaspers. It lay behind his belief that in psychopathology, for reasons of practice if not of principle, we have to be concerned as much with meanings as with causes (Jaspers 1913). Modern psychopathologists, by and large, share this view. Andrew Sims, for example, whose *Symptoms in the Mind* (1988) is a contemporary classic of psychopathology, has argued forcefully that even the operationally defined symptoms of the PSE, let alone the symptoms identified less formally in everyday practice, cannot be adequately assessed diagnostically in isolation from their meanings for the individuals concerned (Sims 1997; see also the discussion of Case 4.3, Simon Greer).

In psychiatry, though, we are concerned not only with the psychology and sociology of mental disorders, but with their biology. This gives us a second kind of causal story — a biological–causal story. And Jane Gillespie's case indeed shows clear signals of 'biology at work'. First, she may well have had a constitutional predisposition to depression: affective disorders are in part genetically determined, and her father, although not described as suffering from depression, may well have done so (male aggression towards women is not uncommonly combined with low self-esteem, and he may anyway have suffered an atypical grief reaction following the death of his wife). Second, Jane Gillespie had at least one 'biological' symptom: her early waking, observed on the ward, is likely to have been an important factor behind the consultant, Henry Walsingham's diagnosis of endogenous depression. Third, she responded to physical treatments: she did not 'do well' on antidepressants (though given their untoward side-effects and Jane Gillespie's independent frame of mind, it is likely that they were not trialled sufficently); but Dr Tannenbaum, her 'key clinician', was making little progress with 'talking therapies'; and ECT (the most physical of physical treatments) gave at least temporary relief.

In contrast to our understanding of the social origins of depression, we have as yet no well-worked-out theory of the biology of the condition. However, hypotheses abound, and with recent dramatic advances in the neurosciences few would lay money on there not being a credible account of the brain basis of the emotions within, say, fifty years. As we have already noted, the diagnostic concept of 'endogenous depression' (and its modern cognate, 'major depression') are promissory on such an account. Suppose, then, we are fifty years on. Suppose it is Jane Gillespie's granddaughter who is depressed and (psychiatry, too, running in families) Dr Tannenbaum's granddaughter who is the doctor. Could the future Dr Tannenbaum resolve her dilemma with a brain scan?

Such a possibility is implicit in the assumption that 'brain trumps mind' which, as we outlined in the introduction of this chapter, lies behind much bioethical and legal as well as medical thinking. On questions of legal responsibility, we noted that the courts are much impressed by the production of brain scans, EEGs, and so forth. We also cited the newspaper report of a patient with anorexia nervosa who welcomed the discovery of an enlarged temporal gyrus in such cases because this at last proved to everyone that there is something biologically wrong. As we also noted in the introduction, we are at risk here of slipping into the deep metaphysics of determinism and the nature of human freedom. This is a high-class risk in the sense that psychiatry, so long as it is to do with real people, cannot avoid being concerned with these metaphysical deeps — this is part of what makes psychiatry so difficult. But we do not need to get involved in these metaphysical deeps to see that, as a way of resolving Dr Tannenbaum's (or her granddaughter's) dilemma, 'brain trumps mind' thinking cannot be right. This is essentially because a causal account of the brain basis of pathological depression depends, for its cogency, on an account of the brain basis of non-pathological depression. If this were not so, how else could the account be subject to experimental demonstration (or, critically, falsification)? Hence, the *mere* demonstration of a brain cause for a depression cannot distinguish pathological from non-pathological depressions: it cannot resolve Dr Tannenbaum's dilemma.

It is necessary to add that 'brain trumps mind' thinking is no more coherent in physical medicine than in psychiatry. Indeed, as with so many aspects of the philosophy of medicine, this is a point which, though writ large in psychiatry, signals important lessons for medicine as a whole. We return to this theme in our concluding chapter. But the lesson for medicine, from the transparent incoherence of 'brain trumps mind' thinking in psychiatry, is that it is equally, and for partly the same reasons, incoherent to think that 'disease trumps illness'. Just as the woman with anorexia, in the newspaper report noted above, felt vindicated when a brain lesion was demonstrated, so, conversely, patients feel cheated when their doctor, unable to find a recognized lesion, denies that they are ill. From 'I can find no recognized underlying causal disease process' doctors jump all too readily to 'there is nothing medically wrong with you'. Of course, it *may* be that there is nothing medically wrong, but this does not follow, diagnostically, from the failure to find a recognized abnormality. Yet all too often this is precisely what is suggested. And in its denial of the reality of the patient's experience, the suggestion is highly abusive in effect.

The assumption that 'disease trumps illness' is pervasive in physical medicine essentially because we have well worked-out causal disease theories of physical illnesses. Such theories allow diagnostic short cuts in the form of blood tests, ECGs, or other tests. But the diagnostic relevance of such tests — what makes them short cuts to a *diagnosis* — is their already established status as valid markers of the underlying causes of recognized illnesses. This is a difficult idea which relies on an understanding of the complicated (logical) process by which causal disease theories are derived (see Fulford 1989, Chapter 4, for a detailed account). The basic point against 'disease trumps illness', however, is the same as that against 'brain trumps mind'. *All* experience, whether of health or illness, depends (in some sense) on bodily causes. As you read this book, for example, there are causal processes going on in your brain. Hence it cannot be causation, as such, which marks out pathological from non-pathological experience. On the contrary, if we follow the logic through carefully, it is clear that it is the patient's experience which has to come first. As Fig. 5.1 illustrates, while the causal story runs from disease first to illness second, the logical story (the flow of meaning) runs the other way, from illness first to disease second. It is our

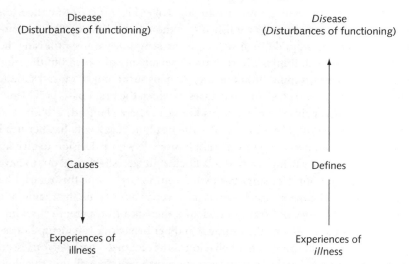

Figure 5.1 The different directions of the causal and conceptual links between disease and illness. Experiences of illness are caused by diseases which are, typically, underlying disturbances of bodily and mental functioning. But all experiences, pathological and non-pathological alike, are caused by such underlying states. Hence, which particular states of bodily and mental functioning are states of *bad* functioning (rather than states of functioning which are merely different or even better than usual) is not defined by the causal process as such. The negative value judgement essential to defining a state of functioning as a *dys*function (and hence as a *dis*ease) is derived from the negative value judgement by which experiences are (partly) marked out as experiences of *ill*ness. (See Fulford 1989, Chapter 4 for a more extended account of the concept of disease, including asymptomatic lesions.)

experiences of illness which, ultimately, mark out underlying causal processes as *disease* processes, not vice versa.

The flow diagram in Fig. 5.1 begs an important question: if illness is not marked out by disease, how is it defined? One element in the definition of illness, as we have seen in the preceding two chapters, is values. It follows, therefore, that just as neglect of the values involved in symptom-based diagnoses may be abusive in effect in psychiatry (because of the inherent diversity of values in the areas with which psychiatry is concerned), so too will 'disease trumps illness' thinking be abusive (because, if disease is defined by illness, then disease no less than illness is defined (in part) by values).

As we noted a moment ago, 'disease trumps illness' thinking is far from benign even in physical medicine (recall the 'nothing really wrong with you' scenario where the doctor fails to identify an established disease). But in psychiatry, the dangers are indeed writ large, for, as we noted in the last chapter, we are constantly vulnerable to the values of the majority being imposed on the minority behind a mask of scientific theory. 'Disease trumps illness' thinking provides just such a mask.

In the case of depression, to return to Jane Gillespie, our scientific theories, as already noted, are not well established — although this has never been a barrier to 'brain trumps mind'! In the UK at the present time we are witnessing the re-emergence of such thinking in relation to personality disorder. But the dangers of 'brain trumps mind' thinking are, perhaps surprisingly, most dramatically illustrated by so-called 'organic' cases in which the brain basis is evident.

One of us has analysed a case of this kind elsewhere (Fulford, 2000b). The story was reported in *The Times* under the headline 'Lazy wife has her head examined'. The woman in question was a housewife whose decision to give up housework led to her being referred to a doctor! In fact, she turned out to have a frontal lobe tumour. Her story has two lessons for us — one theoretical, the other practical. The theoretical lesson is that even in as obvious an organic case as this, brain still does not trump mind. Yes, there is a transparent causal link between 'Mrs Lazy's' brain (the tumour) and her behaviour (giving up housework); yes, the brain cause of her behaviour is a recognized *pathological* lesson (frontal lobe damage makes people less conscientious); but still, no, this does not make her change of behaviour necessarily pathological. Nothing in the mere description of Mrs Lazy's brain, still less in the merely causal connection between brain and behaviour, can, in itself, determine whether her giving up housework is pathological. It was assumed by those concerned that the brain tumour caused a pathological change in behaviour (laziness). But the 'brain' story is equally consistent with the tumour having cured a previously pathological pattern (being over-conscientious about housework).

As already noted, this begs the question of how illness in general is to be distinguished. But the relevance of 'Mrs Lazy's' values to the distinction in this case (that is, between causing and curing pathology) is essentially the same as that in Simon Greer's case in Chapter 4 (between psychosis and spiritual experience). In both cases, the patient's values, if not sufficient, are at least necessary to mark out pathology. And this is also the nub of the practical lesson from Mrs Lazy's story. For however sensitively her case may have been dealt with in practice, in the report in *The Times*, *her* values, and more generally the meaning of her decision to give up housework to *her*, figured not at all. Mrs Lazy, as a person, disappears from the story as soon as the tumour is discovered. The key practical point from her story, then, is that even (perhaps especially) in an obvious 'organic' case like Mrs Lazy's, it is crucial to good clinical care that the patient's perspective, their values and beliefs, should not be allowed to drop out of the clinical picture. Jane Gillespie's is not an obvious organic case. But the lesson from 'Mrs Lazy' is that in fifty years, when the brain basis of affect is the subject of an established causal theory, the dilemma for Dr Tannenbaum's granddaughter will be no less acute.

We anticipated at the start of this discussion that we would not be seeking to resolve Dr Tannenbaum's dilemma. In fact, the discussion, so far from resolving her dilemma, has endorsed it; it has shown it to be well founded. The discussion, though, also points the practical way forward. For in demonstrating the central (and ineliminable) importance of meanings, it shows that Dr Tannenbaum is right to take seriously the meanings of the different management options to her patient. There are no short cuts here. Taking these meanings seriously involves everything that goes into good communication. As we noted in Chapter 2, an important feature of psychiatric ethics is the extent to which ethical reasoning and good communication are woven together in the practice skills on which good clinical care critically depends. In this, moreover, not just psychiatry but medicine generally has an increasingly helpful partner in ethics. For in ethics, as we also noted in Chapter 2, we are witnessing the emergence of a number of new approaches emphasizing, in different ways, the importance of individual meanings interpreted in the context of real relationships between real people in real-life situations. Narrative ethics (Parker 1996 and 1999), discursive ethics (Gillett 1999), hermeneutic ethics (Widdershoven, forthcoming), and feminist ethics (Adshead, forthcoming), all offer precisely this crucial point of contact between ethics and the realities of everyday clinical practice.

It is important to add, though, a final caveat. Emphasizing the importance of meanings should in no way be taken to undermine the importance of causes. If brain does not trump mind, neither does mind trump brain. This caveat is important because of a tendency among those who deal in the humanities to denigrate biology. This kind of inverted snobbery involves seeing 'biological psychiatry' as intellectual 'new money' — flashy and successful, but shallow, and, it is fondly hoped, evanescent. According to this picture, those concerned with the meaningful aspects of mental disorder — not only ethicists, but psychologists, psychoanalysts, and even social psychiatrists — are involved in a defence of humanistic medicine against a dehumanizing technology. The snobbery, it should be said, is not all one way. Modern American psychiatry, although often bowdlerized as exclusively biological, is built on a biopsychosocial approach (see McHugh and Slaveney 1983; also the introduction to DSM–IV, APA 1994). Properly understood moreover, biological psychiatry, as John Wing among others has argued (Wing 1978), must incorporate psychological and social processes. But less thoughtful enthusiasts for biological psychiatry have been openly dismissive of what they take to be non-biological approaches. The most ideologically driven of such enthusiasts, it should be said, are often not professional scientists (for example, Shorter 1997)! But there is considerable crossfire, nonetheless, and as we saw in Chapter 3, it is, ultimately, patients who get hurt in this crossfire.

Meanings, then, are important in psychiatry, but alongside rather than in place of causes. This gives a final twist to Dr Tannenbaum's dilemma. We have seen that the acuteness of her dilemma arises in part from a pressure, derived in turn from the diagnosis of endogenous depression, to see Jane Gillespie as a patient rather than an agent. The pressure is to deny the meaning for Jane Gillespie of a further episode of involuntary admission. The diagnosis of endogenous depression implies that this is merely a symptom of Jane Gillespie's depression, a causal consequence of a disease process beyond her control, and hence something which ought to be overriden out of Dr Tannenbaum's responsibility as a doctor to provide treatment.

But there is also an opposing pressure, arising, in this case, from Dr Tannenbaum's expressed preference for cognitive–behavioural therapy. There may be good clinical reasons for recommending this. Such therapy, where it is successful, helps to restore agency by giving the person concerned new skills of self-management. Cognitive–behavioural therapy, moreover, starting as it does from the values and beliefs of the subject, engages directly with his or her *meanings*. But in Jane Gillespie's case, her priority, of retaining control, is served rather by *physical* treatments. There should be no surprises here. After all, firsthand accounts of depression often spell out the value of being able to think of the condition in strictly medical terms, as symptomatic of, say, a biochemical deficiency which an antidepressant can make up. The biologist Louis Wolpert (1999) expresses this view forcefully. Recent feminist psychology has also suggested that silence is itself a form of control for women (Mahoney 1996), and control is central to Jane Gillespie.

Jane Gillespie, we are told, did not respond well to antidepressants, but it was the lithium-induced tremor to which she objected since she thus risked giving herself away at work and hence of destroying what, in her scale of values, was more important than life itself. A further trial of a different antidepressant regime, therefore, in which Jane Gillespie is given control of the assessment of outcome, allowing the medication to be directly titrated to her particular needs, would be one way forward. She might be encouraged to persevere with such a trial by the evidence that while ECT gives more immediate relief, in the longer term antidepressants are equally effective. We might still be thrown back on ECT, of course, and as both Dr Walsingham and Dr Tannenbaum would have pointed out to Jane Gillespie, this may have untoward effects in the long term — untoward indeed in *her* scale of values, in that it might affect her memory and thus undermine her competence at work. There could come a point, therefore, at which neither doctor could recommend further ECT. But the risks here would be, as in the case of physical disorders, a matter, at least partly, for Jane Gillespie to judge. And once she felt that she had control of her treatment, and with it a degree of lightening of mood, she might begin to engage successfully with cognitive–behavioural therapy or even a psychotherapeutic approach (given her childhood experiences this is far from being a clinical long shot).

But the key to all this is to start from respect for the validity of Jane Gillespie's values and beliefs — the meaning of the situation to her as an agent in her own right. Ironically, this is true above all in this case, where respect for Jane Gillespie's meanings (her preference for ECT) conflicts with Dr Tannenbaum's clinical instinct for a meaningful (cognitive–behavioural) rather than causal (ECT) approach to treatment.

Practitioner commentary (CASE 5.1)

Jeremy Holmes Consultant Psychotherapist, North Devon District Hospital

Medical ethics is necessary because medical methods are never purely technical: they involve persons as well as procedures. For the most part, the technical and the ethical domain can be clearly separated — the ethics of abortion, for example, bear little relation to the specific techniques used by the gynaecologist to terminate a pregnancy. Psychotherapeutic ethics is different in that psychotherapy is a technique whose subject is persons (Holmes 1999). For example, 'motivational interviewing' is an effective way of getting people to think about giving up illicit drug use — the patient's thought process can be influenced in a direction desired by the therapist. So what is at stake is not just the choices open to the patient, but her capacity to make those choices.

This takes us straight into the case of Jane Gillespie. We are told that Jane 'made little progress with "talking cures" '. Was this simply because she was, as the authors query, 'unsuitable' for therapy, or was there a failure on the part of the therapist to make an adequate assessment, assign Jane to an appropriate modality of therapy, to engage her in an effective working alliance, hold her in therapy, and to move her in a mutative direction? Severely depressed patients can be very difficult to engage in therapy, but there is also evidence that in real clinical situations, as opposed to psychotherapy trials which often exclude complex patients such as Jane, some forms of therapy are much more effective than others. In a recent study, marital therapy outperformed both pharmacotherapy and cognitive therapy, mainly thanks to a lower drop-out rate (Leff *et al.* 1999). Perhaps Jane's husband was not sufficiently included in the therapeutic process.

This suspicion is supported by the very unusual situation in which Jane is compulsorily detained despite her husband's wishes to the contrary. The reasons for this are not given. Occasionally, the next of kin's wishes are overruled in order not to jeopardize a fragile marital relationship — this procedure may have been a way of reassuring Jane that her husband was still 'on her side'. Psychodynamic aspects of the use of the Mental Health Act are often highly significant. To 'section' a patient is to invoke an external power that overrides everyday relationships. In conventional family structures power is invested in the father. Where the father has abused or abrogated that power, a vacuum is left that may have to be filled by instruments of the State. In Jane's case, the sectioning process paralleled her father's cruel treatment of her in that it rode roughshod over her expressed wishes, but it also represented an attempt by a 'good father' to restore her to health. Incidentally, the implication that ECT and cognitive therapy are incompatible is incorrect: in severe cases like Jane's, physical and psychological methods of treatment are often necessary. Indeed, the idea of benign collaboration may also have dynamic reverberations for Jane: her mother died when she was eight, her father was a brute, and she may never have had the experience of a loving 'combined parent' which she could internalize.

The case nicely brings out the ways in which psychiatric diagnoses are used to further ideological ends. The distinction between 'endogenous' and 'reactive' depression has relatively little scientific basis, yet each can be used to justify a particular therapeutic approach. There may be good clinical reasons for this. A coherent treatment philosophy — of whatever variety — is reassuring for patients and their families and may in itself aid recovery. The 'social–causal' story is essentially a psychodynamic one. Jane's history powerfully illustrates the influence of a formative story in shaping a life and the impact of apparently random events on it — phenomena that any 'narrative ethics' would have to take into account. She absents herself from her family through depression just as her mother had done so through death. The violence of the distressed father on the neonatal ward reactivated her feelings of helplessness and terror when attacked by her own father. Trauma becomes 'traumatic' when it touches on a pre-existing vulnerability. The secure base inside her psyche, to which she could have retreated when faced with the onslaught, was itself sullied by her experiences as a child. Feelings of hopelessness, helplessness, failure, and utter vulnerability — all characteristic of depressive illness — were a logical consequence.

The brain–mind debate is important because it reminds us of the limitations of our contemporary models and understanding. But it can also be used destructively to harden polarized ideological positions. Faced with uncertainty, it takes courage — and the secure intellectual base which it is the job of psychiatric training to provide — to live on the boundary of knowledge and exploration, rather than to cling to simplistic and splitting explanations. John Bowlby (Holmes 1993) always insisted that psychotherapy was no less 'biological' than biochemistry, since human behaviour and relationships are just as much the product of evolution as neurotransmitters. Equally, every brain event has a meaning — Jane's illness cannot be divorced from her life story, however much we elucidate its biochemical architecture.

The chapter rightly ends with the importance of the 'patient's perspective'. From a psychotherapeutic angle, the patient's viewpoint is all-important, both in itself, and as a target of therapy. Therapy will aim to help patients achieve a 'meta-perspective' on themselves and their values — Jane needs to think about *why* she was so keen on the 'quick' (and anaesthetized) 'fix' of ECT. Was it that, once her mother died when she was eight, her feelings died too, and she became an instrumental rather than an affective being, an efficient ward sister for whom emotions like fear and rage were as threatening as the father who evoked them? But good therapy is always pragmatic: it starts from where the patient is, and is keenly aware of what can and cannot be achieved, given the patient's philosophy, severity of illness, and the therapeutic resources available. Psychiatric ethics is practical or it is nothing.

References (CASE 5.1)

Adshead, G. (forthcoming) A different voice in psychiatric ethics. In *Healthcare Ethics and Human Values* (ed. Fulford, K.W.M., Dickenson, D., and Murray, T.H.). Oxford, Blackwell Science.

American Psychiatric Association (1994) *Diagnostic and statistical manual of mental disorders* (4th edn). Washington, DC: American Psychiatric Association.

Brown, G.W. (1989) Life events and measurement. In *Life Events and Illness* (ed. Brown, G.W. and Harris, T.O.), pp. 49–94. New York, Guildford Press; London, Unwin and Hyman.

Brown, G.W. and Harris, T.O. (1978) *Social Origins of Depression: a Study of Psychiatric Disorders in Women.* London, Tavistock Publications, New York, Free Press.

Fulford, K.W.M. (1989, reprinted 1995; 2nd edn forthcoming) *Moral Theory and Medical Practice.* Cambridge, Cambridge University Press.

Fulford, K.W.M. (2000*a*) Philosophy meets psychiatry in the twentieth century— Four looks back and a brief loof forward. In Louhiala, P., Stenman, S. (eds.): Philosophy Meets Medicine. Helsinki: Helsinki University Press; p. 116–34.

Fulford, K.W.M. (2000*b*) Disordered minds, diseased brains and real people in Philosophy, Psychiatry and Psychopathy: Personal identity in mental disorder. (ed. Heginbotham, C.), Chapter 4 Avebury Series in Philosophy in association with The Society for Applied Philosophy. Aldershot (England): Ashgate Publishing Ltd.

Gillett, G. (1999) *The Mind and its Discontents.* Oxford, Oxford University Press.

Holmes J. (1993) *John Bowlby and Attachment Theory.* London, Routlege.

Holmes J. (1999) Ethical aspects of the psychotherapies. In *Psychiatric Ethics* (3rd edn) (ed. Bloch, S., Chodoff, P., and Green, S.A.). Oxford, Oxford University Press.

Jaspers, K. (1913) Causal and meaningful connexions between life history and psychosis. Reprinted in 1974 in *Themes and Variations in European Psychiatry* (ed. Hirsch, S.R. and Shepherd, M.), Chapter 5. Bristol, John Wright and Sons Ltd.

Leff, J., Vearnals, S., and Brewin, C. (1999) The London depression intervention trial: an RCT of antidepressants versus couple therapy in the treatment and maintenance of depressed people with a partner: clinical outcome and costs. *British Journal of Psychiatry.* ???

McHugh, P.R. and Slaveney, P.R. (1983) *The Perspectives of Psychiatry.* Baltimore (USA), The Johns Hopkins University Press.

Mahoney, M.A. (1996) The problem of silence in feminist psychology. *Feminist Studies,* **22**, 602–25.

Parker, M. (1996) Communitarianism and its problems. *Cogito,* **10**:3.

Parker, M. (ed.) (1999) *Ethics and Community in the Health Care Professions.* London, Routledge.

Shorter, E. (1997) *A History of Psychiatry.* New York, John Wiley and Sons.

Sims, A. (1988) *Symptoms in the Mind: An Introduction to Descriptive Psychopathology.* London, Baillière Tindall.

Sims, A. (1997) Commentary on 'Spiritual experience and psychopathology'. *Philosophy, Psychiatry, and Psychology,* **4/1**:79–82.

Widdershoven, G. (forthcoming) Alternatives to principlism. In *Healthcare Ethics and Human Values* (ed. Fulford, K.W.M., Dickenson, D., and Murray, T.H.). Oxford, Blackwell Science.

Wing, J.K. (1978) *Reasoning about Madness*. Oxford, Oxford University Press.

Wolpert, L. (1999) *Malignant Sadness*. London, Faber and Faber.

CASE 5.2
Francesca Gindro — motivated self-deception or delusion?

Synopsis A 27-year-old woman with Turner's syndrome is referred for psychotherapy after repeated failures of IVF. The therapy seems to be going well: she talks for the first time about her abuse as a child. Then the therapist receives a letter from Francesca thanking him for offering to donate his sperm which would make everything fine because the problem had always been her husband's infertility rather than hers.

Key dilemma Should the therapist continue to see her?

Main topics Delusion and self-deception.

Other topics Infertility; IVF; ethics of psychotherapy; transference; Hinshelwood's principle of integration; personal identity; abuse (child); rationality; prudence; Plato; Sartre; agency; Kantianism; utilitarianism; Parfit; unity of consciousness; Locke; Radden; Gardner.

Francesca Gindro is a 27-year-old accounts clerk, fourth in a family of seven siblings whose parents were first-generation Italian immigrants to the UK. Her father died when she was ten, and she was sent temporarily to live with relatives near Verona, as her mother found it difficult to cope with all the children on her own. During her stay with her mother's family, she was sexually abused by a cousin, but never told anyone what happened.

At nineteen, Francesca asked her GP whether she needed any contraception, given — as it transpired in the course of a reticent and difficult consultation — that she had never had a menstrual period. Investigation revealed that she had a variant of Turner's syndrome, a genetic disorder characterized by the absence of one of the two X chromosomes present in the normal female. Francesca's case involved a mosaic pattern: about two-thirds of her cells lacked the second X chromosome, and the remainder comprised structurally incompetent X chromosomes. Thus she had no normal cells, and was completely infertile. Although Francesca received genetic counselling, she seemed to have only vaguely understood the implications of the diagnosis. She was actually quite pleased to have no periods to impede her life, she said, and not having children would also be a relief, for someone from such a large family.

When Francesca married Joseph five years later, he was not quite so sanguine: he very much wanted children, and Francesca too seemed to have changed her mind. The couple were re-investigated for infertility, which confirmed that Joseph's sperm count was normal but that Francesca's primary amenorrhoea did indeed have a genetic basis. They were told that although IVF did occasionally succeed in patients with Turner's syndrome, there had been no reports to date of success in patients without any normal cells, such as Francesca.

After further counselling, the couple decided to pursue infertility treatment, despite the low probability of success. They were accepted on a private basis for IVF with donor oocytes, and four fertilized ova were implanted. Unexpectedly, this resulted in a quadruple pregnancy, but Francesca and Joseph were adamant against selectively aborting any of the foetuses. The pregnancy was maintained by hormone supplements and monitored carefully, but at twenty weeks Francesca was admitted to hospital on an emergency basis with pre-eclampsia. Two male and two female foetuses, three with severe abnormalities, were born by emergency Caesarean section; all died.

Francesca had always been a regular attender at her GP's clinic, but now her attendance increased by leaps and bounds. After two further private attempts at IVF, both unsuccessful, she requested as many as a hundred consultations with the GP, Catherine Wark, in one year. Catherine referred Francesca to a psychiatric out-patient clinic for psychotherapy. Francesca also attended these sessions faithfully, apparently developing what her psychotherapist, Mike Callahan, considered to be a good therapeutic relationship. She called him by his first name and told him about her childhood sexual abuse, the first time she had mentioned it to anyone — even including Joseph. She had wondered if it was all in her mind, she said, but now she was beginning to realize it really had happened.

After six months, however, Mike was shocked to receive a letter from Francesca thanking him for offering to donate his sperm for a further attempt at IVF: 'so this time it should work', she wrote, 'because it was really Joseph's problem all along'. What stunned him was not so much the sexual nature of the letter — 'that's just classic transference stuff,' he shrugged — but what he now began to see as a much deeper form of irrationality and self-deception. Mike had believed that Francesca understood that her infertility had nothing to do with Joseph's sperm count; he had thought that her depression sprang from her realization of how intractable it really was. This was a necessary stage, he thought, in adjustment to the full implications of Turner's syndrome. But this did not seem to be the course the therapy was now taking.

At their next session, Mike wanted to discuss the possibility of transferring Francesca to another member of the team, but Francesca became very upset when the subject was raised; she accused Mike of rejecting her because he thought she was a bad mother. Everybody believed she had caused the deaths of her 'babies', she wept, and some people in her family even thought she was sexually abusing her sister's children, to whom she was very close. Mike was more dismayed than ever by the turn the discussion took; he began to feel he had lost all grip on what was giving rise to Francesca's problems — that they were not anything like what he had thought they were. His consternation deepened when, two days later, Francesca took an overdose, with suicidal intent. She survived, barely, and was admitted to a psychiatric hospital on a compulsory basis under the Mental Health Act.

Mike Callahan, the psychotherapist, was rightly dismayed by the depths of impenetrability and irrationality in this case; there is a sense of a Greek tragedy, hastening suddenly and unexpectedly to an implacable and fatal end. Worse still, it was hastening to an end which, he felt, he had totally failed to foresee. His dilemma, then, was deep indeed. On the one hand, his failure to anticipate the course of events, and the overtly sexual nature of the ideas Francesca had developed about him, suggested that he should arrange for her to be transferred to another therapist. But her reaction to this suggestion — a nearly fatal suicide attempt — implied that he could be ducking his clinical responsibilities by failing to take her therapy forward and work through the present crisis.

As with the previous case of Jane Gillespie, we will not be tackling Mike's dilemma directly. Rather, we will be looking at the implications for his decision of different ways of understanding Francesca's ideas about him. Are these delusions, as perhaps seems at first glance most likely? Or is this a case of self-deception? Could it be, even, malingering — a conscious attempt to manipulate Mike or perhaps Joseph (Francesca's husband)?

Consider delusion then. One interpretation of Francesca's ideas is that she has developed some form of psychotic illness, an atypical form of erotomania perhaps. Her beliefs certainly appear mistaken: Mike, we must suppose, is hardly likely to have volunteered his sperm; professional niceties aside, the fact that Francesca has Turner's syndrome and that attempts at IVF had proved disastrous would have made the offer futile. Francesca's persecutory beliefs, moreover, about people thinking she was a 'bad mother', who had 'caused the deaths of her babies' and was 'sexually abusing her sister's children', would be consistent with the delusions typical of a major depressive illness. A psychotic reaction, anyway, in circumstances of this kind, would not be particularly surprising. Francesca had coped with her diagnosis in the past by denial (she only 'vaguely understood' its implications despite genetic counselling; and she was 'actually quite pleased to have no periods'). But as she proceeds in therapy, and with the failure of IVF, denial is less and less possible. A strategy of complete escape from reality, then — a psychotic withdrawal — may be all that is left.

A diagnosis of psychosis, of one kind or another, might seem at first sight to solve Mike Callahan's dilemma. Like the diagnosis of endogenous depression in Jane Gillespie's case, it suggests a 'disease process', beyond the control of the patient, which explains her beliefs and behaviour merely as the cause–effect consequences of an abnormality of brain functioning. As such, delusional psychosis would be the moral equivalent of an epileptic fugue: something for which the patient is not responsible, a condition in relation to which he or she is, literally, a passive patient rather than an active agent. Mike's course then, on this interpretation of Francesca's case, might seem to be clear — Francesca should be treated with neuroleptics and then, if further psychotherapy is felt appropriate, this should be with a new therapist to obviate any suggestion, however ill-founded, of impropriety in his dealings with her.

Closer inspection, however, shows that matters are not so straightforward. In the first place, the moral status of delusion, and of psychotic disorders generally, is a matter of continuing theoretical debate. Intuitively, as we saw in Chapter 2, delusion is the paradigm case of mental disorder involving loss of responsibility. (Recall the central place of psychotic disorder in the conceptual map of psychopathology; see Chapter 2 and Table 2.1). This intuition, moreover, is neither a recent nor a local invention: it has deep historical roots (going back at least to classical times) and it is found in many very different cultures around the world (Fulford 1993).

Yet if the intuition that delusion undermines responsibility is well established, its basis is far from clear. Mike need not be concerned with this as such. He could, if he is satisfied that Francesca is suffering from a psychotic illness, simply rely on the received ethical status of delusion to justify transferring her to another therapist. Indeed, in the case of involuntary treatment for someone who is, say, suicidally depressed, a failure to rely on the ethical intuition that delusion radically undermines responsibility could lead to a charge of negligence!

But *can* Mike be satisfied that Francesca is deluded? Most textbooks define delusions broadly as false beliefs which are culturally atypical and incorrigible. But Francesca's beliefs are not culturally atypical; incorrigible beliefs are not always delusions, even if false; and delusions (as identified clinically) are not necessarily false beliefs. As one of us has shown elsewhere (Fulford 1989, Chapter

10), delusions may be true beliefs (as in the Othello syndrome) and paradoxical (as in the delusion of mental illness). Moreover, they may be value judgements, positive (as in hypomania) or negative (as in depression).

In the past, philosophers, noting the difficulty of defining delusions, have tended to rely on gross falsity of belief (for example, 'I have a nuclear reactor inside me') in justifying the ethical intuition of loss of responsibility (for example, Glover 1970; Flew 1973; Quinton 1985). But Francesca's beliefs, even if delusional, are certainly not grossly false. Joseph's sperm, for example, might appear normal but the failure of her pregnancy with donor ova could suggest that it was not so. On this construction, then, combining donor sperm (Mike's) with donor ova might result in a successful pregnancy. And while it is very unlikely that Mike volunteered his sperm, it is not unlikely that Francesca mistakenly inferred this from something he said. That she was a 'bad mother', moreover, who had caused the deaths of her babies, is, biologically speaking, true. And the accusations of sexual abuse could easily arise if someone in her family is 'psychologically minded' and aware of stereotypes of the abused becoming an abuser. All this is unlikely, perhaps very unlikely, but none of it is beyond the bounds of possibility.

The recognition that delusions are not (necessarily) false factual beliefs has led recent writers in psychiatry (for example, Gelder *et al.* 1989), as well as philosophy, to define delusions as 'unfounded' beliefs. This, however, in the absence of a criterion of falsity, begs the relevant meaning of unfounded (that is, not all unfounded beliefs are delusions). The most straightforward interpretation is that in this context unfounded means that the belief in question is a product of a disturbance of cognitive functioning. This interpretation assumes that delusions are on a par with the disturbances of functioning by which bodily diseases are constituted; hence that they are beyond the person's control and are indeed the ethical equivalent of an epileptic fugue (in our parallel already mentioned). Yet despite extensive efforts over many years, no such disturbance of cognitive functioning has been demonstrated (see Garety and Freeman, 1999, for a recent comprehensive review). Delusions certainly occur in conditions in which cognitive functioning is disturbed, but in these conditions, delusional and non-delusional beliefs are affected equally. (In dementia, for example, delusional beliefs, like normal beliefs, are minimally elaborated, often lack emotional 'charge', and are poorly sustained over time.) The 'best-quality' delusions actually occur in cases (like Francesca Gindro's) in which cognitive functioning is to all appearances intact.

The difficulty of defining delusions in terms of disturbed cognitive functioning is at the heart of the wider difficulty, noted in the last chapter, of using established bioethical criteria of incapacity derived from physical medicine as the basis of judgements of competence in patients with psychotic disorders. It could certainly be argued, in terms of these criteria, that Francesca lacks the capacities for autonomous choice. It could be said, for example, that she has failed to understand the information given to her or, perhaps, failed to weigh this information. But as with Cases 4.1 and 4.3, in the absence of criteria of incapacity which are independent of the content of her beliefs, we have no way of deciding whether she is deluded or merely mistaken. She *could* be deluded, certainly; but she could have simply made a mistake — and this indeed assumes that her beliefs are false. For as Ian Kennedy has pointed out (Kennedy 1997), bioethical (and legal) criteria of incapacity, or at any rate those criteria currently advocated, provide no way of distinguishing between someone who lacks the capacity for autonomous choice and someone whose choice is merely different from everyone else's.

One theoretical approach to the problem of defining delusion is to seek to interpret it, not in terms of impaired cognitive functioning, but rather of impaired practical reasoning (of the reasons people have for their actions). A full account of the justification for this approach would take us beyond the scope of this book (see Fulford 1989, Chapter 10). The evidence for it is partly psychopathological: that delusions have the same phenomenology as reasons for action — both may take the form of factual beliefs, true as well as false; both may take the form of value judgements, positive as well as negative. The approach has construct validity to the extent that it explains the psychopathology of delusions consistently with an account of the experience of illness generally, bodily as well as mental, in terms of failure of (a particular kind of) action. Most importantly for our present purpose, it also has face validity, for it accounts directly for the ethically central place of delusion without relying on a (still putative) disturbance of cognitive functioning. Again, the details of this are beyond our scope here, but the argument runs thus:

1 Practical reasoning is the form of rationality characteristic of moral agents capable of intentional actions.

2 Intentional actions are defined by our reasons for doing something (waving my arm is signalling a bid or saying 'hello' or hailing a taxi, according to the reasons I have for waving my arm; see Austin 1956/7 for a clear account of this).

3 Actions can fail in different ways.

4 But a failure of practical reasoning is the most *radical* failure. This is because, since our actions are *defined* by our reasons, a failure of practical reasoning is a *constitutive* rather than merely executive failure of action.

Delusion, then, emerges from this account as an illness in which there is, literally, no action, hence no intention, and hence no responsibility for what is done by the person concerned.

The implications of this theory, in the present state of our understanding of delusions, are as much theoretical as practical. The theory provides at least an approach to understanding the ethically central place of delusions (Fulford 1989, Chapter 10); it connects the psychopathology of delusions with work in the philosophy of mind, including the philosopher John McDowell's call for an expanded 'space of reasons' (Thornton, 2000); and this in turn connects with work in neuroscience on the need for whole-brain, rather than part-function, interpretations of the results of dynamic brain imaging. The practical implications of all this for Mike Callahan, reflecting on his dilemma about how to proceed in his work with Francesca, are, broadly, that he is thrown back on exploring her 'space of reasons'. If delusions are or arise from a failure of practical reasoning, then far from writing off her beliefs, he must (at least in the first instance) take them seriously and must treat her as (at least potentially) a semiotic subject — an agent whose (apparently odd) beliefs and actions may in fact be meaning-driven rather than merely symptoms of a disease process. Therefore, Francesca's ideas and her reaction to Mike's psychotherapy cannot be simply written off as the effects of a causal disease process. Francesca may be deluded but this has to be established *within*, rather than outside, the space of reasons.

We return to Mike's practical dilemma, and how he might proceed, later. For now, the point is that on this account of delusions, as involving a failure of practical reasoning, even if Francesca is deluded there is no escaping meanings in favour of causes. And once we take seriously the possibility that Francesca's ideas are meaningful, this opens up a whole series of further possible interpretations of them. One possibility, perhaps, is conscious malingering. As a manipulative strategy, directed at Mike or Joseph or Francesca's wider family, her behaviour seems sadly misconceived. But people do behave foolishly — against what might seem to everyone else to be in their best interests — when they are desperate. Even with this interpration, however, Francesca should not be 'written off'. Her behaviour would be a transparent cry for help, though it would not necessarily be Mike who should or could give the help required.

We have no evidence of malingering, however. There are no inconsistencies in Francesca's behaviour and, by way of contrary evidence, her suicide attempt was all too genuine. This suggests a further possibility — what the philosopher Sebastian Gardner has called motivated self-deception (Gardner 1993). As Gardner has pointed out, self-deception is in a sense the most rational irrationality, apparently at the furthest end of the spectrum from madness (Gardner 1993, p. 32). After all, it can be prudent to bring about a condition in which one knows that one will hold a false belief. This notion of 'reasonable irrationality' (Gardner 1993, p. 17) could explain Francesca's about-face, from her studied unconcern about having children at nineteen to her adamant refusal to consider selective abortion of any of the foetuses. On marriage, it might have been prudent for Francesca to believe she could have children and wanted to have children, even so strongly that she could persuade herself, and perhaps Joseph, that her sterility could be overcome.

It is still a step from there to believing — as she now seems to — that she is not sterile at all: Joseph is. But up to this point, motivated self-deception is a possibility. At the very least this would explain why Mike's guard was apparently down. Its surface resemblance to rationality makes motivated self-deception hard to spot; it also makes it hard to understand philosophically, for it seems to involve the apparently self-contradictory idea of deceiving oneself. The motives usually adduced to explain self-deception — such as the painfulness of certain thoughts — are also used to explain rational action; they are not unique to self-deception. This indeed may amount to a logical contradiction: the same factor cannot explain both a phenomenon and its absence, and so the same mode of explanation cannot differentiate self-deception from rational behaviour. But why does the subject's life fail to take a rational course, if it can be explained in rational terms? It is precisely because the motives explaining self-deception are understandable — whilst self-deception is irrational and hence mysterious — that self-deception is philosophically problematic, and clinically problematic in this case as well.

Self-deception then, defined as a motivated failure of self-knowledge (Gardner 1993, p. 16), could help to explain at least parts of Francesca's story. It also shows how it involves a moral problem. Gardner analyses self-deception as involving two sets of beliefs: one 'buried', the other 'promoted'. A strong interpretation of self-deception regards the 'burying' and 'promoting' as intentional, no different ethically from deliberate lying. We have already argued that this is a possible but unlikely interpretation in Francesca's case. A weak interpretation merely requires that the two sets of beliefs be motivated by something else, such as avoidance of painful realizations. But both interpretations view the self-deceiver as an active agent, thus distinguishing self-deception from the passive nature of akrasia (weakness of will) which we encountered in Case 4.2 (Delia Jarrett).

The self-deceiver is thus construed as making an active choice to deceive herself. Such a choice has clear ethical dimensions. It goes against the ethical importance attached to self-knowledge, by many philosophers, as the fount of all other moral behaviour: Plato in classical times ('Know thyself') and Sartre (1943) in our own day (the notion of 'bad faith' — roughly speaking, deliberate falseness to one's inner nature as a subject rather than an object). Partly on this basis, Gardner draws a sharp distinction between self-deception (in which agency is retained) and delusion (in which agency is lost). Broadly in line with the distinction between the constitutive failure of agency involved in delusion (as a disturbance of practical reasoning) and the lesser executive failures of agency involved in all other forms of illness, Gardner suggests that delusion 'implies some impairment of the very faculty of belief-formation, a fault at the level of competence rather than performance' (Gardner 1993, p. 17).

We might interpret self-deception in broadly psychoanalytic terms. Something — perhaps Francesca's experience of childhood sexual abuse — made her want to deny the abnormality of her amenorrhea, which she must surely have realized by then. At the normal age of menarche, as a child of ten or twelve, it might have been plausible that she failed to understand the seriousness of not having periods, but somewhere between then and nineteen she had begun deceiving herself in a way in which, Gardner argues, children tend, in fact, not to do. As he puts it (p. 22), 'Although children can do something much like self-deceive — they can cover themselves by telling lies and then be utterly taken in by what they say — they lack the requisite grasp of the susceptibility of belief to manipulation in the first person case.' At all events, there seem powerful possible motivations for this in Francesca's case: the devastating diagnosis of Turner's syndrome, coupled with inner conflict over her fertility resulting from her mother's example and her own exposure to sexual abuse as a child; and now Joseph's (as well as her own) desire that they should have a family.

Gardner argues that viewing self-deception primarily in psychological or psychoanalytical terms may be a dead end. 'Instead', he says, 'self-deceivers should be seen as mistakenly taking themselves to have solved their real problem in solving their psychological problem; or, put another way, as failing to make a proper distinction between psychological and real problems' (Gardner 1993, p. 18). Perhaps this applies to Francesca's apparent progress in therapy: she thinks she has solved her infertility because she thinks it is all in the mind — as she told herself the abuse was — and she is making great progress with her 'mind' treatment, as Mike has told her. Perhaps this is even more true in her case because there is no somatic treatment for Turner's syndrome. It might indeed be suggested that the psychotherapist is vulnerable to self-deception himself, insofar as he encourages Francesca to concentrate on her psychological problems at the expense of her physiological ones. This could be one reason why the tragic denouement hits Mike so hard. The ethical issues on this construction are thus brought firmly back into Mike's court. As the psychoanalyst Jeremy Holmes and the philosopher Richard Lindley have argued, a central ethical imperative for the therapist is to identify the emotional responses in himself (the counter-transference) which the patient's transference has aroused (Holmes and Lindley 1989, p. 129).

We return to the ethics of psychotherapy, and in particular to the significance of transference and counter-transference, in a moment. First, we need to look briefly at one further interpretation of Francesca's behaviour — that it represents some form of dissociative state. Thus, Francesca's failure to accept the reality of her infertility could be the result of an internal splitting of her mind, the painful knowledge being separated from her conscious mind, walled off like an emotional abscess. Ethically, there is a clear difference between this and Gardner's concept of motivated self-deception. Motivated self-deception involves, at some stage, the intentional denial of the painful material. Dissociative denial is also motivated by avoidance of painful material but is primarily unconscious and, to this extent, beyond the responsibility of the subject.

A more radical version of the interpretation of Francesca's behaviour in terms of dissociation is that it is the manifestation of different 'selves'. In some countries, multiple personality disorder (MPD) or dissociative identity disorder ((DID) in the DSM–IV; APA 1994, p. 484) is a common diagnosis. In this condition, the behaviour of one biological individual seems to reflect, at different times, quite different people. The diagnostic validity of the concept of MPD has been widely disputed, but the phenomena it reflects, however they are interpreted, do involve deep difficulties in the attribution of responsibility (see Radden 1996; Reznek 1997; and Braude 1991 and 1996, for careful discussions of these issues).

Francesca certainly does not meet the criteria for DID. Her contradictions of belief, though, might be considered manifestations of what the Oxford philosopher Derek Parfit has called 'successive selves' (Parfit 1984, p. 305). Rather than reflecting Gardner's notion of 'buried' and 'promoted' beliefs co-existing simultaneously in her mind, the desires of Francesca's nineteen-year-old self (to avoid pregnancy, welcoming amenorrhea and infertility) and those of her pregnant self (to continue the pregnancy at all costs, refusing selective abortion) seem so radically different as to suggest that in some sense they belong to different people.

One difficulty with this approach is that it raises serious problems about the unity of consciousness. Locke's *Essay on Human Understanding* (1690; reprinted in 1979) notes that 'a thinking intelligent being, that has reason and reflection, and can consider itself as itself, the same thinking thing, in different times and places; which it does only by that consciousness which is inseparable from thinking, and, as it seems to me, essential to it' (Book 11, Chapter xxvii, paragraph 11). Psychoanalytic theory, and indeed the unconscious influences on our thought and behaviour which it seeks to explain, suggest that this oversimplifies the case. But unity of consciousness is an important feature, at least of our sense of identity as unique individuals.

With Parfit's theory, treatment of these difficulties involves distinguishing between successive 'selves' of the same person as we would between successive identities or periods in a single nation's history (for example, the Anglo-Saxon,

Norman, and Tudor periods). This notion does not seem immediately helpful in Francesca's case, however. On Parfit's account, each successive self's beliefs would be equally valid. He argues that this is ethically comforting; it avoids an individual being held hostage to fortune by his or her desires and beliefs, and indeed by his or her actions, at an earlier stage of their life. *That* 20-year-old person, we can say when in our 50s, was not *me*! But this is really the converse of Francesca's case. Far from separating her present 'self' more radically from her earlier 'selves', the need is for integration, for reconciliation of her deepest desires (for a family) with the reality of her infertility. The metaphor from history breaks down at this point. The Battle of Hastings settled things between the Anglo-Saxon and Norman 'selves' of English history, but what would be the equivalent in an individual psyche? To say that Francesca's suicide attempt represents the victory of one self over another seems, at best, a rather callous misreading.

Rather than seeking therefore to eliminate the contradictions and conflicts to which Francesca Gindro is subject, our aim, clinically, should be to resolve them. One's view on exactly how this should be achieved, in this and similar cases, will depend on one's theoretical orientation. Even within psychotherapy and psychoanalysis there are widely different approaches, and in Francesca's case it is far from clear that there is no role for other therapies, including, for a period at least, drug treatments.

There are, though, unifying ethical themes. Holmes and Lindley (1989), whose work we mentioned a moment ago, have argued that the core 'value' of psychotherapies (of all kinds) is to restore and extend people's power of choice. This is clearly relevant in Francesca's case: her life choices seem wholly blocked. The psychoanalyst Bob Hinshelwood has taken this idea further through a detailed analysis of the conceptual and ethical implications of the phenomena of splitting, projection, and introjection (Hinshelwood 1995 and 1997*a* and *b*). As he points out, these are phenomena which, though among the technical concerns of psychoanalysis, occur in a wide variety of everyday situations, well beyond the analyst's 'couch'. This suggests that personal identity is more fluid than we generally recognize: it is not a 'given'. It has to be constructed through interpersonal processes. The therapist, as an expert in handling these processes, has a particular ethical responsibility for them. The philosophical notion of rationality, and the bioethical notion of autonomy, he suggests, are unhelpful here — both assume a unique and indivisible individual. Hence, he argues for a 'principle of integration' as the key to psychotherapeutic ethics: as he puts it, 'those practices are ethically beneficent that aim to minimise the distortions of identity and interpersonal spreading; and those are unethical which aim to fragment the personality and to enhance the interpersonal spreading' (Hinshelwood 1997*a*, p. 137); or again, 'those practices are ethical, in which the professional minimises the distortions of his own identity;

and those practices are unethical in which he colludes with his client to distort both their personalities' (Hinshelwood 1997*a*, p. 138).

Hinshelwood's concern here — of the danger of 'a collusive situation (arising), perhaps to mutual relief, but with mutual distortion of each other' (1997, p. 138) — seems clearly relevant to the situation between Mike Callahan and Francesca Gindro. Just how Hinshelwood's principle is applied here will depend, partly, on technical considerations specific to the particular school of psychotherapy to which Mike belongs. Ethically, it connects with a number of general points about psychiatric ethics that are beginning to emerge from our cases. Hinshelwood's principle shows, first, that in Francesca's case, as in several of the cases in preceding chapters, there is a central connection between ethics and communication; there is no 'exploring the space of reasons' without good communication. Second, in so far as this reveals differences of value, cross-referencing of perspectives is essential. As we noted in Case 4.3, this implies a new and crucial role for the multidisciplinary team. Psychotherapists often work in relative isolation (or perhaps only with a supervisor who, after all, reflects the same orientation); but perhaps this is an ethically vulnerable model of practice. We will suggest later, in Chapter 8, that different perspectives are crucial, not just to balancing values but also, more widely, to the processes by which, in the absence of determinate criteria, we apply the high-level concepts, such as rationality, on which psychiatry depends.

We have reviewed a number of possible interpretations of Francesca Gindro's story. The common theme, running from delusion through deception and self-deception to various forms of dissociation, is that meanings, as well as causes, are essential to a proper understanding of her case. The importance of meanings in psychotherapy may seem self-evident. It is in 'organic' cases, some may say, that meanings are at risk of being eclipsed by causes. Correspondingly, it has been mainly 'organic' treatments — drugs, ECT, and psychosurgery — which have been considered most problematic ethically in psychiatry. Francesca Gindro's story, and the dilemma in which Mike Callahan finds himself, show that the so-called 'talking treatments' — psychoanalytic, psychotherapeutic, or psychological — are certainly no less problematic ethically than the more obviously intrusive physical methods of treatment.

Practitioner commentary (CASE 5.2)

Professor R.E. Hinshelwood Centre for Psychoanalytic Services, University of Essex

The psychotherapist described is in an ethical dilemma over whether to continue therapy with someone he has misdiagnosed, and who has produced a sudden erotic delusion about him (and is therefore in the midst of a very intense transference), or whether to discontinue on the basis that there is a sexual situation between them, and he could be accused of unprofessional behaviour.

My sense is that to take action in the way Mike did, on the basis of a transference manifestation, is not professionally correct (indeed, might itself be unethical). If I were to see his dilemma in my own psychoanalytic terms (as a dilemma over integration) it would go like this.

First of all, we should not see the patient's delusions in isolation; they erupt in the context of a relationship, a relationship with the therapist — this is very clear. The patient's delusions about the relationship point us towards what is happening between them. Secondly, a psychoanalyst would not take false beliefs as completely false, and would consider that they have a rational enough meaning, but a hidden meaning that is distorted and concealed inside the delusional meanings presented at face value. The unconscious meaning, in other words, is more important than the overt articulation of the delusion.

Working from these two premises, we can see that something very powerful has happened in the relationship; the psychotherapist has to absorb the impact of something going terribly wrong in his therapy when his patient demonstrates an unsuspected psychotic state. Mike seriously questions his own competence to continue this therapy. Now I think we have a very stark situation here:

- On one hand, Francesca denies her fertility and the competence of her body to produce fruitful results in the form of babies. Something is missing from her mental state — her sense of failure is denied.

- On the other hand, Mike is filled with a sense of incompetence; one might say he is over-filled since he considers an abandonment of his therapy altogether. Even to discuss the ending seems disastrously hasty, provoking a suicide attempt.

It may be right that Mike should reconsider his competence with this patient; but he seems to be more than considering it — in fact, jumping to a conclusion that he has failed. I would want to explore his excessive feelings of failure, which, together with Francesca's strategy (successful at the point of the appearance of the delusion) of denying her sense of failure, lead me to conclude that a projection of some intensity has occurred. The sense of failure, which she might feel, has disappeared, and it would seem to have entered Mike instead, combining with his own bewilderment to result for him in a double dose, as it were. This projection of the patient's sense of failure directly on to the therapist, joining his own sense of failure, creates a different dilemma for the therapist, albeit one that is active at an unconscious level. The therapist needs to 'do' something with the patient's projection which the therapist has introjected. Previously, Mike had seen his job as helping to raise Francesca's awareness of her feelings of failure, but now he has to do a different job — actually to feel and tolerate the depth of failure.

We can follow what actually happens in terms of the projected part of the patient's mind. Crucially, we need to see this *from the patient's point of view*. Unconsciously, Francesca has relocated a part of herself into Mike, out of a desperate feeling she cannot cope with her own experience. This is the intense transference. Then she hears that Mike wants to finish with her. This leaves her, potentially, with no therapist in which to locate her intolerable experience. Unwittingly, he has, from her point of view, told her he will no longer accept the projection she wishes (needs) for her own intolerable experience; and she must do so without him and on her own, as he leaves her. Her state is now desperate:

1 She has lost hope.
2 Her mind must cope with something she believes cannot be coped with (and which perhaps she now believes her therapist confirms cannot be coped with).
3 She must do it on her own.

This makes a particular sense of her next act — her suicide attempt. It is understandable in terms of the hopelessness that she believes is confirmed; and it may also include a cry for help, by demonstrating with the death of her body that her mind is also being destroyed by coping with the intolerable. In other words, the therapist has in effect sought to drop the introjected failure, and the patient is very abruptly left to pick it up. This amounts to a rather forceful projection back into the patient who seems to have little alternative but to introject it into herself again — with intolerable and catastrophic results to her mind.

In this account, delusions are in the context of a relationship (they are 'object-related' in psychoanalytic terms). The effect of the delusion on the therapist is the main meaning for the patient.

Also, this meaning which I have adduced tends to ignore the overt sexual interpretation. This is in order to understand a hidden, unconscious level to the transference/counter-transference encounter: one which is played out in terms of the projective and introjective psychic acts that relocate parts of a disturbed and divided mind. In fact, it seems to me one could extend the understanding of the patient's experience by interpreting the therapy as a replay of an infertile and eventually miscarried intimate relationship (repeated from her parenting as a child, and her actual sterility with her husband).

So, there are two acts in this drama:

1 A projection from the patient into the therapist, who reacts with bewilderment and feels in some sort of crisis.

2 A secondary, abrupt projection from the therapist into the patient, who feels overwhelmed by a crisis, hopeless, and in fear of the 'death' of her mind.

The understanding of transference leads to a considerable complication for professional ethics: an understanding at just the conscious level is inadequate. There are profoundly important, hidden aspects to conducting psychotherapy — ones which may be difficult for the therapist to recognize precisely because he is emotionally carried along by the relationship as well as the patient. However, as the illustrations indicate, to ignore that level of the professional relationship could itself be ethically dubious — and lead to downright dangerous professional behaviour.

References (CASE 5.2)

American Psychiatric Association (1994) *Diagnostic and statistical manual of mental disorders* (4th edn, revised). Washington DC, American Psychiatric Association.

Austin J.L. (1956/7) A plea for excuses. *Proceedings of the Aristotelian Society* 57:1–30. Reprinted in White, A.R., ed. (1968) *The Philosophy of Action*. Oxford: Oxford University Press.

Braude, S.E. (1991; 2nd edn, 1995) *First Person Plural: Multiple Personality and the Philosophy of Mind*. London, Routledge.

Braude, S.E. (1996) Multiple personality and moral responsibility. *Philosophy, Psychiatry and Psychology*, 3:37–54. (Commentary by Clark, S.R.L., 55–8 and Shuman, D.W., 59–60.)

Flew, A. (1973) *Crime or Disease?* New York, Barnes and Noble.

Fulford, K.W.M. (1989, reprinted 1995; 2nd edn forthcoming) *Moral Theory and Medical Practice*. Cambridge, Cambridge University Press.

Fulford, K.W.M. (1993) Value, action, mental illness and the law. In *Action and Value in Criminal Law* (ed. Shute, S., Gardner, J., and Horder, J.), pp. 279–310. Oxford, Oxford University Press.

Fulford, K.W.M. (2000a) Philosophy meets psychiatry in the twentieth century— Four looks back and a brief loof forward. In Louhiala, P., Stenman, S. (eds.): Philosophy Meets Medicine. Helsinki: Helsinki University Press; p. 116–34.

Fulford, K.W.M. (2000*b*) Disordered minds, diseased brains and real people in Philosophy, Psychiatry and Psychopathy: Personal identity in mental disorder. (ed. Heginbotham, C.), Chapter 4 Avebury Series in Philosophy in association with The Society for Applied Philosophy. Aldershot (England): Ashgate Publishing Ltd.

Gardner, S. (1993) *Irrationality and the Philosophy of Psychoanalysis.* Cambridge, Cambridge University Press.

Garety, P. A. and Freedman, D. (1999) Cognitive approaches to delusions: a critical review of theories and evidence. *British Journal of Clinical Psychology*, **38**:113–54.

Gelder, M.G., Gath, D., and Mayou, R. (1989) *The Oxford Textbook of Psychiatry* (2nd edn). Oxford, Oxford University Press.

Glover, J. (1970) *Responsibility.* London, Routledge.

Hinshelwood, R.D. (1995) The social relocation of personal identity as shown by psychoanalytic observations of splitting, projection and introjection. *Philosophy, Psychiatry, and Psychology,* **2**:185–204.

Hinshelwood, R.D. (1997*a*) Primitive mental processes: psychoanalysis and the ethics of integration. *Philosophy, Psychiatry, and Psychology,* **4/2**:121–44.

Hinshelwood, R.D. (1997*b*) *Therapy or Coercion? Does Psychoanalysis Differ from Brainwashing?* London, Karnac Books Ltd.

Holmes, J. and Lindley, R. (1989) *The Values of Psychotherapy.* Oxford, Oxford University Press.

Kennedy, I. (1997) Consent: adult, refusal of consent, capacity. Commentary on Re MB [1997] 2 F.L.R. 426. *Medical Law Review,* **5**:317–25.

Locke, J. (1979) *An Essay Concerning Human Understanding* (ed. Nidditch, P.H.) Oxford, Clarendon Press.

Parfit, D. (1984) *Reasons and Persons.* Oxford, Clarendon Press.

Quinton, A. (1985) Madness. In *Philosophy and Practice* (ed. Griffiths, A.P.), Chapter 2. Cambridge, Cambridge University Press.

Radden, J. (1996) *Divided Minds and Successive Selves: Ethical Issues in Disorders of Identity and Personality.* Cambridge(Mass.), MIT Press.

Reznek, L. (1997) *Evil or Ill? Justifying the Insanity Defence.* London and New York, Routledge.

Sartre, J.-P. (1943) *L'être et le néant.* Trs. H.E. Barnes. New York, Philosophical Library.

Thornton, T. (2000) Mental Illness and Reductionism: Can Functions be Naturalized? *Philosophy, Psychiatry, and Psychology,* **7/1**:67–76.

Reading Guide

Causes and meanings

The distinction between meanings and causes goes back a long way. Jasper's 1913 paper, from which the title of this chapter is taken, was published just before the first edition of *General Psychopathology*. Jaspers was in turn influenced by the *Methodenstreit* — a debate which raged through much of the nineteenth century about whether the human sciences were in principle different from the physical sciences.

The modern counterpart of this debate is an exchange in philosophy of mind about whether reasons can be reduced to causes. A useful collection on this is J. Heil and A. Mele, *Mental Causation* (1993). A widely influential argument for reasons being causes was developed by the American philosopher Donald Davidson in his essay 'Actions, reasons and causes' (1980) in *Essays on Actions and Events*. Davidson was attacking philosophers such as A. I. Melden (in Melden's *Free Action*, 1958). Davidson deploys the possibility of the rational and the causal coming apart to explain weakness of will in his 'Paradoxes of irrationality' in *Philosophical Essays on Freud* (1982). A recent attack on the idea that reason explanation is really causal is given in Chapter 6 of Tim Thornton's *Wittgenstein on Language and Thought* (1998).

In their influential *Mind, Meaning and Mental Disorder* (1996), Derek Bolton (a philosopher and psychologist) and Jonathan Hill (a psychiatrist) have brought the debate about meanings and causes back to psychopathology. For a brief account of this see Bolton's 'Encoding of meaning: deconstructing the meaning/causality distinction' (1997). For an analysis and review of Bolton and Hill's work, see T. Thornton's 'Reasons and causes in philosophy and psychopathology' (1997). Steven Sabat and Rom Harré (1997) have made a careful philosophical case for the clinical importance of continuing to treat people even with advanced dementia as semiotic (that is, meaning-driven) subjects.

For a thorough philosophical treatment of the interpersonal and constructed nature of personal identity, see Rom Harré and Grant Gillett's *The Discursive Mind* (1994). Harré has applied his work in this area to the problem of understanding violently sadistic behaviour in forensic psychiatry in an article on 'Pathological autobiographies' (1997). Grant Gillett has recently published an extensive and very readable treatment of the discursive approach in psychiatry, including ethical issues, in his *The Mind and its Discontents* (1999).

Reading Guide: references

Bolton, D. (1997) Encoding of meaning: deconstructing the meaning/causality distinction. *Philosophy, Psychiatry, and Psychology*, **4/4**:255–68.

Bolton, D. and Hill, J. (1996) *Mind, Meaning and Mental Disorder: the Nature of Causal Explanation in Psychology and Psychiatry*. Oxford, Oxford University Press.

Davidson, D. (1980) *Essays on Actions and Events*. Oxford, Oxford University Press.

Davidson, D. (1982) Paradoxes of irrationality. In *Philosophical Essays on Freud* (ed. Hopkins, J. and Wollheim, R. Cambridge, Cambridge University Press.

Gillett, G. (1999) *The Mind and its Discontents*. Oxford, Oxford University Press.

Harré, R. (1997) Pathological autobiographies. *Philosophy, Psychiatry, and Psychology,* 4:99–110.

Harré, R. and Gillett, G. (1994) *The Discursive Mind*. London, Sage.

Heil, J. and Mele, A. (1993) *Mental Causation*. Oxford, Oxford University Press.

Jaspers, K. (1913) *Allgemeine Psychopathologie*. Berlin, Springer. In translation in 1963 as *General Psychopathology* (translated by Hoenig, J. and Hamilton, M.W.). Manchester, Manchester University Press. New edition in 1997, with a new foreword by McHugh, Paul R. Baltimore, The Johns Hopkins University Press.

Jaspers, K. (1913) Causal and meaningful connexions between life history and psychosis. Reprinted in 1974 in *Themes and Variations in European Psychiatry* (ed. Hirsch, S.R. and Shepherd, M.), Chapter 5. Bristol, John Wright and Sons Ltd.

Melden, A.I. (1958) *Free Action*. London, Routledge and Kegan Paul.

Sabat, S.R. and Harré, R. (1997) The Alzheimer's Disease sufferer as semiotic subject. *Philosophy, Psychiatry, and Psychology,* 4/2:145–60.

Thornton, T. (1997) Reasons and causes in philosophy and psychopathology. *Philosophy, Psychiatry, and Psychology,* 4/4: 307.

Thornton, T. (1998) *Wittgenstein on Language and Thought*. Edinburgh, Edinburgh University Press.

CHAPTER 6

Treatment: trick or treat?

Deep theoretical issues in moral philosophy and philosophy of mind underpin many dilemmas of treatment choice in psychiatry

With treatment, we come full square to those issues that are at the heart of traditional bioethics — autonomy, consent, confidentiality, equal access, dual (indeed multiple!) responsibility, rationing, advance directives, and so forth.

Besides an extensive general literature, a good deal has been written about the ethical problems of treatment choice specifically in psychiatry (see Reading Guide to Chapter 2 and at the end of this chapter). One 'big issue' for psychiatry is involuntary treatment. Psychiatry is ethically unique in that it is only for mental disorders that treatment without the consent of a fully conscious adult patient of normal intelligence is sometimes justified, not just for the protection of others, but in the interests of the person concerned. This is a 'big issue' practically: the boundary between justified and unjustified uses of involuntary treatment is the boundary between good practice and some of the worst abuses of psychiatry as a means of social control. It is also a 'big issue' theoretically: a full justification of involuntary treatment would take us from the debate about the basic concept of mental illness, through the nature of delusion, and from there into the metaphysical deeps of freedom, responsibility, and the relationship between mind and brain.

In Chapter 2, we started from a paradigmatic case for involuntary psychiatric treatment — a person with a major depressive illness and evidence of suicidal intent. Mr Able, on whose story we focused, is the kind of patient for whom, most would feel, involuntary treatment is fully justified, ethically as well as legally. Mr Able's case was thus an appropriate one in which to explore both the value and the limitations of standard bioethics in psychiatry. The value was that bioethical reasoning — a combination of principles, casuistry, and perspectives — helped to map out the issues. The limitation was that, in psychiatry, the issues became ethically critical just where traditional bioethics left off! There have been important exceptions (some of which we noted in Chapters 1 and 2), but bioethics has largely taken for granted the nature of such concepts as rationality, personal identity, true wishes, voluntariness, and even 'the patient', which are often at the very heart of the ethical dilemmas we face in our everyday practice in psychiatry.

The cases we consider in this chapter take up issues raised by some of these underlying concepts. Each case involves a standard bioethical problem. But discussion of these issues leads us into an examination of one or more of the problematic concepts crucial to psychiatric ethics.

Thus, our first case is one of dual responsibility. 'Captain Ahab', as we call him, is a man of 38, an abuser of drugs and alcohol, who finds himself unexpectedly left responsible for his daughters when his wife dies. He has never actually abused his daughters, and it seems right that they should stay with him, but he becomes violent when drunk. The dilemma for the psychiatrist arises when 'Ahab' 'negotiates' for an increase in his methadone prescription in return for a promise not to drink. The psychiatrist feels that Captain Ahab is using his daughters in a kind of emotional blackmail. But should she go along with this (which would probably be good for his daughters) or deny him the methadone (which in the long run she believes would be better for him)?

Of course, psychiatry offers a wide variety of more high-profile cases of dual responsibility. In forensic psychiatry, doctors often find themselves taking decisions on behalf of 'the state' rather than their patients. Similar dilemmas can arise for psychiatrists working in the armed forces. Captain Ahab's story illustrates how these tensions in the responsibility of the psychiatrist permeate everyday practice. They turn, as we have seen in Chapters 3 and 4, partly on how we understand the concept of mental illness. This raises difficult theoretical issues about the role of a professional, the relationship between professional and client, and the scope of psychiatry as a specifically medical discipline.

Traditional bioethics, which has been developed largely on a model of rational individualism, offers little help here. Instead, the discussion draws on recent developments in ethical theory —feminist, Hegelian, and communitarian ethics — which make *embeddedness in relationship* a hallmark of the rational, and hence autonomous, person (for example, Held 1993; Brody 1992; Adshead, forthcoming; Sandel 1998). This understanding of autonomy has come directly from challenges to traditional bioethics' narrow concentration on negative rights and instrumental rationality. As one of us has argued elsewhere (Dickenson 1997), it is precisely this challenge which makes a conception of autonomy embedded in relationships, at one and the same time, more clinically relevant *and* more philosophically persuasive.

A further issue, which we explore in relation both to Captain Ahab and his daughters, is how we should understand 'best interests'. This is one of the anchors of traditional bioethics. Even in physical medicine it may be difficult enough to define in a given case; in psychiatry it is further complicated by dif-

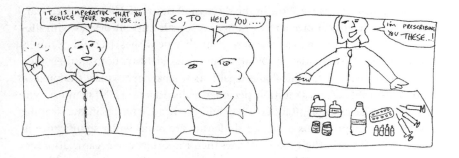

ferent kinds of psychopathology. Absent psychopathology, the most reliable guide to best interests, at least for adult patients, is generally assumed to be what a patient says he or she wants. But addiction, our intuitions suggest, makes people want (or desire) things that are plainly not in their best interests. On the other hand, though, if an addiction is not affecting anyone else, and if the addict does not want (that is, wish) to break their addiction, are we right to impose our values on the addict? We might do this as a friend or colleague but is it right as a *professional?* Are we not at risk of merely imposing our own value system in the guise of medical treatment?

One response to this is that we should be guided, not by the patient's immediate desires, but by their values as expressed in their life as a whole. This was Aristotle's concept of eudaimonia. The New Zealand philosopher Andrew Moore has shown the importance of this concept in relation to the ethical problems raised by mild and fluctuating hypomania in which a person's immediately expressed values may change rapidly over a short period of time (Moore *et al.* 1994). In Captain Ahab's case, we explore the relevance of eudaimonia to the ethical issues raised by dual responsibility in psychiatry.

Best interests is an issue, too, in our second case. Ida Harbottle was a 69-year-old woman with moderate dementia who was determined to remain living independently but was causing considerable upset and stress by her repeated calls on her neighbours. As with Captain Ahab, one issue for the psychiatrist was whose interests — the patient's or the neighbours' — should be paramount. But in this case, balancing these interests depends critically on the view one takes of the 'present Mrs Harbottle'. Is 'independence' on these terms what the original, pre-dementia Mrs Harbottle, would have 'really' wanted? This is a familiar bioethical problem which, here in Ida Harbottle's case, makes unavoidable one of the 'big issues' in philosophy of mind — that of the nature of personal identity and its continuity over time.

Personal identity, as we show in the discussion of Ida Harbottle's case, bears directly on the ethical problem of how to reconcile current desires with life-long attitudes in coming to a view of someone's 'true wishes' (see, for example, Parfit 1984). In psychiatry, problems of personal identity, both in their own right and in relation to ethical and legal issues, have been widely explored in such high-profile cases as multiple personality disorder and false memory syndrome (see, for example, Radden 1996, and further references in the Reading Guide). But the problems of personal identity are of far wider significance in psychiatry. Ida Harbottle's case illustrates their importance in organic disorders in which there is marked loss of cognitive functions. The Oxford psychiatrist and ethicist Tony Hope has shown the significance of the emotional and cognitive changes in dementia in this context (Hope 1994).

At the other end of the organic–functional scale from Ida Harbottle, issues of personal identity may be crucial to valid consent in relation to the quite different ethical problems raised by psychotherapy. There is something of an ethical paradox here, that in psychotherapy a 'client' gives consent from within a value system which it may be part of the very object of therapy to change! The psychoanalyst Bob Hinshelwood came hard up against this paradox in his work as Director of the Cassel Hospital (for Forensic Psychotherapy). Is psychotherapy then, as the title of his recent book asks, therapy or brainwashing? (Hinshelwood 1997a). In the case of Kleinian therapy, as Hinshelwood has shown elsewhere, the phenomena of identification, projection, and introjection point directly to the importance of personal identity at the heart of this key distinction (Hinshelwood 1995). As we noted earlier (in Case 5.2, Francesca Gindro), this led to Hinshelwood's conclusion that a principle of 'integration' should replace the standard bioethical principle of autonomy as the basis of valid consent in all forms of psychotherapy (Hinshelwood 1997b).

Our third case is of a rather different kind in that it is concerned with screening rather than treatment. Robin is a teenager who requests screening for Huntington's Disease when her father is found to test positive for the disorder. Her family and the psychiatrist believe she has the maturity to make this choice, but the guidelines adopted by the local genetics clinic restrict screening to those of 18 and above. This opens up a whole plethora of issues about consent — the impact of new technology and the special position of those responsible for its delivery in practice; the role of law, and of conflicts between legal and moral issues; the use of the UK's Children Act in psychiatry; the dangers of over-rigid codes (important as they may be in other respects); the gap between the right to consent and the freedom to reject treatment; and so on. These issues, severally and together, lead inexorably to the need for a more sophisticated framework for issues of consent in everyday psychiatric practice.

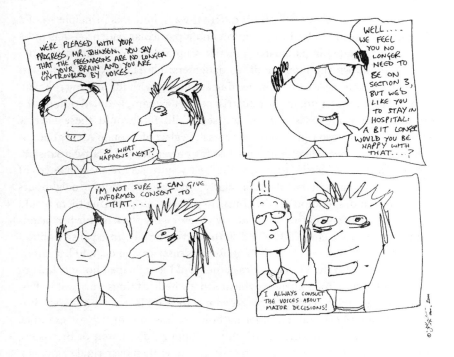

One of us has explored this in detail elsewhere in relation to children's consent to treatment: 'true wishes' — the term at the heart of the Children Act's attempt to shift the balance of decision making in favour of the child's best interests — turns on deep issues of rationality and personal identity (Dickenson and Jones 1995). But the practical bottom line to which this theoretical work leads is that autonomous choice is not just a precondition for consent; it is also an outcome of the experience of being allowed to choose. It is through the experience of choosing that we gain the capacities for autonomous choice.

A common theme linking these cases is how we should understand 'the patient' in psychiatry. The rights, obligations, and duties of doctors to offer treatment have traditionally (and in our view rightly) been closely linked with the notion of a patient— that is, some *particular* person to whom a doctor has a *particular* relationship and who needs treatment for a *medical* problem. With someone who is suicidal, for example, as we noted in Chapter 2, a psychiatrist may intervene like anyone else on humanitarian grounds, but specifically *medical* interventions (admission to hospital and/or treatment) require a specifically *medical* problem.

The cases in this chapter show, in different ways, how this principle — of a close link between medical intervention and a particular patient — has to be diluted and adapted in psychiatric practice. Captain Ahab's psychiatrist could have played down the interests of his daughters; Ida Harbottle's psychiatrist could have taken the 'easy option', leaving autonomy with Ida and the problem with her neighbours; Robin's psychiatrist could have simply opted out, on the grounds that Robin was not, in any sense, ill. But would these narrow approaches have been right? At the very least, neglect of Captain Ahab's daughters would have been an opportunity lost for preventive psychiatry: a satisfactory resolution of his situation was the best way to secure their chances of sound mental health in the future. Similarly, leaving Ida Harbottle's neighbours to fall back in desperation on the courts to prevent her pestering them would have been needlessly harsh: it would have been highly stressful for her neighbours, highly distressing for Ida, and, at the end of the day, an expensive option for both Health and Social Services! In Robin's case, leaving her and her family to fight it out with the local genetics clinic would have helped no one, least of all the staff at the clinic. There is evidence that whether things work out well or badly with genetic screening is governed not by *what* is done but by *how* it is done (Brandt 1994), though other authors are less optimistic (for example, Bloch *et al.* 1993; Scourfield *et al.* 1997). Support, discussion of the issues, counselling, in other words, 'human contact', rather than over-rigid principles, are what matter clinically.

Our discussion of involuntary treatment in Chapter 2 highlighted the dangers of psychiatrists allowing their skills to be used for non-medical purposes, for political and social ends rather than for the treatment of illness. The cases examined in this chapter remind us of the opposite danger, of psychiatrists adopting a narrowly legalistic restriction of their area of concern, excluding those whose interests they might legitimately serve.

References

Adshead, G. (forthcoming) A different voice in psychiatric ethics. In *Healthcare Ethics and Human Values* (ed. Fulford, K.W.M., Dickenson, D., and Murray, T.H.). Oxford, Blackwell Science.

Bloch, M. *et al.* (1993) Diagnosis of Huntington's disease: a model for the stages of psychological response based on experience of a predictive testing program. *American Journal of Medical Genetics,* 47:368–74.

Brandt, J. (1994) Ethical considerations in genetic testing: an empirical study of presymptomatic diagnosis of Huntington's disease. In *Medicine and Moral Reasoning* (ed. Fulford, K.W.M., Gillett, G.R., Soskice, J.M.), pp. 41–59. Cambridge: Cambridge University Press.

Brody, H. (1992) *The Healer's Power.* New Haven, Yale University Press.

Dickenson, D. (1997) *Property, Women and Politics.* Cambridge, Polity Press.

Dickenson, D. and Jones, D. (1995) True wishes: The philosophy and developmental psychology of children's informed consent. *Philosophy, Psychiatry, and Psychology,* 2:287–304.

Held, V. (1993) *Feminist Morality: Transforming Culture, Society and Politics.* Chicago, University of Chicago Press.

Hinshelwood, R.D. (1995) The social relocation of personal identity as shown by psychoanalytic observations of splitting, projection and introjection. *Philosophy, Psychiatry, and Psychology,* 2:185–204.

Hinshelwood, R.D. (1997a) *Therapy or Coercion? Does Psychoanalysis Differ from Brainwashing.* London, Karnac Books Ltd.

Hinshelwood, R.D. (1997b) Primitive mental processes: psychoanalysis and the ethics of integration. *Philosophy, Psychiatry, and Psychology,* 4/2:121–44.

Hope, T. (1994) Personal identity and psychiatric illness In *Philosophy, Psychology and Psychiatry,* (ed. Phillips Griffiths, A.). *Royal Institute of Philosophy Supplement,* 37:131–43. Cambridge, Cambridge University Press.

Moore, A., Hope, T., and Fulford, K.W.M. (1994) Mild mania and well-being. *Philosophy, Psychiatry and Psychology,* 1:165–78.

Parfit, D. (1984) *Reasons and Persons.* Oxford, Clarendon Press.

Radden, J. (1996) *Divided Minds and Successive Selves: Ethical Issues in Disorders of Identity and Personality.* Cambridge (Mass.), MIT Press.

Sandel, M. (1998) *Liberalism and the Limits of Justice* (2nd edn). Cambridge, Cambridge University Press.

Scourfield, J., Soldan, J., Gray, J., Houlihlan, G. and Harper, P.S. (1997) Huntington's disease: psychiatric practice in molecular genetic prediction and diagnosis. *British Journal of Psychiatry,* 178:144–9.

CASE 6.1
'Captain Ahab' — dual role psychiatry

Synopsis A 38-year-old unemployed man, with a history of inveterate alcohol and drug abuse, and who is violent when drunk, becomes the principal carer for his three daughters when his divorced wife dies suddenly from a cerebral aneurysm. He bargains with his psychiatrist that he will avoid street drugs and alcohol if she increases his methadone.

Key dilemma Should the psychiatrist: (1) go along with this, provided 'Captain Ahab' accepts family counselling and regular tests for alcohol and drugs; (2) try to establish a more conventional contract; or (3) adopt a *laissez-faire* attitude.

Main topics Dual responsibility; autonomy, personal and rational.

Other topics Doctor–patient relationship; best interests; protection of others; alcohol/drug abuse; rationality; virtue theory; setting limits; feminist ethics; Aristotle; MacIntyre; Plato; altruism; Hume; Hobbes; contract; Hegel; Locke; autonomy; responsibility.

George MacKinnon is a 38-year-old unemployed man, trained as an electrician but out of work because of his history of drug and alcohol abuse. With his first use of alcohol at the age of ten, and regular drinking established as a pattern by sixteen, he began using injected morphine, cocaine, diconal, amphetamines, and barbiturates in his late teens. He has not declared himself available for work since his apprenticeship: by the age of nineteen he was making several thousand pounds a month from drug dealing and burglary, having committed his first break-in at the age of ten with a gang of older boys. He also developed a talent for 'spotting' doctors who would prescribe drugs which he could sell illegally.

His wife Carol, who died six months ago of a cerebral aneurysm at the age of 34, was also dependent on substances. Before their divorce two years ago, they had three daughters, now aged fourteen, eleven, and eight. After the divorce the girls lived with Carol, who would not allow George to see them, but they returned to him after their mother died. There are no other relatives with whom they could live.

George's only periods of abstinence from drugs and alcohol took place when he was in approved school or prison, for burglary and robbery with violence. Conventional treatment programmes have had little effect: three early attempts at heroin withdrawal through methadone maintenance programmes all failed. George has been admitted for alcohol detoxification several times, most recently four weeks ago, after he was taken into hospital for injuries sustained in a fight. (Alcohol results in violence with him, giving him social problems in a way that drugs do not.) He had severe withdrawal symptoms, including agitation, sweating, marked tremor, tactile hallucinations, and incipient seizures. Discharged a week later, he began attending the out-patient clinic, where he demanded a minimum 'treatment' of injectable methadone ampoules (40 mg daily), chlordiazepoxide (60 mg daily), and ibuprofen (800 mg daily). His average alcohol meter reading over the past three weeks has been 300 g/l, and he is also using street heroin.

At George's first out-patient attendance, his clinician, Justine Nelson, wrote: 'I knew I had met him before: he was Captain Ahab. He came in the room in a dark grey overcoat. I soon realised it had once been cream. He had a limp, and staggered from side to side. When he stared, his eyes had a menacing quality. His beard was infested with ants, and he had an odour about him that made me wish I had a cold. In his slow, monotonous voice, he asked whether I would be a good doctor and never try to reduce his medication. In fact, his price for not drinking or using street drugs was a large increase in injectable methadone.'

Should Justine accept this Faustian bargain? She is concerned to stop George using street drugs in addition to his prescribed medication; to prevent the violence which results from his misuse of alcohol; and to keep him on the right side of the law. There are three possible management strategies:

1 Bargain with George: for example, increasing his methadone prescription only if he agrees to return the used ampoules (to prevent his selling them on), to undergo an alcohol breath test three times a week, and to participate in weekly family counselling (to capitalize on his feelings for his family and to mobilize his daughters to support him). The advantage of this management plan is that it is pragmatic, accepting George's addiction rather than trying to reform it. The disadvantage, Justine thinks, is that this is still a form of playing God, manipulating George to do what the clinicians think best. On balance, however, this is her preferred method of management.

2 Adopt the traditional model of a limit-setting contract for the substance misuse and a supportive problem-solving approach to social difficulties. George is capable of understanding the terms of such a contract: his cognitive abilities are not impaired, and neither does he have any mental illness. But there is no evidence that this standard method has worked in the past, and quite a number of indications that it has not. In addition, Justine is more concerned about George's alcohol abuse than his substance misuse. When he becomes violent with alcohol, his behaviour is beyond the power of a problem-solving approach.

3 Try a *laissez-faire* approach in the hope that George's new-found family responsibilities will encourage him to change his behaviour. This strategy respects his 'right' to remain an addict, relies on his 'better nature', and encourages him to take responsibility. But it leaves Justine in the likely position of merely presiding over George's further decline.

Before we can decide which is the best strategy for management, we have to decide who it is that is being managed. Justine is very sensitive to the issue of whether she is manipulating George in her preferred first strategy, but oddly unaware of the way in which her proposed treatment plan can be said to manipulate George's daughters. There is a risk of either using them as a means to George's rehabilitation, or of ignoring them altogether. These girls have just lost their mother — shouldn't their welfare come first? Justine might well reply that the girls are not her patients; their father is. But this seems unduly narrow, although there is no duty of care to anyone other than George. Still, it is hard to see how this treatment strategy could be ethical if the charges about manipulating or ignoring the girls are correct.

Generally, the moral reason for putting the patient's welfare first is that the patient is in a vulnerable position and needs to be protected from possible abuse of the physician's power (Lindemann Nelson and Lindemann Nelson 1995, p. 2). If the doctor puts other considerations first, including the demands of family members, the patient's welfare may be compromised. But in this case George is actually in quite a powerful position, with regard to both Justine and his daughters. He does not need extra protection; the girls do. With this caveat about the children's welfare in mind, let us examine the ethical implications of the three possible forms of management, beginning with bargaining with George.

There is a risk that George might use his responsibilities for his children as a bargaining weapon, to allow him to maintain his dependence, and Justine needs to be sensitive to that possibility. Keeping George able to function means keeping the children at home, rather than in care. Because George functions reasonably well on methadone (it is alcohol which makes him violent), the first strategy is probably the most likely to allow the girls to remain with their father. But is this necessarily the best thing for them? The Children Act 1989 operates on the presumption that it would be in most cases, but is this an ordinary case? The Act uses a 'reasonable parent' standard: an order to prevent significant harm to a child, for example, must compare the care which a child is currently receiving (or is likely to receive, if the order is not made) with what it would be reasonable to expect a parent to give. One could certainly argue that any reasonable parent would be primarily concerned with the needs of his bereaved children, rather than his own drug access.

This raises wider questions about George's rationality. He is rational in the narrow sense that he is pursuing a consistent, coherent strategy for maximixing his preferences — like Tom Benbow (Case 3.2). Tom's project was getting Social Services to rehouse him; George's is maximizing the availability of his preferred drugs. On the face of it, both are pursuing rational goals, if rationality is defined in the conventional economic manner as maximization of personal preferences. With this underlying presumption about what constitutes rationality, a bargaining strategy might well be appropriate: a rational agent can be expected to make valid, durable bargains in pursuit of rational goals.

But if we take a less narrowly instrumental view of rationality, we have to doubt whether George's project is really rational. A profound critique of rational instrumentalism has proceeded apace in philosophy, and even in economics, allowing for plural rational strategies and the revival of altruism (for example, Collard 1978; Gauthier 1990; Dancy 1993; Hurley 1989; Blum 1980; Gibbard 1990). Increasingly, in philosophy, rationality is being redefined in terms not of consistently ordered and relentlessly maximized egotistic preferences, but of understanding what it means to be a fully flourishing human being.

The 'good life' for such a person includes connectedness, responsibility to others, and relationship, in accounts ranging from Aristotle's — resurrected by modern 'virtue' theorists such as Alasdair MacIntyre (1981 and 1988) — to that of feminist writers who emphasize the centrality of relationships and not just of individual rights (Gilligan 1982 and 1993; Held 1993). The picture of rationality as merely the tool of the individual's desires is not timelessly true or factually incontrovertible. The classical view, found in Plato, is that reason should actually be construed as a moral motive, intimately linked to the altruistic desire to do good; rationality has a natural affinity for finding out the truth, and the truth is intertwined with the good (Green 1995, p. 155). Recent moral philosophy, feminist and 'mainstream', rediscovers that model of reason as linked to altruism and virtue, rather than as 'the slave of the passions' — the dominant view found in Hume.

The point here is not that it is the clinician's job to make George a virtuous person — that really would be playing God. Rather, what we want to demonstrate is that Justine's first strategy rests on unexamined and probably untenable assumptions about rationality. As is inevitably the case, clinicians operate with certain philosophical presuppositions, which they may not recognize as such. Justine's assumptions turn out to come from Hobbes, who allowed for no natural altruism, as well as from Hume. But if rationality is construed in non-Humean fashion, the clinical implications for developing a management plan are quite different.

We might still want to leave the door open for following this first strategy, however, once we have examined the underlying presuppositions of the other two in an equally critical manner. However, on both philosophical and pragmatic grounds, it begins to look less appealing. The philosophical grounds have already been stated. The practical ones have to do with the limited success one can expect in bargaining with an irrational person, if rationality is construed in the wider sense as awareness of relationship. Someone with little or no sense of relation to others is unlikely to be motivated to keep promises, such as the ones Justine wants George to make in return for increasing his methadone. He will

not experience guilt at letting others down or breaking his word. Nor is he likely to be moved by the threat of the girls being taken into care, if it conflicts with
his first priority of ensuring his free access to drugs. If this is an accurate picture, the first strategy will not work.

One can only bargain with someone who has a certain degree of rationality;
but George's object in life and his style of achieving it do not clearly match the
more rigorous model of rationality which we have traced here. The fact that he
is more concerned with getting his drugs than thinking about his daughters'
welfare shows that. Captain Ahab, too, is a stranger to parental concern: he
refuses the request for help of another captain who is searching for his twelve-
year-old son, stranded in a dinghy. Just as Ahab took all the crew of the *Pequod*,
except Ishmael, down with him in his obsession, so George may well destroy his
daughters' lives. There may be a good reason why his dead wife would not let
him see them while they lived with her.

Ahab, too, goes about on an artificial support — a leg made of whale jaw
ivory to replace the one the white whale ripped off him. The white whale —
drugs, to extend the metaphor to George — cannot kill him. He laughs deri-
sively, 'I am immortal, then, on land and sea.' Is there an element of this same
hubris in George? After all, he has always got what he wanted, by one means or
another. Why should he bargain?

What about the second strategy then, of following the traditional limit-setting model of a contract for the substance misuse, together with a supportive,
problem-solving approach to social difficulties? Justine is sceptical about the
efficacy of this approach for two reasons: it has not worked in the past, and
George's alcohol abuse results in greater social problems than does his injected
methadone — violence which is beyond the scope of problem-solving counselling. So even if George kept to a contract for limiting his use of drugs, the
more serious problem would remain.

There is at least one solid, pragmatic argument in favour of this approach,
and again, it is one which is only obvious if the girls' welfare is kept firmly in
mind. Our scepticism about George's capacity for relationship may be ill-
founded or premature. Because he puts drugs first does not necessarily mean
he is completely blind to his daughters' needs, although we still maintain that a
reasonable parent would put them first. Now that the girls are living with him,
he has new child-rearing dilemmas to contend with, and he might actually welcome the problem-solving advice on offer, for the first time. Similarly, a limit-
setting contract could use the threat of the girls being taken into care as a
weapon. This is not manipulating the girls or using them as means, because it
is very likely consistent with their best interests. Although children almost
always prefer to stay with the natural parent, no matter how inadequate, the
child's wishes and preferences are only one factor to be considered (Children

Act, Section 1). In short, there is a new stick and a new carrot available to Justine now. So what has not worked in the past might work under George's changed circumstances.

That is the pragmatic argument: the philosophical argument in favour of the second course is twofold. The first part of it has already been sketched — George is not so obviously rational as Justine seems to assume, and bargaining is not appropriate with someone whose rationality is so impaired. The second part has to do with the widespread tendency to view contract as something of a dirty word. We have been alerted to the hypocrisy of the term 'marriage contract' by the feminist movement, which correctly pointed out the imbalance of power in this supposedly freely made contract — at least under older Anglo–American law of coverture (Pateman 1988). Similarly, patients' rights organizations and others have highlighted misuse of 'contracts' in mental health care, when a patient is in no position to refuse.

But there is also an older view about contract in political philosophy, one found primarily in Hegel, which views it as the first stage in the agent's development of social awareness — something George lacks. In Hegel's developmental account, contract is not merely the means by which property is protected (as the liberal contractarians such as Locke would argue). In contract, two isolated individuals transcend their own individuality (Dickenson 1997, p. 101) As Hegel puts it in the *Philosophy of Right* (1967) 'A person by distinguishing himself from himself relates himself to another person…This is *contract*' (Section 40, original emphasis). That is, contract represents the first progress beyond the stage of utter self-absorption, requiring the agent to 'distinguish himself from himself' by limiting his inchoate desires in conformity with his own deferred, higher-order desires and his agreement with another person. For George to agree to a contract limiting his substance use would not only be in his medical interest: it would actually make him more of an autonomous moral agent. We have already argued that he is not fully rational or autonomous as things stand, and that Justine has been too quick to assume that he is.

The third strategy, *laissez-faire*, can be dismissed fairly quickly if these arguments are accepted. Allowing George to continue as he is means presiding over his medical and mental decline, Justine rightly fears. On a Hegelian view, it also means presiding over his further decline as an autonomous moral agent. The more he is made to recognize his interrelatedness to others — his daughters and the clinicians — the more autonomous he will become. Since it is presumably his autonomy and his rights which would justify a *laissez-faire* approach, the third strategy is self-contradictory. George cannot be allowed to do what he likes on the grounds that he is an autonomous agent, because the more he is simply allowed to do what he likes, regardless of others' welfare, the less of an autonomous agent he becomes. This is an important point about autonomy in general, not just in a Hegelian account. Autonomy means 'self-rule', in its original derivation, but it has widely been misconstrued as 'doing whatever you please'.

This is a case about the scope of the clinician's responsibilities — to whom and for how much. The 'to whom' question is the one that raises the issue of whether the management plan needs to consider the welfare of others, besides the patient. The 'how much' query concerns what it is that the clinician is responsible for. Justine is aware that George's behaviour is ultimately his responsibility, that she is not responsible for it. But she has made a logical jump from there to the less defensible position that any concern on her part for the consequences of George's actions is nothing but 'playing God'.

Practitioner commentary (CASE 6.1)

Phil Robson Consultant Psychiatrist, Drug and Alcohol Unit, Warneford Hospital, Oxford

This case certainly represents an everyday dilemma from my out-patient clinic in a busy drug and alcohol treatment centre.

There are two concerns that I have with the approach to rationality. The first lies in the nature of addiction and its influence on autonomy, which, of course, remains highly controversial. One of the many possible elements of the matrix which underpins 'addiction' is a genetically linked, biological deficiency of one or more neurotransmitters. In George's case, for example, it is conceivable that his unusually positive response to opiates (and to alcohol too) may be related to an inherent lack of endorphins. His deficit thus resembles that of a diabetic, who cannot reasonably be expected to abstain from insulin. So if this is part of George's problem — and who can say for certain that it is not — it would be entirely rational for him to seek to get his deficiency legally sorted out so that he could move on to giving the girls his full attention.

The other issue not considered is the rationality of Justine's position. Her dilemma is a twentieth-century artefact created by the Misuse of Drugs Act (1971) and its predecessors. She is the ill-equipped gatekeeper to the derivatives of a natural substance that she doesn't really understand, and the agent of a prohibition which has made a monster out of George and millions like him (Robson 1999).

Accepting that the world we inhabit is not rational, I would approach the case from the entirely pragmatic viewpoint that the children's interests are paramount, and that a positive outcome for them and, if possible, for George justifies the means. The 'care' system poses more risk and heartbreak than even a fairly incompetent biological parent. Predicting the outcome of any interaction with George is very unreliable, and it is better to rely on the outcome of practical experiments. His rationality, whatever that is, like mine, is not an all-or-nothing entity, and it may ebb and flow. He will probably respond well to a frank and informal therapeutic alliance based openly on a carrot-and-stick formula guided by unambiguous objective criteria (Robson 1992). So, a combination of (1) and (2) is the practical answer.

A further interesting question is why not give him heroin? since that is the drug he actually wants and methadone has not proved helpful. In my experience, the prospect of a heroin prescription (albeit rigorously supervised) can provide a powerful incentive for real lifestyle changes, and a recent controlled trial confirms its utility in treatment-resistant subjects (Perneger *et al.* 1998).

As a final point, Justine could be considered remiss in continuing to prescribe injectables to a man who persists in abusing both alcohol and street drugs — she is already part of the problem rather than the solution, and no wonder George thinks doctors are mugs!

References (CASE 6.1)

Blum, L.A. (1980) *Friendship, Altruism and Morality*. London, Routledge and Kegan Paul.

Collard, D. (1978) *Altruism and Economy: A Study in Non-Selfish Economics*. Oxford, Martin Robertson.

Dancy, J. (1993) *Moral Reasons*. Oxford, Blackwell.

Dickenson, D. (1997) *Property, Women and Politics*. Cambridge, Polity Press.

Gauthier, D. (1990) *Moral Dealing: Contract, Ethics and Reason*. Ithaca and London, Cornell University Press.

Gibbard, A. (1990) *Wise Choices, Apt Feelings: A Theory of Normative Judgment*. Oxford, Clarendon Press.

Gilligan, C. (1993) *In a Different Voice: Psychological Theory and Women's Development* (2nd edn, 1st edn 1982). Cambridge (Mass.), Harvard University Press.

Green, K. (1995) *The Woman of Reason: Feminism, Humanism and Political Thought*. Cambridge, Polity Press.

Hegel, G.W.F. (1967) *Hegel's Philosophy of Right*, H.T.M. Knox. Oxford: Oxford University Press.

Held, V. (1993) *Feminist Morality: Transforming Culture, Society and Politics*. Chicago and London, University of Chicago Press.

Hurley, S.L. (1989) *Natural Reasons: Personality and Polity*. Oxford, Oxford University Press.

Lindemann Nelson, H. and Lindemann Nelson, J. (1995). *The Patient in the Family: An Ethics of Medicine and Families*. London, Routledge.

MacIntyre, A. (1981) *After Virtue*. London, Duckworth.

MacIntyre, A. (1988) *Whose Justice? Which Rationality?* Notre Dame, University of Notre Dame Press.

Pateman, C. (1988) *The Sexual Contract*. Cambridge, Polity Press.

Perneger, T.V., Giner, F., del Rio, M., and Mino, A. (1998) Randomised trial of heroin maintenance programme for addicts who fail in conventional drug treatments. *BMJ*, **317**:13–18.

Robson, P. (1992) Opiate misusers: are treatments effective? In *Practical Problems in Clinical Psychiatry* (ed. Hawton, K. and Cowen, P.). Oxford, Oxford University Press.

Robson, P. (1999) Drug policy — a time for change? In *Forbidden Drugs* (2nd edn). Oxford, Oxford University Press.

CASE 6.2

Ida Harbottle — dementia, true wishes, and personal identity

Synopsis A 69-year-old divorced woman, whose son is in Australia, has moderately severe Alzheimer's disease. She refuses all help from Mental Health and Social Services because she wants to be independent. But in practice she is making her neighbours' lives impossible by asking for help up to twenty times a day.

Key dilemma Should she be 'helped' by Mental Health and/or Social Services against her expressed wishes?

Main topics Ethical relevance of 'true wishes' and 'true self' in issues of consent and control.

Other topics Consent; competence; dementia; involuntary treatment; personal identity; hypotheticals; casuistry; principlism; Nussbaum; Rawls; reflective equilibrium; Williams; successive selves; Aristotle; Descartes; Locke; Hume; memory; consciousness; best interests; paternalism.

Ida Harbottle, a divorced woman of 69, lives alone in a small house in a 'respectable' suburb. Her only child, a son, lives in Australia. Mrs Harbottle is a former hospital personnel officer and has retained a sympathetic interviewing manner which she presents to professionals involved in her care. Dementia of the Alzheimer's type, however, is rapidly eroding her short-term memory. In addition, she has recently been bereaved of a 'gentleman friend' who took her out to tea dances and provided her with companionship.

Ida's neighbours, Ken and Annie Baines, had always asked Ida if she needed anything whenever they went to the shops. This has developed into a situation in which Ida knocks on Ken's door at least a dozen times a day, asking for items which she already has, or requesting other kinds of help. Ken and Annie are fond of Ida, admiring her independence, but they were hoping that their retirement would be a peaceful time. In addition, they have travel plans which they feel must be deferred for the time being, given Ida's condition. They are willing to do what they can: 'Auntie Ida' used to babysit for nothing when their children were small. But whenever Ida calls, she insists it is the first time that day — even if it is the tenth. Nor does she recall when people have visited her. When her television set is turned on, she believes that people are in the house, and she is more likely to 'remember' these non-existent 'visits'.

Ida's son, Gerald, flew over six weeks ago to try to sort out his mother's situation. Uncharacteristically, his once impeccably polite mother began shouting at him as soon as he raised the issue of moving into a nursing home. She furiously refused any help, claiming that she was managing perfectly well on her own. Gerald found his mother's condition very distressing and was stunned by the apparent change in her personality. Before he was sent to Australia by his firm three years ago, they had been quite close. Through Ida's GP he asked for a psychiatric referral, much to his mother's annoyance. It was decided that every effort should be made to enable Ida to remain at home, but to reduce dependence on her neighbours. After all, Gerald reasoned, if he could arrange a home help and 'meals on wheels', the burden on Ken and Annie would be reduced. But as soon as Gerald had left, three weeks ago, Ida dismissed all the domiciliary services. She is a house-proud woman, and resented 'having to tidy up for all these visitors'. On top of the 'visits' she believes to be going on when voices are on the television, it was all too much for her. Anyway, she said, she preferred her neighbours' help to the company of strangers.

'I've known Ida over twenty years,' Annie remarked recently. 'She'd hate to see herself now, you know. This isn't like her, banging on our door all the time. Used to keep herself to herself, so independent. This isn't really what she wants, I don't think, but then, I don't know what she really does want.'

The community psychiatric team are left with a dilemma. Ida has a known organic cerebral impairment, affecting her ability to assess her own need for care. She furiously refuses offers of help, but in practice seeks help constantly from Ken and Annie. In interviews, however, she can still be polite, even charming, and apparently rational. So long as she is treated in a gentle,

non-threatening manner, she accepts visits. But any mention of formal assessment procedures or admission to another environment provokes an angry
refusal and an unwillingness to accept any further visits. Yet they are uncertain about whether, deep down, she really wants help. At their most
recent meeting, two issues dominated their discussion. First, what are Ida's
wishes at present — her 'true choice'? Second, what would her previous
self's wishes have been?

In contrast to the floridly literary style of the case of 'Captain Ahab', Ida's
case may seem quite pedestrian and ordinary. This does not make it any less of
a dilemma. Everyday cases are too often downplayed in medical ethics, which
thrives on the dramatic hypothetical or the courtroom clash. This style has
become a sort of formula in medical ethics — in part because it compels attention; in part because the exception tests the rule. But any formula is ultimately
counter-productive. 'The problem with clinical ethics arises when the genre
becomes formulaic, when it forces us to look only at those aspects of the case
decided in advance to be significant: at that most constricted of literary genres,
the medical record.' (Murray 1995, p. 30)

The inductive approach, exemplified by casuistry or case analysis — in contrast to the deductive approach of principlism — can only work if it is based on
the widest possible range of beginnings. To narrow our base down to the
dramatic instance and the precedent-setting case automatically prejudices our
chances of success in deriving balanced clinical judgements and reaching some
sort of moral 'reflective equilibrium' (to use John Rawls' phrase). As Martha
Nussbaum has written:

> Moral knowledge...is not simply intellectual grasp of propositions; it is not even
> simply intellectual grasp of particular facts; it is perception. It is seeing a complex
> concrete reality in a highly lucid and richly responsive way; it is taking in what is
> there, with imagination and feeling. (Nussbaum 1991, cited in Murray 1995, p. 30)

It is important to be sensitive to what kinds of case studies we look at, as well as
to what we find in them.

In fact, we will use the everyday example of how to manage Ida's care in order
to explore some of the most persistently troubling problems in philosophy,
concerning personal identity. Senile dementia actually illustrates two different
types of problem, both subsumed under the heading of personal identity:

1 Identification — what it takes to be a person: a difficulty which also arises in
relation to psychopathy and severe retardation.

2 Reidentification — whether A is the same person as B: an issue in hysteria,
fugue, and multiple personality states as well (Wilkes 1988).

We will mainly be concerned with reidentification.

Dissimilar as they may look on the surface, the first two case studies in this section both remind us of the need to site the patient in relationship when developing a management plan. In discussing 'Captain Ahab's' case, we tried to keep the interests of his children to the fore. Here, in the case of Ida Harbottle, it is equally vital to bear the interests of others in mind — Ken and Annie, clearly, and Gerald. This is true not merely because they, like Ida, have rights as individuals, but because of the special bonds of intimacy.

> ...all the conflicts that may go on within families aren't necessarily conflicts between individuals or subgroups of individuals: some will be clashes between what an individual family member needs or wants, and the things a family needs so that it can do its special job of conveying the goods of intimacy. (Lindemann Nelson and Lindemann Nelson 1995, p. 86)

When family members clash, as Ida and Gerald have done, something more is going on than conflicts of individual rights. It is more productive to understand the tension in terms of Ida's rights versus Gerald's duties of care, which he is trying to fulfil. This means that Ida's rights do not necessarily 'trump', as they would in a purely patient-centred view.

Taking a family-centred view, therefore, is the first caveat we want to suggest before launching into the main part of our discussion. (We might want to extend the notion of family to Ken and Annie, too.) The second also concerns understandable but perhaps excessive concentration on the patient's rights. Because psychiatric illness is commoner in old age, but a psychiatric diagnosis actually harder to make, clinicians normally tend to play safe by over-diagnosing mental illness in the elderly (Oppenheimer 1991, p. 367). Sensitive clinicians will be aware of this tendency, and may therefore consciously tend to under-diagnose or under-treat. This could be particularly true in conditions for which effective treatment is hard to find, such as dementia. Is something of this sort going on in the management of Ida's case?

This may well be true, but there is also another possibility, likewise especially linked to the management of dementia. 'In dementia, it is difficult to make the same clear distinction between a person and her illness that we make when we compulsorily treat functional illness.' (Oppenheimer 1991, p. 373) To put it another way, the management of dementia raises philosophical issues about identity and true wishes, and it is on these that we shall concentrate the rest of our discussion. Ida's clinicians are concerned about whether her refusal of consent to assessment or any further steps represents her true wishes. As Annie points out, Ida's present state is not at all likely to be what her past self would have wanted. At the present time she is totally dependent on Ken and Annie, although she claims to be managing entirely on her own. A clear-sighted woman, Ida would probably have hated to see the tangle of contradictory beliefs and anger at her son which she has become. Her words indicate one thing, her actions another. Her 'previous self' might well have wanted help to be given, the clinicians' questions imply; perhaps her very independence of character actually suggests that.

But can we be so sure that Ida's 'true' identity is her past, pre-demented self? We need to be very sparing in our use of the 'previous self' notion. Bernard Williams has underlined

> ...the basic importance for our thought of the ordinary idea of a self or person which undergoes changes of character, as opposed to an approach which, even if only metaphorically, would dissolve the person, under changes of character, into a series of 'selves'. (Williams 1981, p. 5)

Perhaps it is all the more important that we should cling to a unified sense of identity throughout life, because we no longer see identity as conferred at birth — by social status, gender, or rank in the 'great chain of being'. Our identity is no longer legislated by divine authority but, in a post-modern or an existentialist analysis, created through the decisions which we take. The Aristotelian and medieval view of the world as populated with fixed essences was largely overturned by Descartes, and subsequently by Locke and Hume.

In his *Treatise of Human Nature*, Hume questioned 'whether in pronouncing concerning the identity of a person, we observe some real bond among his perceptions, or only feel one among the ideas we form of them'. Hume opts for the latter — the felt bond — which arises from the causal relations which a person perceives among his or her own experiences (Vesey 1987). Hume's analysis does not necessarily entail that someone's successive sets of perception can be labelled the experiences of different people. It merely calls into question — in quite a radical way — whether the notion of coherent identity is itself coherent. Rather than seeing past and present selves as separate, it undermines the notion of the self altogether. Hume does not think of identity as continuous or of consciousness as unified. 'The true idea of the human mind,' he wrote, 'is to consider it as a system of different perceptions or different existences, which are linked together by the relation of cause and effect, and mutually produce, destroy, influence and modify each other.' The implications of this view were so vertiginous that Hume wrote, in the appendix to the *Treatise*: 'Upon a more strict review of the section concerning personal identity, I find myself in such a labyrinth, that, I must confess, I neither know how to correct my former opinions, nor how to render them consistent.'

If instead we do see the person as a series of selves, the problem of whose wishes should take precedence becomes one of political theory, of deciding who among the selves should rule over the others. None of their wishes can be identified as 'true wishes' which should constrain the others. There is no innate reason why any one of these 'selves' or 'individuals' should be allowed to legis-late for the others. However, the 'selves' with better powers of foresight and self-governance might be presumed to have an edge over the others; a prudent, rational, past 'self' should be allowed to determine what happens to a present confused and irrational one.

The foundational notion of autonomy, if defined as the capacity to govern oneself, is threatened if we admit that there can be multiple identities and mul-tiple selves (Adshead 1997). Then it becomes impossible to identify what it would mean to lack autonomy: even if I manifestly cannot govern myself, even if I flit from one set of contradictory actions and beliefs to another, I can sim-ply claim that I am merely embodying a series of desires and a series of selves. But if that is so, then I cannot claim that my preferences should be respected because they are the preferences of an autonomous agent. So, accepting the notion of a past self and a present self in Ida's case gives no reason for thinking that we should respect the wishes of the past self above that of the present self.

The alternative, which maintains the notion of the autonomous self with a single identity, would be to identify Ida's pre-dementia personality with her true and only self. That means that the present 'Ida' is not really a self at all. But this seems quite a harsh conclusion, beset with further difficulties: exactly when, for example, did she stop being a self? Perhaps one might want to argue that she will have lost her selfhood when she loses her memory of the incidents and people who make up her identity. To the extent that our identity is consti-tuted through social interaction and buoyed up by memories (Lindemann Nelson and Lindemann Nelson 1995), the 'person' who has lost memories that constitute selfhood (for example, where my house is, what my relatives and friends mean to me) is not so much a different person as not a person at all. As one woman in the early stages of Alzheimer's disease put it, 'I feel like half a person. Where's the rest of me?' (Shapiro 1989). Note that she does not say, 'Where's the other me?'

If this is so — if Ida is no longer a person, rather than a different self — then balancing her interests against those of her carers becomes much easier: she can-not really be said to have any interests. This is clearly an extreme view that belies the clinician's duty of care and would make most of us profoundly uncom-fortable. It is at best a useful reminder that Ida's current wishes ought not auto-matically to dominate over the wishes of her carers. But we already knew that.

Is there no possible compromise between the two positions? Must we say either that Ida is no longer a person, or that her present self is different from her past self? A third possibility is suggested by Locke's argument from the identity of consciousness. Although consciousness can be interrupted by forgetfulness — as in Ida's case — that is not sufficient to undermine personal identity. This seems consistent with commonsense, which recognizes that we can remember things wrongly without losing our identities. By inference, then, if we don't remember them at all, we don't actually stop being the same person. According to this view, even the invasive forgetfulness of dementia is not enough to label Ida either a non-person or a different person: she still has the same identity.

Is the corollary that her current wishes are the ones which count? That really is another matter. There are all kinds of reasons why we might not want to take Ida's current wishes to be the wishes of an autonomous agent, without resorting to the philosophically dubious argument that they are not her wishes at all, or not the wishes of her 'true' self. Her wishes may be irrational or imprudent, but still truly hers. Yet we are not obliged to grant every authentic wish: wishes which are morally wrong, for example, receive no such protection.

It is better if we admit straightforwardly that we are not granting imprudent and dangerous wishes because we judge that they are not in the best interests of the patient. This may be paternalistic, but it is at least honest. It does not resort to the fiction of what the patient's 'real self' would want or what her 'true wishes' are. This is likely to become particularly uncomfortable if the patient's present wishes are perfectly consistent with her past ones, but still ill-advised, in the clinician's judgement. Then it will be necessary to construct an imaginary, past, autonomous self for the patient — a sanitized version of the person before us — to whom we can appeal. Something of this sort seems to be going on more and more often. There is an increasing tendency to trot out the 'true wishes' argument in place of overt paternalism: for example, in the Law Commission proposals on mental incapacity, which suggest that

> A mentally disordered person should be considered unable to take the medical treatment decision in question if he or she can understand the information relevant to taking the decision but is unable because of mental disorder to make a true choice in relation to it. (Law Commission 1993, Section 2.20)

We recognize that there are times when it is appropriate to use the notion of someone's 'true wishes': for example, in the case of a person with learning difficulties who cannot express their wishes readily. In the case of children, too, simple difficulties in communication may obscure what it is that the child really wants (Dickenson and Jones 1995, p. 191). What we want to warn against, however, is too wholesale a use of either 'true wishes' or 'past self'. Both notions raise more philosophical difficulties than they solve; on a pragmatic level, both represent an attempt to avoid having to admit paternalism. In thinking about how to manage Ida's troubling problems, her clinicians might do better to begin by rephrasing what they are. What Ida's 'true wishes' are is not a matter for clinical investigation; thinking about the problem this way raises more difficulties than it solves. Asking what her previous self would have wanted is probably no better.

Practitioner commentary (CASE 6.2)

Julian Hughes Consultant in Old Age Psychiatry, Newcastle General Hospital

At the end of this case history, Dickenson and Fulford suggest that the community psychiatric team have two issues dominating their discussion. First, what are Ida Harbottle's true choices; secondly, what would her previous self's wishes have been? I think that the case history is true to life, but I doubt that many community psychiatric teams would actually bother with these questions for long (and with the second, hardly at all). Instead, clinicians would ask: 'what is it practical to do?' The conceptual notion to support any action taken would be that of 'best interests'. The task for the clinical team, therefore, is to establish Ida's best interests. Whereas philosophy often informs and clarifies clinical practice, this is an example of the traffic going in the opposite direction (Fulford 1991).

What clinical practice ought to show is that the estimation of 'best interests' must (to have practical usefulness) be as broadly based as possible. Moreover, the broad conception of 'best interests' finds some support in philosophy. I have in mind Anscombe's seminal essay 'Modern moral philosophy' (1981), where she suggests that it is not profitable to do moral philosophy until we have an adequate philosophy of psychology. This surely relates to things that Wittgenstein said about 'inner' mental states.

To return to Ida Harbottle, what constitutes her 'best interests' involves what is going on in her mind (her wishes and inclinations), but it also involves her relationships and standing as a person in a unique context. So 'best interests' brings into play her son, her neighbours, as well as her history. A conceptual analysis of 'best interests', therefore, would have practical consequences. First, to establish her 'best interests' we need to meet with as many people as possible who have relevant information concerning Ida. Secondly, the way forward is probably for someone from the team to establish a therapeutic relationship with Ida. That is, someone must enter the nexus of relationships in which Ida's 'best interests' are to be established. The aim of the relationship is to shift her towards a practical outcome, in keeping with her 'best interests'. 'Best interests' is not to be decided, however, by reference to particular 'inner' goings-on in Ida, nor by the goings-on in the mind of her consultant psychiatrist. Rather, her 'best interests' are to be worked out as a practical matter, in public space, taking into account elements from her history and from the situated position (physical, psychological, social, and spiritual) in which she now finds herself.

Wittgenstein moves us towards a broader understanding of mental states. He does this by showing that there are certain features of mental states which are not just 'inner', but decidedly 'outer' too. I am tempted to say (with a stamp of my foot) that I *know* (inwardly) what is best for me. But Ida can undertake this performance as well. If the 'inner' is construed broadly, then 'best interests' cannot simply be a matter of what passes through Ida's mind, or the mind of her doctor. If Wittgenstein impels us in this broadening direction, so too does good clinical practice, which must take a broad view, necessitating wide consultation and a type of expert negotiation if it is to achieve its practical objective.

There is a final point to be made about Ida Harbottle. If we take a broad conception of mental states, then that should lead us to a broader conception of personal identity. My identity cannot just depend upon the 'inner' voice of memory that I happen to be experiencing at this moment. For memory, too, has an outer, shareable aspect. And if this is the case, then personal identity will not disappear with the fading of memory. In *Life's Dominion* (1993), Dworkin concludes, in connection with the severely demented, by talking of dignity and the sacred. My contention is that such concepts are instantiated in the context of good-quality care. The practical business of talking and listening and forming relationships, in order to move a situation forward, is a truer characterization of clinical practice than that of estimating true choices and the previous self's wishes. This makes sense from the philosophical perspective which regards psychological states and personal identity as being constituted not only by the 'inner', but also by the reality of physically embodied, historically and socially situated human beings in the world — a reality which persists even in severe dementia.

References (CASE 6.2)

Adshead, G. (1997) 'All in the mind: autonomy, feminism and the self.' Paper presented at the second Turku workshop of the European Biomedical Ethics Practitioner Education Project, June 1997.

Anscombe, G.E.M. (1981). Modern moral philosophy. In *The Collected Philosophical Papers of G.E.M. Anscombe. Volume 3: Ethics, Religion and Politics*, pp. 26–42. Oxford, Blackwell. (First published in 1958 in *Philosophy*, **33**.)

Dickenson, D. and Jones, D. (1995) True wishes: the philosophy and developmental psychology of children's informed consent. *Philosophy, Psychiatry and Psychology*, **2/4**:287–304.

Dworkin, R. (1993). *Life's Dominion*. London, Harper Collins.

Fulford, K.W.M. (1991). The potential of medicine as a resource for philosophy. *Theoretical Medicine,* **12**:81–5.

Hume, D. (1740) *A Treatise of Human Nature* (ed. Selby Bigge, L.A., 1978). Oxford, Oxford University Press.

Law Commission (1993) *Mentally Incapacitated Adults and Decision-Making: Medical Treatment and Research. Consultation Paper No. 129.* London, HMSO.

Lindemann Nelson, H. and Lindemann Nelson, J. (1995) *The Patient in the Family: An Ethics of Medicine and Families.* London, Routledge.

Murray, T.H. (1995) Attending to particulars. In 'Does clinical ethics distort the discipline?' *Hastings Center Report,* **26**, pp. 28–34.

Nussbaum, M.C. (1991) *Love's Knowledge. Essays on Philosophy and Literature.* Berkeley: University of California Press.

Oppenheimer, C. (1991) Ethics and psychogeriatrics. In *Psychiatric Ethics* (2nd edn) (ed. Bloch, S. and Chodoff, P.), pp. 365–89. Oxford, Oxford University Press.

Shapiro, J. (1989) *Ourselves, Growing Older: Women Ageing with Knowledge and Power.* London, Fontana/Collins. (British version of original text by Doress, P.B., Siegal, D.L., and the Midlife and Older Women Book Project in co-operation with the Boston Women's Health Book Collective.)

Vesey, G. (1987) Personal identity. In *The Oxford Companion to the Mind* (ed. Gregory, R.L.). Oxford, Oxford University Press.

Wilkes, K.V. (1988) *Real People: Personal Identity without Thought Experiments.* Oxford, Clarendon Press.

Williams, B. (1981) Persons, character and morality. In *Moral Luck,* pp. 1–19. Cambridge, Cambridge University Press.

CASE 6.3
Robin and Alex — testing genetic testing

Synopsis Robin, age 15, requests genetic testing, after being told that her father has tested positive for Huntington's disease (which in turn was prompted by the paternal grandmother's death from this condition). Robin and her younger brother, Alex, have recently been returned to the family after a period in care following suspected abuse by the maternal grandfather. The family are getting on well with the support of the local psychiatrist, and Robin's parents support her request. However, the local clinical genetics service will not see children under 18.

Key dilemma Should the psychiatrist support Robin and her parents against the local clinical genetics service?

Main topics Genetic testing in psychiatry; capacity in young people.

Other topics Children's consent; autonomy and beneficence; consent; capacity; ownership of genetic information; 'true wishes'; negligence; professional codes; guidelines; uncertainty; rationality; role of the family; non-maleficence; values; individualism; property in body; Locke.

Robin Parfit, a girl of fifteen, has recently been returned to her family of origin, together with her ten-year-old brother, Alex. Despite protests from their parents, the children had been placed in care after allegations of neglect and suspected sexual abuse by their maternal grandfather. While the children were in foster care, their father Tom was diagnosed with Huntington's disease: he had himself tested after his mother died of the condition. At present Tom is asymptomatic, although clinically depressed.

Tom's diagnosis, combined with the development of an emotionally abusive relationship in the foster home, increased pressure in favour of the children's return home. Things have been going quite well at home, with the family maintaining a good relationship with Fiona Slattery, the consultant child psychiatrist in the case. Fiona was not involved in the abuse investigation, although she had participated in the initial stages of the case.

However, Fiona is now uncertain how to respond to Robin's expressed wish to be tested for Huntington's disease. (The news of her father's diagnosis was broken to the girl by her parents, five months after she returned home, although they have kept the news from Alex.) In one sense there is no dilemma for Fiona: the predictive testing guidelines at her local clinical genetics unit stipulate that a patient must be aged eighteen or over to be tested. (In fact, that is the only part of the information leaflet for families which is printed in bold type.) In the interim, Robin is receiving genetic counselling.

But this raises problems for Robin's long-term management, until she turns eighteen, and risks harming the good therapeutic relationship which Fiona has built up with her and her family. (For Alex, there would be an even longer period to manage.) Although Robin is generally a 'laid-back' young woman, she seems quite firm in her desire to be tested now, though being a quiet and compliant sort of person, she accepts what she has been told about the 'eighteen' rule. Her parents also support her right to be tested, not least because Robin has a boyfriend. Robin's mother, Sally, feels particularly strongly that information should not be withheld from Robin. Sally's older sister has recently developed breast cancer, the condition from which their mother died. Sally is considering having herself tested for the BRCA1 gene implicated in some familial patterns of breast cancer. She has discussed the implications of the test with her husband and daughter.

Fiona wonders whether Robin's request may be mixed with anticipatory grief for her father — with a desire to show solidarity with him. Perhaps she also needs to be the perfect child for her parents, now that she is home from her foster placement. Is she simply too vulnerable, as well as too young, to learn what could be a very ugly truth? A diagnosis of Huntington's disease in Robin might also sever the bond between her and Alex, and increase pressure for the younger child to be told and tested. Finally, testing could upset the parents' attempt to protect both children from future harm (the vulnerable child syndrome). All these seem important (if hypothetical) considerations to Fiona, but deep down she wonders if she is just being paternalistic. Or is it just that she can't endure the idea of knowing for certain that this vulnerable girl carries the Huntington's marker in addition to all her other burdens?

Both evolving law and changing professional guidelines in the UK suggest that the clinical genetic unit's guidelines are too rigid in affirming an 'eighteen' rule, although they do not necessarily come down on the side of definitely allowing Robin to be tested. To some extent, practice may be changing and age cut-offs becoming less common. But the ethical issues in this case remain problematic, not least because they upset the usual pattern of paternalism and autonomy — a point to which we return later.

The main legal question to be considered in this case concerns the capacity of children and young people to consent to treatment or testing (Dickenson 1999). Since 'treatment' includes diagnosis (Family Law Reform Act 1969, Section 8[2]), consent to testing can be considered under the same rubric as consent to treatment. The general legal principle that eighteen is the age of majority was modified in the Family Law Reform Act to allow young persons of sixteen to give consent which would be as valid and effective as an adult's. More recent case law has undermined the ability of young people under eighteen to refuse consent to a procedure. For example, in Re W (1992) the Court of Appeal held that where someone with parental responsibility gave consent to treatment on the minor's behalf, the young person — a sixteen-year-old anorexic girl — could not refuse. However, that is not the case here: both Robin's parents and she give consent, and the young person's right to consent was reiterated in Re W.

It might be objected that Robin is still only fifteen, whereas the dividing line in the Family Reform Act was sixteen (also the age of the girl in Re W). But in the Gillick case (1985), the argument that a fifteen-year-old girl's consent to treatment would be legally ineffective was rejected by the majority in the House of Lords. Instead of an age-specific criterion, a function-specific, flexible test of competence was set down — whether the young person had 'sufficient understanding and intelligence to enable him or her to understand fully what is proposed' (Gillick *v* W. Norfolk AHA (1985), at 423). Although in time-honoured fashion the Law Lords refrained from stipulating exactly what 'understand fully' might mean, Lord Scarman, at least, included the emotional and familial implications of the decision in addition to cognitive criteria. One could certainly argue that Robin is likely to have a fuller understanding than many fifteen-year-olds of the familial implications of genetic disorders, particularly with her mother's decision about being tested for the BRCA1 gene having been shared with the rest of the family. Nor is there any indication that her cognitive functioning is in any way impaired. On balance, we feel, Robin is quite likely to be '*Gillick* competent' to consent. (If this were a Scottish case, she would also probably be able to consent on her own behalf, on the similar grounds that she had sufficient understanding of the issue to make a choice: see Age of Legal Capacity (Scotland) Act 1991, Section 2[4].)

Although Robin was in foster care at the time that her father was tested for Huntington's disease, it seems plausible that her grandmother's and aunt's cancers mean that Robin has been exposed to an atmosphere in which genetic disorder and the risks of testing are everyday subjects — which they are not in most families. According to Christine Lavery, director of the Society for Mucupolysaccharide Diseases and the mother of a seven-year-old boy who died of the genetic disorder Hunter's disease, her younger child Lucy was competent at seven to request the test — three years younger than Alex, and eight years younger than Robin. 'Children in families like ours, with a severe genetic disease, in which you know categorically that the affected child will die young, grow up very fast.' Lucy told her GP: 'No one is making me have this test. I just know that when I grow up, I could not cope with having a child with Hunter's disease.' (Ferriman 1996) Perhaps there is a parallel in children with chronic cardiac or orthopaedic conditions, such as those studied by Alderson (1990 and 1994), who likewise discovered that exposure to long-term conditions creates surprisingly high levels of familiarity with diagnostic procedures, cognitive sophistication about probabilities and prognosis, and strong personal values.

Another strand in the legal position is the Children Act 1989, which introduced 'the ascertainable wishes and feelings of the child considered concerned (considered in the light of his age and understanding)' into the 'welfare check-list' which must be used in deciding on the child's welfare in any case affecting him or his upbringing (Section 1[1][3]). However, the child's wishes are only one of several factors to be considered — albeit the first in the list. The Act also requires the decision to include consideration of 'his physical, emotional and educational needs', 'the likely effect on him of any change in his circumstances', and — perhaps most importantly in Robin's case — 'any harm which he has suffered or is at risk of suffering'. It might be argued that 'inflicting' the near-certainty of developing Huntington's disease on Robin, at such a vulnerable stage of her life, is indeed doing her a harm. But it is debatable whether disclosure of a terminal diagnosis would be regarded as a harm in this context: the definition of 'significant harm' in the Children Act was formulated more with areas such as ongoing abuse in mind.

Overall, however, the impact of the Children Act is not so radical as the doctrine of 'ascertainable wishes and feelings' might suggest (White *et al.* 1991; Eekelaar and Dingwall 1990). 'The principle that decision making should be influenced by the child's wishes is thus explicit in the Children Act, but the Act also leaves scope for courts to find that the child's expressed wishes are not her 'true wishes', those that serve her best interests.' (Dickenson and Jones 1995, p. 289). Certainly there might be grounds for arguing that Robin's expressed wishes are not her true wishes: Fiona has doubts about whether Robin's expressed wish to be tested can be put down to her desire to please her parents now that she has been reintegrated into the family. But as one of us has argued elsewhere (Dickenson and Jones 1995; Dickenson 1994), there is a great risk of paternalistic condescension in taking that line. Are an adult's wishes necessarily any more 'true'— particularly to an observer trained in psychoanalysis? Yet the competence of adults is not legally in doubt.

The last legal consideration which needs to be mentioned is negligence. Could Fiona be subject to a negligence action if Robin were tested and grave consequences resulted from a positive finding? This is a vulnerable young person, after all; what if Robin tried to harm herself as a result? Even if Fiona had merely followed her request, could that be argued to be professionally irresponsible? The probable answer is no if (1) Fiona was acting on her clinical judgement of Robin's best interests and (2) she could show that she was following a responsible body of medical opinion (*Bolam* v *Friern HMC*, 1957).

The first criterion — the Children Act requirement that the best interests of the child should dictate — would depend on clinical evidence about psychological morbidity in patients who test positive for adult-onset, incurable genetic disorders. There is a dearth of such evidence, although Brandt (1994) found no greater psychological morbidity for patients informed that they had tested positive than for those told they had negative status. There was already a high prevalence of affective psychological disorders in persons at risk for Huntington's disease. Certainly this seems applicable to Robin, particularly with the further complications of breast cancer and alleged abuse in the family. Fiona cannot simply turn the clock back to a state of innocence for this girl, much as she might like to.

The second criterion in relation to negligence would hinge on whether a responsible body of medical opinion favours testing for minors in cases of adult-onset, incurable disorder. That requires us to move beyond the law, and look now to professional codes and committees. In the past, whilst the consensus was quite clearly against such testing (meaning that Fiona could indeed be negligent on that count), it was also suggested that 'an over-rigid policy' against testing anyone under eighteen 'might be found negligent because it was not addressed to the particular child's needs and would therefore be unacceptable to professional opinion' (Clinical Genetics Society 1994, p. 789). So is Fiona caught in a 'Catch-22' situation?

Professional guidelines on the predictive testing of at-risk children all seem to share a common limitation: they focus primarily on the situation where parents request testing on the child's behalf, rather than the scenario in which the young person him- or herself wants to be tested. For example, in 1989, a research group of the World Federation of Neurology issued a policy statement on the then-available tests for Huntington's disease, declaring that children should not be tested on their parents' request. The limited applicability of those guidelines to this case is lessened still further by the change in testing procedures since then. The current, highly accurate genetic marker tests based on direct mutation testing, in a single blood test, were not available at that time; instead, what was required was a complicated and less accurate testing process using blood samples from several relations to detect linked genetic markers. The new procedure is based on the number of repeats of the 'gene for' Huntington's disease, which was only isolated in March 1993. The number of repeats of the gene, which the testing procedure ascertains, determines with great predictive accuracy whether an individual will manifest Huntington's disease. One might argue that the uncertainty which the current test removes is a benefit which the earlier working party would not have considered. Nor is it now essential to take samples from numerous family members (which had increased the numbers who might have been harmed without any obvious benefit).

Revision of these guidelines was necessary in the light of the altered testing process, and in 1994 a joint committee of the International Huntington Association and the World Federation of Neurology Research Group on Huntington's Chorea issued new recommendations (IHA/WFN 1994). The committee recommended that the test should be 'available only to individuals who have reached the age of majority (according to the laws of the respective country)', but it introduced a potential conflict by noting that 'it seems appropriate and even essential, however, that the child be informed of his or her at-risk status upon reaching the age of reason'. That raises troubling ethical issues to which we will return later. If the age of reason is thought to be younger than the age of majority, is it just that young people should be thought rational enough to cope with this knowledge, but not rational enough to consent to be tested?

In the same year, the Clinical Genetics Society (UK) issued guidelines produced by a working party chaired by Dr Angus Clarke. The CGS working party concluded that

...predictive testing for an adult-onset disorder should generally not be undertaken if the child is healthy and there are no medical interventions established as
useful that can be offered in the event of a positive test result unless there are
clear-cut and unusual arguments in favour...The more serious the disorder, the
stronger the arguments in favour of testing would need to be. (Clinical Genetics
Society 1994, p. 785)

Although discussion and counselling could and should be offered to minors,
'formal genetic testing should generally wait until the "children" request such
tests for themselves, as autonomous adults.' However, the working party did say
that testing should wait either until the person affected is adult or 'is able to
appreciate not only the genetic facts of the matter but also the emotional and
social consequences'. In this, the working party was apparently following Lord
Scarman's opinion in the *Gillick* case.

That the CGS working party was largely uninterested in cases such as Robin's
is illustrated by its survey of current practices and opinions. On the question,
'Who should have the right to request a test?', the only alternatives given to
interviewees were as follows: parents, extended families, adoption agencies,
and medical practitioners. No mention was made in the question of the mature
minor who wants to know his or her own genetic status. Indeed, the mature
minor was conspicuous by his or her absence throughout the report: younger
children seemed to be the focus. The most extensive breakdown of results in the
survey was a table asking whether clinicians would test a five-year-old child for
various genetic disorders. The survey turned up considerable variance between
geneticists and paediatricians on this question — whereas almost no geneticists
were willing to test the child for Huntington's disease, the majority of paediatricians would have done so. This raises interesting issues in relation to negligence: the responsible body of professional opinion differs from profession to
profession. It also suggests that Fiona Slattery is not alone in finding her local
laboratory's attitude more fixed than her own. The gap was widest on
Huntington's disease: 43 out of 49 geneticists would have tested for Marfan's
syndrome — a more pronounced majority than the 199 out of 260 paediatricians (Clinical Genetics Society 1994, Table 4, p. 796).

A reply to the CGS document by the Genetic Interest Group (GIG) — a
national umbrella organization representing genetic-disorder families —
agreed with the principle that 'children should not be tested for adult-onset
conditions for which there are no pre-symptomatic medical treatments'.
However, it warned that the overall tone of the CGS report was 'patronising to
parents' (GIG 1994, p. 2) and 'overly preoccupied with psychological considerations, and the harm that knowledge of genetic disorders can cause within
families...it seems to reflect more the fears of doctors that they will be held
responsible for negative reactions, rather than the needs of families'. As a

prime example of overreaction to negative risk, the GIG report cited Huntington's disease, claiming that there had only been one suicide after a positive test result in the ten years since testing was introduced, and that one related to failure to follow a protocol. It is worth quoting at some length from the GIG response on the subject of children's competence:

> Whilst we totally uphold the principle that families need counselling and support, we also believe they should be given credit for being responsible and having coping capacities. Although the vast majority would prefer there not to be a genetic disorder in their family, knowledge comes to be accepted as a fact of life in the same way that other issues are recognised to be individual and integral to any family. It is also our experience that children can cope with information about themselves from an early age and that it is much more often the adult who has a problem in giving information. We feel ourselves to be in a strange position in this argument — it is often the role of the voluntary sector to educate the medical profession in the need to understand psychological factors — perhaps the pendulum has swung too far the other way in genetics. (Genetics Interest Group 1994, p. 3)

Following a meeting in June 1996 between the Genetics Interest Group and Euroscreen (an EC-funded project on genetic screening), the BMA set up a working party to report on consent to genetic testing. The report (BMA 1998) did suggest a more flexible, less age-specific approach to testing mature minors: an exceptional case might be made for a young person with very high level of competence. Such BMA guidance itself lessens the chances that Fiona could be at risk of negligence, if she can argue that she is following the BMA line.

To summarize, both legal and professional guidelines appear to be evolving towards a less rigid bar against mature minors who request genetic testing. However, it will still be up to the psychiatrist to help Robin and her family construct a strong case for her *Gillick* competence. What if Fiona feels it would actually be ethically wrong to do so? We come now to our discussion of the properly ethical questions in Robin's case, which we will subdivide into three headings:

1 Paternalism, best interests, and autonomy

2 Consent and capacity

3 Rights in and ownership of genetic information

Paternalism, best interests, and autonomy

Fiona Slattery suspects that she may just be being paternalistic in denying Robin access to genetic testing for Huntington's disease, or, more properly, in relying uncritically on the guidelines which deny it. The paternalism/autonomy chestnut is often useful, but in this case it is too simplistic. Paternalism usually favours treatment on the grounds of best interests, even in the absence of the patient's consent; here we have the reverse. The paternalistic thing to do in Robin's case is not to override her refusal and impose treatment, but to override her consent and withhold the test.

The difference is only superficial, however. In both cases, the underlying rationale of paternalism would be the notion of beneficence (of doing good) as outweighing patient autonomy. The reason why this case is unusual is that generally treatment is presumed to be beneficial, and therefore in the patient's best interests. If there is no possibility of treatment for Huntington's disease, then presumably there is no benefit in knowing that one carries the genetic marker for the disorder — and therefore, testing is not in the patient's best interests. The principle of beneficence would not dictate testing, since no good can be done; the principle of non-maleficence ('first do no harm') might well dictate not testing. It should be noted in passing that this sort of argument applies as much to adults as to children. We will return to the question of why adults are thought competent to consent to genetic testing regardless, whereas children and young people are not. For now, we simply want to examine the argument that no good can be done by genetic testing for incurable adult-onset disorders in young people — that such testing imposes harm with no countervailing benefit.

We have already noted that the jury is out on the question of whether psychological morbidity is affected by a positive test result (see the aforementioned reference to Brandt 1994). So, whether harm is being done is debatable, even in psychiatric terms; and if we extend our discussion beyond the medical and psychiatric, it is even possible that good is being done. The Genetic Interest Group complained, in its critique of the Clinical Genetics Society guidelines, that physicians were too fixated on harm from disclosure of an adverse genetic status because they were too narrowly concerned with medical harms and benefits. There are other kinds of benefits than cure, although it has to be noted that there are non-medical harms from testing, too — for example, opportunities may be denied if a child is felt to have no future (Wertz *et al.* 1997, p. 878). This is merely a hypothesis, counterbalanced by the data in Bloch *et al.* (1993), who reported a sense of relief from uncertainty, even on learning of a high-risk test result — an important benefit. But according to some studies 'a high-risk result merely exchanges the uncertainty of whether HD will develop for that of when it will develop' (Scourfield *et al.* 1997, p. 148).

There is also the benefit of control, especially potent for adolescents. Wanting to take control of one's future, including one's reproductive future, seems to us a perfectly valid and indeed very 'adult' motivation for a young person to request genetic testing for an incurable adult-onset disorder. Although it is unclear whether Robin's request has anything to do with her sexual life —

which seems to be more her parents' concern than hers — that could be an important factor. There is a tension between the age of sexual maturity and that of legal majority, which the law recognizes to some extent: that is certainly a subtext in the *Gillick* decision. Similarly, the 'emancipated minor' doctrine in US law extends to pregnant girls living at home and teenage parents; in fact, some states set the age of fertility as the age of consent to contraception. If a young person is autonomous enough to have a sexual life and reproductive concerns, should that be where paternalism stops?

Consent and competence

Whatever the benefits–harms calculation, adults are allowed to request genetic testing for incurable disorders, subject to limitations of individual protocols; but young people under 18 are generally barred from doing so. Adults are presumed competent to consent to or refuse treatment, whereas children and young people are presumed incompetent unless 'proven' otherwise — by meeting the standards for *Gillick* competence to consent. Does Robin meet those standards? We have already argued that there is a strong case for suggesting that she does; but it might be objected that she is too vulnerable in several senses — her history of abuse, her recent reintegration into the family, and the very fact that she is at risk for Huntington's disease.

But we are all by definition vulnerable at the time we are asked to give an informed consent to treatment: generally, we are ill or facing uncertain results about a possible diagnosis. Why is Robin any different? There are unique factors in this family's dynamics, one might argue, which could make Robin vulnerable in another sense — vulnerable to parental influence. Is she just trying to show solidarity with her afflicted family? Do her parents have particular reasons — reasons which are against her individual best interest — for wanting her tested? If so, we might be entitled to doubt whether her consent meets the crucial legal requirement of voluntariness, and, in ethical terms, whether she is really an independent moral agent.

It may well be true that adolescents are more subject to family influence than adults: studies of 14- and 15-year-olds asked to make hypothetical medical decisions showed that these teenagers frequently deferred to what they saw as their parents' wishes (Sherer and Repucci 1988). But that is just what families are about: studies of adults might equally well show that they did what they thought their spouses or children would want. Again, there is no absolute dividing line between adults and children on the issue of voluntariness of consent or refusal. In *Re T* (1992) a 20-year-old Jehovah's Witness was compelled to receive a blood transfusion on the grounds that her refusal was insufficiently autonomous — that she was too much under the influence of her mother. Conversely, in *Re E* (1993) a judge ordered a 15-year-old Jehovah's Witness to receive a transfusion against his wishes, but the boy exercised his right to refuse transfusions when he turned eighteen, and died; his values and beliefs were coherent at fifteen, and representative of what they would be at eighteen.

We need to guard against the corollary of distrusting any consent to testing given by an adolescent on the grounds that it 'really' represents pressure from his or her parents. If the young person's values and identity seem reasonably coherent and secure, then a consent should be honoured — as should a refusal. But identity only comes with making choices and having them honoured (Dickenson and Jones 1995). We noted earlier that it is odd to distinguish between the 'age of reason' at which a young person should be told that she is at risk for Huntington's disease and the much later age at which she can consent to be tested. If she is rational enough to know the risks, then arguably she is rational enough to know whether they are real for her. The limbo Robin is in now is doing her sense of efficacy and identity no good at all.

Ownership of genetic information: individual or family?

Is it necessarily wrong that families should exert an influence over their members when it comes to genetic testing? The model of ownership of genetic information in our society is individualistic: the individual is the locus of autonomy and rights, and the individual is also an adult. But a growing dissatisfaction with such a narrowly atomistic model has made itself felt both in feminist moral theory (Gilligan 1982; Held 1993; Lloyd 1992; Dickenson 1997) and in medical ethics, where autonomy-centred approaches are under fire from more communitarian alternatives.

Rights in genetic information hinge on rights in the body, but although it is usually assumed that we own our bodies unequivocally, the genesis of this notion is ambiguous. Classical Lockean liberal theory is usually thought to be the source, but in fact Locke does not claim that we have a property in our bodies (Waldron 1988; Dickenson 1997). What we do have is property in our person, in our moral agency and identity. We do not own our bodies unequivocally because we did not labour to create them — God did, according to Locke. Since property rights are created by labour, we have no such property rights over our bodies.

It is plausible, if speculative, to argue that to the extent that families give birth to and labour to bring up their children, they have some sort of mutual property rights in their genetic information that pertains to them. Less controversially, we might well want to argue that the negative claim, at least, is true: even if families do not have a positive claim to ownership and control over their members' genetic data, the individual member is not the sole owner. The excesses of such a view must be avoided, of course. Families do not have an unequivocal right to have their children tested, when those children cannot give an informed consent. But in this case, where both the young person and the family agree, we must be equally careful not to impose a conflictual, individualistic model based on the premise that individual and family interests necessarily collide.

Practitioner commentary (CASE 6.3)

Hilary Henderson Consultant Child Psychiatrist, Barnet Healthcare NHS Trust

I was quickly drawn into identifying with the child psychiatrist in this case, Dr Fiona Slattery. Many of the issues raised are akin to my everyday work on the front line: not the genetics testing as such or Huntington's disease — I have virtually no direct experience in either of these — but more the task of teasing out beliefs, wishes, and hidden agendas, to try and help children and families towards the nearest best solution to whatever predicament they face. A recent similar experience of my own involved a young teenager seeking a breast reduction operation; another involved choosing a live donor from within family members for a child in end-stage renal failure. Cases as difficult as these do not come up every day, but I believe that our training as child psychiatrists in both physical and psychological aspects of medicine, coupled with experience in complex family systems, equips us with a good grounding for this kind of work.

In reading the story of Robin and Alex, a number of key questions immediately sprang to mind. How has Dr Slattery become involved in the genetics testing issue in this case? Has it just emerged in the course of therapeutic work around other concerns? Or has another professional made a specific formal request? What exactly is her brief? And — most crucially — is it actually appropriate for her to take on this task given her existing relationship with the family? These children do not appear to have fared well at the hands of 'responsible' adults to date: the last thing they need is a muddle about Fiona Slattery's role.

The background to the case seems particularly complicated: suspected abuse by grandfather, history of neglect, the children's reception into care, subsequent emotional abuse within the foster home, grandmother's death from Huntington's disease, father's positive testing for this condition, his depression, and now, emerging concerns about the family risks for breast cancer on the mother's side. Again the detail is somewhat sparse and my curiosity was aroused. What was the nature of the suspected abuse? How did this come to light? Did one of the children make allegations?

What happened to Grandfather? And, most perplexing, why were these children taken into care? It was presumably thought to be in their best interests. Was it in line with their wishes? I found this particularly hard to understand given their ages and the circumstances described. The position of the local child psychiatrist, however, would be somewhat different. Dr Slattery was already involved in the case and would therefore know all these details and would probably be in close touch with colleagues in Social Services and other professionals from health and education.

When I first read the story, I was a little alarmed at the portrayal of Dr Slattery. She seemed to be going round and round in ever-increasing circles of organized speculation. I found myself wanting to say 'keep calm, just do a straightforward careful assessment, make sure you have brushed up your knowledge in all the relevant areas, and it's very probable that the "right" way forward will emerge. And if it doesn't, arrange a consultation with a colleague. It's such an interesting and challenging case: many psychiatrists would welcome the opportunity to share their thoughts with you.'

Reading on, though, I began to see the dilemma! I realized that I had already jumped the gun and positioned myself on the paternalistic side. This was on the basis of minimal information and my declaration about the importance of doing a proper assessment! It was quite sobering to note that I had already formed a clear picture of Robin inside my head and decided that I must protect her from acquiring the awful knowledge that she would go on to develop this appalling incurable condition. I was interested to see later on in the chapter that this is not uncommonly the stance of the medical profession, and then to read the counter-arguments put forward by the Genetic Interest Group, together with the very pertinent comments about the inconsistencies in age of 'majority', age of 'reason', and the almost magical acquisition of 'competence' from the legal point of view as soon as an individual becomes an adult.

There were some aspects of the debate which I was not able to follow, or with which I was not familiar, for example, the 'vulnerable child syndrome' and theories of Locke. As a practitioner, though, I was particularly interested in the fact that the Clinical Genetics Society appear to have omitted considering the position of the mature minor in their guidelines about genetic testing. I found myself wondering if this was by accident or design. In my experience it can be easier in some ways to present difficult information to younger children than to their teenage siblings. This allows them to grow up with the knowledge. Children are invariably aware when there is a family secret and I have all too often seen the adverse outcome in young children who have been misinformed in a misguided attempt to protect them from the truth. Given that the peak age for acts of self-harm is in the mid-teens, one could argue that it is less straightforward for adolescents, some of whom are at their most vulnerable and impulsive at around this time.

Another issue that is of particular interest to me is that of ascertaining the true wishes of children or indeed of adults for that matter. Again, based on my own clinical practice, it has been my experience that stated beliefs and wishes are not necessarily true ones. This is not to claim that psychiatrists have skills in reading people's minds. It is more to acknowledge the complexity of human communications. And I think that in situations as difficult as the one described we could be doing our young patients and their families a disservice if we simply accept what they say at face value.

Back to Robin and Alex. What would I do in Fiona Slattery's place? I think the first thing is to decide whether or not it is appropriate to take on this problem at all, given my existing therapeutic relationship with the family. I would see the genetics testing issue as a separate and important task, and not something which could just be slotted in, in the course of an ongoing family meeting. There is the need to obtain consent to collect and share information, to brush up on any unfamiliar areas, and to undertake a very careful assessment in whatever combination of meetings with individuals and members of the family seems appropriate. I would expect to see Robin on her own, and with her parents. And what about Alex?

In spite of my awareness of my positional change whilst reading the discussion, I still think it is probable that Dr Slattery, or I, would be able to reach a joint decision with Robin and her parents about Robin's best interests. This is also a situation in which wider discussion, with Robin and her parents' agreement, with other members of a multidisciplinary team may be very helpful. However, I do think it is important to hold on to whatever professional opinion one reaches, even if this appears to be at odds with the family's stated wishes. I was concerned by the notion that Dr Slattery might consider compromising her view in order to safeguard the therapeutic relationship which she had built up with the family.

Finally, I am left with an overriding impression of Dr Slattery's aloneness with her dilemma. This is not and should not be the case, but it is not uncommon. Sometimes reluctance to share decision making is determined by concerns about breaching confidentiality. More worryingly, in some fields of medicine there is a culture in which acknowledging uncertainty risks the designation 'wimp'.

References (CASE 6.3)

Alderson, P. (1990) *Choosing for Children*. Oxford, Oxford University Press.

Alderson, P. (1994) *Children's Consent to Surgery*. Buckingham, Open University Press.

Bloch, M., Adam, S., Fuller, A., *et al.* (1993) Diagnosis of Huntington's disease: a model for the stages of psychological response based on experience of a predictive testing program. *American Journal of Medical Genetics*, **47**:368–74.

Bolam v. Friern HMC (1957) 2 All ER 118.

BMA (1998) *Human Genetics: Choice and Responsibility*. Oxford, Oxford University Press.

Brandt, J. (1994) Ethical considerations in genetic testing: an empirical study of presymptomatic diagnosis of Huntington's disease. In *Medicine and Moral Reasoning* (ed. Fulford, K.W.M., Gillett, G.R., Soskice, J.M.) pp. 41–59. Cambridge, Cambridge University Press.

Clinical Genetics Society (1994) The genetic testing of children: report of a working party. *Journal of Medical Genetics*, **31**:785–97.

Dickenson, D. (1999) Can children and young people consent to testing for adult-onset genetic disorders? *BMJ*, **318**:1003–5.

Dickenson, D. (1994) Children's informed consent to treatment: is the law an ass? Guest Editorial, *Journal of Medical Ethics*, **20/4**:205–6.

Dickenson, D. (1997) *Property, Women and Politics*. Cambridge, Polity Press.

Dickenson, D. and Jones, D. (1995) True wishes: The philosophy and developmental psychology of children's informed consent. *Philosophy, Psychiatry, and Psychology*, **2**:287–304.

Eekelaar, J. and Dingwall, R. (1990) *The Reform of Child Care Law: A Practical Guide to the Children Act 1989*. London, Tavistock/Routledge.

Ferriman, A. (1996) A cruel inheritance. *Guardian*, 11 June.

Genetics Interest Group (1994) *GIG Response to the Clinical Genetics Society Report, 'The Genetic Testing of Children'*. GIG, London.

Held, V. (1993) *Feminist Morality: Transforming Culture, Society and Politics*. Chicago and London, University of Chicago Press.

Gilligan, C. (1982) *In a Different Voice: Psychological Theory and Women's Development*. Cambridge (Mass.), Harvard University Press.

IHA (International Huntington Association) and WFN (World Federation of Neurology Research Group on Huntington's Chorea) (1994). Guidelines for the Molecular Genetics Predictive Test in Huntington's disease. *Neurology*, **44**:1533–6.

Lloyd, G. (1992) *The Man of Reason: 'Male' and 'Female' in Western Philosophy* (2nd edn). London, Routledge.

Re E (1993) 1 FLR 386; (1994) 2 FLR 1065, 1075.

Re T (1992) 4 All ER 649.

Re W (1992) 4 All ER 627.

Scourfield, J., Soldan, J., Gray, J., Houlihan, G., and Harper, P.S., (1997) Huntington's disease: psychiatric practice in molecular genetic prediction and diagnosis. *British Journal of Psychiatry*, **178**:144–9.

Sherer, D.G. and Repucci, N.D. (1988) Adolescents' capacities to provide voluntary informed consent. *Law and Human Behaviour*, **12**:123–41.

Waldron, J. (1988) *The Right to Private Property*. Oxford, Clarendon Press.

Wertz, D.C., Fanos, J.H., and Reilly, P.R. (1997) Genetic testing for children and adolescents: who decides? *Journal of the American Medical Association*, **272/11**:875–81.

White, R., Carr, P., and Lowe, N. (1990) *A Guide to the Children Act*. London, Butterworths.

Reading Guide

Ethical issues of treatment choice, being one of the areas on which traditional bioethics has particularly focused, have generated a substantial literature. In this Reading Guide we indicate a few of the main sources for the headline topics in this literature — the closely related concepts of autonomy, capacity, competence, and consent. In psychiatry, though, as we have seen, the issues raised by these concepts beg deeper theoretical issues. We provide further reading here on one such issue, critically important in psychiatry — the nature of personal identity.

Autonomy, capacity, competence, and consent

A classic development of the principle of autonomy from a USA perspective is Tom Beauchamp and James Childress' *Principles of Biomedical Ethics* (1994). Beauchamp gives a brief and very clear account of autonomy, setting it in its philosophical–ethical context, in 'The philosophical basis of psychiatric ethics' (Chapter 3 in Bloch *et al.*'s *Psychiatric Ethics*, 1999). The strengths and limitations of the principles approach in psychiatry are discussed in K.W.M. Fulford and T. Hope's 'Psychiatric ethics: a bioethical ugly duckling?' (1993). Articles, with cross-disciplinary commentaries, exploring the theoretical underpinnings of consent in psychiatry, appear regularly in *PPP – Philosophy, Psychiatry and Psychology*: see, for example, Moore *et al.* (1994) on mania; Dickenson and Jones (1995) on children; Charland (1998) on the importance of emotion; and Savulescu and Dickenson (1998) on advance directives.

There is a growing volume of empirical work on consent, building on such examples as C.W. Lidz *et al.*, *Informed Consent: A Study of Decision Making in Psychiatry* (1984), and S. Wear's *Empirical Studies of Informed Consent* (1993). Work in this tradition is regularly reviewed in *The Bulletin of Medical Ethics* and in *Current Opinion in Psychiatry*. Valuable insights into the operation of psychiatry from the point of view of the user of services are given in *Experiencing Psychiatry: Users' Views of Services* by A. Rogers *et al.* (1993). Although not dealing specifically with psychiatry, G.J. Agich (1993) provides a highly relevant discussion of autonomy in *Autonomy and Long-Term Care*. Principles and casuistry are compared as approaches to ethical issues of consent in psychiatry in Fulford and Hope's (1993) chapter in Gillon's *Principles of Healthcare Ethics*. Priscilla Alderson's *Choosing for Children* (1990) shows the value of qualitative research.

Recent legal guidance on the assessment of capacity (in England and Wales) is given in a joint report of the British Medical Association and the Law Society, *Assessment of Mental Capacity* (1995). (Competence is the legal counterpart of capacity.) Issues of consent to treatment have been succinctly reviewed recently by the Medical Defence Union (1997).

Autonomy: recent approaches

Donna Dickenson (1998) has pointed out that bioethicists have often conflated the very different approaches to these issues which are taken by people in different parts of the world. Alternatives to the dominant principles-based approach include feminist ethics (for example, Adshead, forthcoming), narrative ethics (Widdershoven, forthcoming), and Hegelian ethics (for example, Dickenson 1997). These approaches emphasize aspects of consent, such as relationship, emotion, and the social context, which are likely to be particularly important in psychiatry.

The feminist challenge to the dominance of autonomy in bioethics, with its ensuing ambivalence about the concept's political uses against medical paternalism, is ably summarized in Susan Sherwin's chapter, 'Paternalism' in *No Longer Patient: Feminist Ethics and Health Care* (1993). Other feminist ethicists include Virginia Held, *Feminist Morality: Transforming Culture, Society and Politics* (1990) and Karen Green, *The Woman of Reason: Feminism, Humanism and Political Thought* (1995). This challenge has also been taken up by non-feminist writers, often from a viewpoint of dissatisfaction with the narrow view of rationality taken by games theory in the 1960s and rational choice theory in the 1990s. Authors who present a more nuanced view of rationality as intertwined with emotion rather than as opposed to it include Lawrence Blum, *Friendship, Altruism and Morality* (1980); Martha C. Nussbaum, *The Fragility of Goodness* (1986); and Allan Gibbard, *Wise Choices, Apt Feelings: A Theory of Normative Judgement* (1990).

Consent to psychiatric treatment in relation to children and young people is discussed from a legal, ethical, and practical viewpoint by Dickenson in a review article, 'Consent in children' (1998). A summary of the position in relation to Huntington's disease also appears in 'Can children and young people consent to testing for adult-onset genetic disorders?' in the *BMJ* (17 April 1999), which uses a version of the Robin and Alex case in this volume.

Personal identity

An excellent general introduction to issues of personal identity in psychiatry is Jonathan Glover's *I: The Philosophy and Psychology of Personal Identity* (1988). This book covers psychoanalytic as well as other psychological theories and a wide range of the philosophical topics traditionally included under personal identity. Ian Hacking in *Rewriting the Soul* (1995) offers a readable and very thorough recent survey, setting the subject in the context of the history of psychiatry (topics include child abuse, memory, schizophrenia, and false consciousness, as well as multiple personality disorder). Also excellent is Stephen Braude's *First Person Plural* (1991; 2nd edn 1995). George Graham's *Philosophy of Mind* (1993) has a very useful chapter on 'Inside persons'.

A useful collection of articles on personal identity is Peacocke and Gillett's edited volume *Persons and Personality* (1987); contributors include Swinburne, Parfit, Harré, Macquarrie, and Wiggins. Goodman's edited collection, *What is a Person?* (1988) also includes excellent chapters relevant to medicine and psychiatry (see especially Tristram Engelhardt's on 'Medicine and the concept of person'). A number of recent edited collections in philosophy and psychopathology include articles on personal identity: Graham and Stephen's *Philosophical Psychopathology* (1994); Sadler *et al.*'s *Philosophical Perspectives on Psychiatric Diagnostic Classification* (1994); Spitzer and Maher's *Philosophy and Psychopathology* (1990); and Phillips Griffith's *Philosophy, Psychology and Psychiatry* (1995). Jennifer Radden's *Divided minds and successive selves* (1996) brings together ethics with the philosophy of mind in a detailed explanation of the ethical and legal issues raised by dissociative disorders.

Among journal articles, there have been many on Multiple Personality Disorder (Braude's book, already mentioned, is a good source of references): note especially Stephen Clark (1998) and Grant Gillett (1986). The first volume of *PPP – Philosophy, Psychiatry and Psychology* (1994) — included two articles on thought insertion and personal identity: Stephens and Graham on 'Self-consciousness and mental agency'; and Ruth Chadwick on Kant, Strawson, Kitcher, and the transcendental self. Note also Stephen Sabat and Rom Harré (1994) on Alzheimer's disease. Peter Binns' article on 'Affect, agency and engagement' (1994) explores the issues more generally, drawing on continental as well as analytic philosophy. Hinshelwood's two articles in *PPP* (1995 and 1997) explore the links between personal identity and ethics specifically in relation to splitting, projection, and introjection. He explores these ideas further in his book, *Therapy or Coercion?* (Hinshelwood 1997).

Reading Guide: references

Adshead, G. (forthcoming) A different voice in psychiatric ethics. In *Healthcare Ethics and Human Values* (ed. Fulford, K.W.M., Dickenson, D., and Murray, T.H.). Oxford, Blackwell Science.

Agich, G.J. (1993) *Autonomy and Long-Term Care*. Oxford, Oxford University Press.

Alderson, P. (1990) *Choosing for Children: Parents' Consent to Surgery*. Oxford, Oxford University Press.

Beauchamp, T. (1999) The philosophical basis of psychiatric ethics. In *Psychiatric Ethics* (3rd edn) (ed. Bloch, S., Chodoff, P., and Green, S.A.), Chapter 3. Oxford, Oxford University Press.

Beauchamp, T.L. and Childress, J.F. (1994) *Principles of Biomedical Ethics* (4th edn; 1st edn, 1989). Oxford, Oxford University Press.

Binns, P. (1994) Affect, agency and engagement: conceptions of the person in philosophy, neuropsychiatry, and psychotherapy. *Philosophy, Psychiatry and Psychology,* 1:11–26. (Commentary by Caws, P.).

Bloch, S., Chodoff, P., and Green S.A. (1999) *Psychiatric Ethics* (3rd edn; 1st edn 1981). Oxford, Oxford University Press.

Blum, L. (1980) *Friendship, Altruism and Morality*. London, Routledge and Kegan Paul.

BMA and the Law Society (1995) *Assessment of Mental Capacity — Guidance for Doctors and Lawyers. A Report of the British Medical Association and the Law Society*. London, BMA.

Braude, S.E. (1991; 2nd edn, 1995) *First Person Plural: Multiple Personality and the Philosophy of Mind*. London, Routledge.

Chadwick, R. (1994) Kant, thought insertion and mental unity. *Philosophy, Psychiatry, and Psychology*, 1:105–14. (Commentary by Stephens, G. Lynn and Graham, G., 115 – 16.)

Charland, L.C. (1998) Is Mr Spock mentally competent? Competence to consent and emotion. *Philosophy, Psychiatry, and Psychology,* 5/1:67–82.

Clark, S.R.L. (1996) Minds, memes and multiples. *Philosophy, Psychiatry and Psychology*, 3:21–8. (Commentary by Bavidge, M., 29–30 and Sprigge, T., 31–6.)

Dickenson, D. (1997) *Property, Women and Politics: Subjects or Objects?* Cambridge, Polity Press.

Dickenson, D. (1998) Consent in children. *Current Opinion in Psychiatry*, 11/4:389–93.

Dickenson, D. and Jones, D. (1995) True wishes: the philosophy and developmental psychology of children's informed consent. *Philosophy, Psychiatry, and Psychology*, 2:287–304. (Commentaries by Eekelaar, J., McCormick, S., Murray T.H., Parker M., and Wells L.A.)

Engelhardt, H.T. Jr. (1988) Medicine and the concept of person. In *What is a Person?* (ed. Goodman, M.F.) Clifton, The Humana Press Inc.

Fulford, K.W.M. and Hope, R.A. (1993) Psychiatric ethics: a bioethical ugly duckling? In *Principles of Health Care Ethics* (ed. Gillon, R. and Lloyd, A.), Chapter 58. Chichester (England), John Wiley and Sons.

Gibbard, A. (1990) *Wise Choices, Apt Feelings: A Theory of Normative Judgement.* Oxford, Clarendon Press.

Gillett, G.R. (1986) Multiple personality and the concept of a person. *New Ideas in Psychology,* **4 (2)**:173–84.

Glover, J. (1988) *I: The Philosophy and Psychology of Personal Identity.* London, The Penguin Group.

Goodman, M.F. (ed.) (1988) *What is a Person?* New Jersey, The Humana Press Inc.

Graham, G. (1993) *Philosophy of Mind; An Introduction.* Oxford, Blackwell Publishers.

Graham, G. and Stephens, G.L. (ed.) (1994) *Philosophical Psychopathology.* Cambridge (Mass.), MIT Press.

Green, K. (1995) *The Woman of Reason: Feminism, Humanism and Political Thought.* Cambridge, Polity Press.

Hacking, I. (1995) *Rewriting the Soul.* Princeton, Princeton University Press.

Held, V. (1993) *Feminist Morality: Transforming Culture, Society and Politics.* Chicago, University of Chicago Press.

Hinshelwood, R.D. (1995) The social relocation of personal identity as shown by psychoanalytic observations of splitting, projection and introjection. *Philosophy, Psychiatry, and Psychology,* **2**:185–204.

Hinshelwood, R.D. (1997) Primitive mental processes: psychoanalysis and the ethics of integration. *Philosophy, Psychiatry, and Psychology,* **4/2**:121–44.

Hinshelwood R.D. (1997) *Therapy or Coercion? Does Psychoanalysis Differ from Brainwashing?* London, H. Karnac (Books) Ltd.

Lidz, C.W., Meisel, A., Zerubavel, E., Carter, M., Sestak, R.M., and Roth, L.H. (ed.) (1984) *Informed Consent: A Study of Decision Making in Psychiatry.* London, The Guildford Press.

Medical Defence Union (1997) *Consent to Treatment* (rev. edn.). London, MDU.

Moore, A., Hope, T., and Fulford, K.W.M. (1994) Mild mania and well-being. *Philosophy, Psychiatry, and Psychology,* **1/3**:165–78.

Nussbaum, M.C. (1986) *The Fragility of Goodness.* Oxford, Oxford University Press.

Peacocke, A. and Gillett, G. (ed.) (1987) *Persons and Personality.* Oxford, Basil Blackwell Ltd.

Phillips Griffiths, A. (ed.) (1995) *Philosophy, Psychology and Psychiatry.* Cambridge, Cambridge University Press (for the Royal Institute of Philosophy).

Radden J. (1996) *Divided minds and successive selves: ethical issues in disorders of identity and personality.* Cambridge, Mass: MIT Press.

Rogers A., Pilgrim D., and Lacey R. (1993) *Experiencing Psychiatry: Users' Views of Services.* London, The Macmillan Press.

Sabat, S.R. and Harré, R. (1994) The Alzheimer's disease sufferer as semiotic subject. *Philosophy, Psychiatry and Psychology,* 1:145–63. (Commentaries by Hope, T. and Greenberg, W.M.)

Sadler J.Z., Wiggins, O.P., and Schwartz, M.A. (ed.) (1994) *Philosophical Perspectives on Psychiatric Diagnostic Classification.* Baltimore, John Hopkins University Press.

Savulescu, J. and Dickenson, D. (1998) The time frame of preferences, dispositions, and the validity of advance directives for the mentally ill. *Philosophy, Psychiatry, and Psychology,* 5/3:225–46.

Sherwin, S. (1993) *No Longer Patient: Feminist Ethics and Health Care.* Philadelphia, Temple University Press.

Spitzer, M. and Maher, B. (1990) *Philosophy and Psychopathology.* New York, Springer–Verlag Inc.

Stephens, G.L. and Graham, G. (1994) Self-consciousness, mental agency, and the clinical psychopathology of thought insertion. *Philosophy, Psychiatry, and Psychology,* 1:1–10. (Commentary by Wiggins, O.P.)

Wear, S. (1993) Empirical studies of informed consent. *Informed Consent: Patient Autonomy and Physician Beneficence Within Clinical Medicine,* Chapter 3, Subsection II. Dordrecht (Netherlands), Kluwer Academic Publishers.

Widdershoven, G. (forthcoming) Alternatives to principlism. In *Healthcare Ethics and Human Values* (ed. Fulford, K.W.M., Dickenson, D., and Murray, T.H.). Oxford, Blackwell Science.

CHAPTER 7

Prognosis: luck and judgement

Moral luck as well as sound judgements of probability drive
current issues of risk management in mental health

Many of the most pressing problems of current clinical practice turn on questions of risk — balancing care and control in the management of suicide, maintaining unstable patients in the community, steering a path between taking advantage of new treatments and waiting for the benefits of hindsight, stepping into the unknown with research. In all these and a host of related ways, psychiatry is a risky business. As we put it in the introduction to this book, in psychiatry uncertainty is the norm.

In this chapter, we explore two of the more common ethical problems arising directly from the uncertainty of prognostic judgements of dangerousness, concerned respectively with confidentiality and clinical practice guidelines.

Case 7.1, Alan Masterson, illustrates an inherent conflict, where questions of dangerousness are concerned, between our obligations to maintain confidentiality and our responsibility to protect third parties from harm. Alan Masterson was an 54-year-old man who was about to be discharged from hospital after being treated for depression. There was prima facie evidence, though no proof, that when depressed he had tried to electrocute his three children in their swimming pool. Social Services wanted to be notified when he was to be discharged, but the hospital team felt this would breach their obligations of confidentiality and hence threaten Alan Masterson's trust in them.

The classic cases in this area, notably the American *Tarasoff* case of 1974 (see Appendix for details), have been concerned with people with asocial or psychopathic personality disorder. The legal guidance based on these cases is that the psychiatrist responsible should only reveal confidential information about their patient where there is a clear and immediate danger to one or more specific people. Such guidance, whatever one thinks of it ethically, is workable to the extent that the behaviour of people with personality disorders is by definition relatively fixed and hence, reasonably predictable. Alan Masterson, by contrast, had an inherently (but not fully predictably) treatable condition (that is, depression) and there was no overt or even proven risk of danger to himself or his children. Moreover, it was far from clear that his children's interests would be secured by breaching confidentiality, since if Alan Masterson lost faith in the hospital team, he might opt out of treatment altogether, thereby increasing the risk of harm to the children. In this case, therefore, 'playing for safety' (that is, breaching confidentiality by informing Social Services) might have the opposite of the effect intended.

This is a 'Catch 22'. If the hospital staff fail to warn Social Services and something goes wrong, they are likely to be severely criticized — reports on homicides by mentally disordered patients regularly emphasize the importance of interagency co-operation. But in this case, warning Social Services might be the key factor leading to a tragic outcome. In Jane Gillespie's case (5.1), for example, involuntary admission to hospital was indicated on the general grounds of her symptoms of major depression combined with suicidal intent; but in her particular case, the ensuing loss of control could have increased rather than decreased the risk of suicide.

We have come across similar 'Catch 22s', where general guidance conflicts with the contingencies of the particular situation, several times in this book; they are all too familiar to forensic psychiatrists. In the treatment of sex offenders, for example, an admission of the offence may be a key step towards reducing the risk of re-offending, but reporting such an admission (of a criminal offence) to the police is one of the legally obligatory breaches of confidentiality; and reporting the offence will greatly reduce the likelihood of an admission, thus increasing the risk of re-offending.

Case 7.2, Philip Caversham, illustrates this 'Catch 22' especially sharply, arising where official guidelines governing the practice of psychiatry conflict with an individual psychiatrist's clinical judgement of what is required in a particular situation. Philip Caversham was a 40-year-old man with a diagnosis of paranoid schizophrenia and a history of indecent assault. He was barely co-operating with treatment and the guidance under the UK's Care Programme Policy clearly indicated that he should be put on the Supervision Register (an official register used in the UK to attempt to keep track of those who are considered in special need of supervision). Those involved, however, felt that if Philip knew he had been put on the Register, he would opt out of treatment altogether and disappear. They could put him on the Register without his knowledge, but the risk of him finding out was such that, even if this were ethically acceptable (see Jim Birley's comments, Chapter 11), it would be clinically hazardous. Again, then, we have a situation in which following the rules, however sound they may be in general, would, in the judgement of those directly concerned with this particular case, increase rather than decrease the risk of harm.

The ethical dilemmas in both these cases arise in part from uncertainty over the clinical outcomes. In Alan Masterson's case, had there been a 'clear and present danger' to his children (that is, to specific people), current law and practice justify (indeed require) breach of confidentiality in so far as this is necessary to forewarn relevant third parties (in this case, including the Social Services). Obligatory breaches of confidentiality pose a particular kind of ethical issue, where ethics and law may be in direct conflict. This is graphically illustrated by some of the problems raised by mandatory reporting of sexual abuse of children (Trowell, 2000).

Philip Caversham's case, similarly, would be straightforward practically if it were clear that putting him on the Supervision Register would obviate the danger of re-offending. This is an example of the conflict between what in moral theory is called 'act utilitarianism' and 'rule utilitarianism'. The guidance under the Care Programme Policy that people like Philip Caversham should be put on the Supervision Register (if necessary without their knowledge and hence consent), is based on the view that, as a rule, this will reduce the rate of offending sufficiently to justify the infringement of liberty involved. The *rule* is thus justified by the overall balance of utilities. But in Philip Caversham's case, those concerned believed that putting him on the Register could have the opposite effect — of increasing the risk of offending. Hence the *act* is not justified by the overall balance of utilities. Yet if practitioners break the rules in cases like this, it could make it less likely that they will be followed in other cases. So the knock-on effect could lead back to an argument for sticking to the rules even though in a particular case their effects might be adverse (for a valuable discussion of act and rule utilitarianism, see Smart and Williams 1973).

The law in many countries has traditionally recognized that there is wide scope for differences of view about the 'best' course of action in medicine. The relevant test in England and Wales is still the 'Bolam principle' — the so-called 'prudent doctor' test — that a course of action is justified (technically, it is 'non-negligent') provided it is one that a group of peers would consider appropriate. A number of factors are putting pressure on the legitimate diversity of professional opinion allowed by this principle: the growth of 'practice guidelines', from trust managers as well as professional bodies (constraining professional freedom); a change in ethics towards patient choice (the 'prudent patient' test, limiting professional authority); the growth of 'evidence-based' medicine (undermining the value of individual experience); and so forth. In practice, it is still the case that individual doctors have considerable discretion. The courts, and indeed most practice guidelines, defer to individual clinical judgement, leaving it open to practitioners to breach the guidelines if they consider this appropriate in the given circumstances. The sting in the tail, though, is that if you depart from the guidelines, you have to be prepared to support your judgement with some very solid arguments if things go wrong!

In the case of judgements of risk, supporting arguments generally turn on the balance between *subjective* (clinical) assessments of a particular case and *objective* (actuarial) risk factors derived from general clinical experience, epidemiological studies, and the like. In Alan Masterson's case, Social Services considered cases of this kind to be highly dangerous; whereas his doctors' clinical judgement was that he did not represent a sufficiently clear danger to his children to bring him within the mandatory breach of confidentiality required by the 'Tarasoff' principle. Similarly, in Philip Caversham's case, the team's clinical judgement was that notwithstanding the Care Policy Programme Guidance, putting this particular man on the Register would increase the risk of re-offending. But this whole area of subjective and objective risk is one in which myths and misunderstandings abound. Before turning to our cases, therefore, we will look briefly at three of these. We will call them the myth of the amazing coincidence (affecting mainly subjective judgements of risk), the myth of 'billiard-ball' causality (affecting mainly objective judgements of risk), and the myth of value-free risk (affecting both subjective and objective judgements). As we will see, simply being aware of these myths can help us to come to a more balanced assessment of risk in a given case.

The myth of the amazing coincidence

The principal myths and misunderstandings in the area of subjective risk assessments are concerned with coincidences. The biologist, Jack Cohen, and the mathematician, Ian Stewart, gives an entertaining account of these in their *Figments of Reality* (1997). What they amount to is that we tend to overestimate the significance of coincidences: finding someone at a party with the same birthday as yourself seems an 'amazing coincidence'; we feel there 'must be more to it'. In fact, the chances of this are better than 50:50 in a group of 20 or more people! Similarly in clinical work, we will be impressed more than we should be, on strictly probabilistic grounds, by the particular cases we have encountered.

This tendency to overestimate the significance of coincidences may have evolutionary advantages — in the natural environment you may not get more than one chance at 'learning from experience'! Moreover, as we have several times emphasized, implicit knowledge (the 'know how' of professional experience) is a rich resource for both technical and ethical aspects of clinical problem solving (see, for example, the discussion of casuistry in Chapter 2). But against this, when it comes to judging risk, we need to be aware of the limitations as well as the strengths of intuition. This is crucial to clinical assessment in psychiatry. It is also important to wider public policy issues. The public perception, for example, of the dangerousness of people with mental disorders is driven by the occasional high-profile cases of homicide. Whilst these certainly are tragedies, the reality is that although there may be a slight excess of risk of homicide by people diagnosed as suffering from schizophrenia, the realtive rate of homicide by people with mental disorders in the community has fallen in recent years roughly 3 per cent per annum, year on year, in the UK (Taylor and Gunn 1999).

The myth of billiard-ball causality

If subjective judgements of probability are prone to myths of coincidence, objective judgements are prone to myths of causality. The most important of these clinically is the idea that every event is in principle predictable, provided we have enough information. Politicians, health service managers, the press, and even some practitioners, often behave as though risk assessment were just a matter of feeding the right variables into a cause–effect equation (a 'tick the boxes' checklist approach), obviating the need for individual clinical judgements. Human behaviour, so this attitude implies, could be predicted in the same mechanical way as the movement of billiard balls, if only the 'experts' knew enough. The implication is that psychiatrists, social workers, and others responsible for clinical risk assessment, are somehow *inexpert* in failing to come up with the same hard-wired predictions as their counterparts in physics and engineering.

The fact, though, is that even in the physical sciences, the billiard-ball model of causality is well past its sell-by date. It was certainly an assumption of physical science right up to the end of the nineteenth century. Pascal believed that if only we had enough information, specifically if we knew the position and momentum of every particle at a given time, we could predict the future course of the universe into the indefinite future. But we now know that the behaviour of a given atom, electron, light quantum, and so on, is indeterminate not just in practice but in principle. However much we know about it, we can only give a series of probabilities that it will behave in one of a number of possible ways. This is counter-intuitive to many people. Einstein himself, one of the founders of quantum mechanics, never accepted it: 'God', he said, 'does not play dice!'. Yet the inherently probabilistic nature of the physical world has been borne out by every conceivable test, including several devised by Einstein himself. Of course, people are part of the macroworld rather than the microworld of quantum physics, and there are unresolved problems of scale here. There are also unresolved problems of moving from causes to reasons (see generally, Chapter 5). But the point is that the myth of billiard-ball determinism has lost its prominent place — even in the physical sciences from which it was derived.

The importance of the myth of billiard-ball determinism for psychiatric ethics cannot be overstated. The popular view of an 'expert' is someone who can tell you what is going to happen. This is derived from the nineteenth-century belief that science can in principle predict everything. Psychiatrists, like other doctors, have sometimes fed the myth of determinism by making exaggerated claims for their subject. Such claims are driven by a number of factors: competition for research funds, interprofessional rivalry, and so forth. We end up promising 'quick fixes' from the neurosciences, a Prozac for every problem. One downside of evidence-based medicine (important as it is in other respects) has been to reinforce the illusion that if only we knew enough we could remove uncertainty.

At all events, the end result of the myth of billiard-ball determinism, as we noted a moment ago, is that every tragedy is treated, by the press and the public if not by one's peers, as a *failure* of expert judgement. Practice, therefore, can become defensive. This in turn, can lead to worse outcomes. The vicious cycle is reinforced by the witch-hunt which follows these tragedies. Nigel Eastman (1996), who is a barrister as well as a forensic psychiatrist, has argued that the mandatory public inquiry which follows homicides by people with mental disorders strongly reinforces the assumption that there is always someone 'to blame'. Practice must be monitored, certainly; and where it is found wanting, there should be redress. But in the area of risk and dangerousness, Eastman has suggested, systematic audit would be more appropriate to the professional context, more informative, and, ultimately, more likely to improve the quality of risk management procedures.

Neither subjective nor objective measures of risk are without their myths, therefore, and being aware of these is important to clinical reasoning in psychiatric ethics. However, there is a further myth which infects both measures of risk. This myth takes us back to one of the themes running through this book — the importance of values as well as facts in all aspects of clinical work and research in psychiatry.

The myth of value-free risk

In the risk assessment literature, 'dangerousness' has often been distinguished from 'risk' by being a more context-dependent concept (Madden 1998). What this means is that what counts as dangerous to one person in a given context may not count as dangerous to another person in a different context. There are clear signals here, therefore, of an evaluative element in the meaning of 'danger'. But is the concept of 'risk' itself value-free? Probability, perhaps, is value-free: the chances of a coin coming up 'heads' are independent of what it means to the person who tosses it that it *should* come up heads! But risk is the combination of probability with *utility*. Hence the myth of value-free risk is the idea that risk, like danger, is context-independent. In contrast with tossing a coin, the point is that the outcomes with which we are concerned *clinically* are *never* value-neutral.

The whole academic industry of 'games theory' has grown up around this idea. Used especially in economics, games theory aims to base 'rational choices' on a combination of objective probabilities weighted with values. But the basic principle, that values as well as (probabilistic) facts drive clinical decisions in the area of risk management, remains important, if only to improve communication. We will be returning to this point in the next chapter when we consider teamwork. But in Alan Masterson's case, the stand-off between the psychiatrists and Social Services was a direct reflection of the difference between the concerns of the former for 'the patient' and of the latter for his children: the psychiatrists were more concerned about the breakdown of the therapeutic alliance if confidentiality *was* breached; Social Services were more concerned about the dangers to the children if confidentiality was *not* breached. Merely agreeing on the probability of Alan Masterson killing himself and/or his children would not, therefore, have resolved the difference between them. There was a difference of utilities, and hence of *risk* perception to be resolved. As we describe more fully in the discussion of this case, there are issues of moral luck here. But recognizing the differences of utilities is crucial in circumstances of this kind to mutual understanding as a basis for co-operative clinical decision making.

We will return to what all this means in practice in the next chapter — to how we can balance different utilities without becoming paralysed by indecision! A number of factors make it likely that problems of the kind discussed in the present chapter, however we resolve them, will become increasingly prominent over the next few years — the community treatment orders likely to be included in any new 'mental health act' (giving psychiatrists legal powers of compulsion and hence obligations without the practical power or resources to compel), the possible inclusion of people with personality disorders under such powers, and the direct conflict between the demands of medical ethics for patient autonomy and expectations of an all-powerful medicine!

In this climate, psychiatrists will have to tread warily between claiming too much and appearing to deny clinical responsibility. In moral theory it is generally held that 'ought' implies 'can' — that is, that we should not be held responsible for outcomes over which we have no control. It is one of the deepest paradoxes of 'moral luck', however, that although being responsible for an outcome is certainly a *sufficient* condition for being praised or blamed for that outcome, it is very far from being a *necessary* condition. For this reason alone (leaving aside the more banal motives of political expediency) we must anticipate that psychiatrists will continue to be blamed for the actions of their patients, whether or not they are responsible for them! Luck, then, as well as judgement, is the theme of this chapter.

References

Christopher Clunis Report: North East Thames and South East Thames Regional Health Authorities (1994) The Report of the Enquiry into the Care and Treatment of Christopher Clunis. London, HMSO.

Cohen, J. and **Stewart, I.** (1997) *Figments of Reality.* Cambridge: Cambridge University Press.

Eastman, N.L.G. and **Hope, R.A.** (1988) Ethics of enforced medical treatment: the balance model. *Journal of Applied Philosophy,* **5**:49–59.

Eastman, N.L.G. (1996) Inquiry into homicides by psychiatric patients: systematic audit should replace mandatory inquiries. *British Medical Journal,* **313**:1069–71.

Gillon, R. (1985) *Philosophical Medical Ethics.* Chichester, John Wiley.

Madden, A. (1998) *Risk Assessment and Management in Psychiatry. CPD Psychiatry* (Rila Publications), **1/1**:8–11.

Smart, J.J.C. and **Williams, B.** (1973) *Utilitarianism: For and Against.* Cambridge, Cambridge University Press.

Tarasoff v. the Regents of the University of California (1974) 118 California Reporter 129, 529, P2d 553.

Taylor, P. J. and **Gunn, J.** (1999) Homicides by people with mental illness: myth and reality. *British Journal of Psychiatry,* **174**:9–14.

Trowell, J. (2000) Confidentiality and Child Protection. Ch 5 in *Confidentiality and Mental Health* (ed. Cordess, C.) London, Jessica Kinglsey Publishers.

CASE 7.1
Alan Masterson — clear and present danger?

Synopsis A 54-year-old man, suffering from depression and suicidal thoughts, came close to electrocuting his sons in their swimming pool. It was not clear whether this was accidental. He was admitted to hospital. However, he has shown little response to treatment and is now due for discharge. Social Services, who are responsible for the children, want advance warning of his date of discharge. The psychiatrist feels this would be a breach of confidentiality which could prejudice the therapeutic relationship and that it is up to his wife to inform Social Services when he is discharged.

Key dilemma Should the psychiatrist tell Social Services Alan's discharge date or would this be an unwarranted breach of confidentiality?

Main topics Confidentiality and dangerousness; teamwork among services (interagency working).

Other topics Moral luck; professional ethics; duty of care; doctor–patient relationship; role of the family; responsibility; child protection; medical model in psychiatry; guidelines; best interests; paternalism; rationality; consent; goals of medicine; contract; Hegel; Nagel.

Alan Masterson, aged fifty-four, was referred to psychiatric services for depression the year after he lost his management job following a corporate 'restructuring'. His GP was concerned about his serious weight loss, which had no physiological cause. Alan reported fleeting suicidal wishes, along with sleeplessness and marital tension. Although he felt guilty about having lost his job, he thought that was not the only factor in his mental state. Depression seemed to 'run in the family', he said: his mother also suffered from it, and had become more or less a recluse in her later years, refusing even to see her grandchildren.

He described himself likewise as 'a bit of a loner, not a team player'. 'I suppose I was never really cut out for management, it's a wonder I lasted as long as I did.' Luckily there was no immediate financial pressure: Alan had received a sizeable redundancy payment from his well-paid position, and his wife Valerie worked as an architect's receptionist. Nevertheless, he was very pessimistic about the financial future, repeatedly predicting that his wife and sons would end up in a council house and he would wind up in a cardboard box at Waterloo station. The senior registrar working with Alan, Anya Washansky, decided that he should be maintained on antidepressants, with a referral to marriage guidance and follow-up in the out-patients department.

Six months later, however, Alan was admitted to a psychiatric ward after his three sons were very nearly electrocuted. The children were swimming in the family pool, and the eldest, thirteen-year-old Tom, had left a portable CD player plugged in, to recharge, on a long lead attached to the electrical point in the machinery which housed the pool heater. As Tom told the story, his father deliberately threw the CD player into the pool; as Alan told it, he tripped over the wire and the player catapulted into the water. By great good fortune the CD player, which had only been loosely plugged in, flew out of the electrical point just before it fell into the water. No one else saw the incident; the two younger boys were rough-housing together, with their backs to their father, and Alan's wife Valerie was out at work. She believed Tom's version of events, and was of course greatly distraught — and very angry with Anya for failing to protect the boys from Tom. She had immediately phoned the police, and child protection machinery was set in motion, including referral to Social Services.

Alan denied to Anya that he had tried to kill the boys, although he did say that his sons would be 'better off dead than stuck with a loser like me for a dad'. However, he did agree to emergency admission on an informal basis, admitting that he had not been taking his antidepressants: 'I can't be bothered, maybe it's better if you make me do it.' In the ward Alan was given a further trial of a tricyclic antidepressant, but without much apparent benefit: he still had depressed mood and suicidal thoughts. He continued to deny that he had tried to kill the boys: 'Kids have accidents all the time, don't they?'

During Alan's period in hospital, Social Services and the police both requested further information from the mental health team. The police requested a psychiatric opinion on Alan's fitness to be interviewed, in the presence of a psychiatric nurse. Their opinion was that it was unlikely that Alan would be prosecuted; at most, a formal caution might be given, but more likely there would be insufficient evidence to prosecute. However, they requested a forensic opinion on the risk posed to the children. The mental health team was willing to grant this latter request, although they did not consider that Alan was yet ready to be interviewed by the police.

In contrast, the Social Services request for more detail on the swimming pool incident and on Alan's previous treatment in out-patients met with a refusal from the psychiatrists, on grounds of patient confidentiality. Nor would they reveal Alan's discharge date to Social Services: on the advice of her consultant, Paul Glover, Anya informed Social Services that it was the responsibility of Alan's wife Valerie to do so, when Alan returned home. Paul felt that it was the mental health team's duty to put Alan's medical needs first, whereas Social Services' primary responsibility was to protect the children. Whilst Paul realized the possible risks to the boys, he felt that their future lay in making Alan well again. And his primary duty was to respect the therapeutic relationship, which would be shattered if Alan believed that the psychiatrists were not fully on 'his' side and if information which he had revealed in confidence was divulged.

Alan was not the easiest person to engage in conversation: he was often morose and taciturn. And after all, he had been admitted informally — so he could discharge himself at any time. Surely the best long-term protection for the boys, too, lay in maintaining an atmosphere in which Alan voluntarily accepted help. In his letter to Social Services, Paul took what he thought was a conciliatory tone, agreeing that Alan was 'certainly a risk to himself'. He assured them that treatments were in hand, although he did not specify that Alan was due to have an MRI scan soon and a course of electroplexy if the scan proved to be normal.

This response occasioned a swift written protest from the Social Services Department, sent in the first instance to Paul, but with copies to senior Social Services, hospital trust and health authority management. The service manager, Kathy McAllister, viewed this as a totally improper interpretation of patient confidentiality and as unreasonable withholding of information necessary for Social Services to carry out its statutory child protection responsibilities. Social Services had decided to defer putting the children on the 'At risk' register so long as Alan was in hospital and the children therefore safe. But there was still an urgent need for full exchange of information. And why was the mental health team only concerned that Alan was a risk to himself, when vulnerable children were in danger?

One clinical psychologist believes that cases like Alan's are chronic: child protection is a 'forgotten problem' in treatment of mentally ill adults. According to this argument, within mental health services there is a serious lack of awareness about child protection issues, matched by a lack of understanding about mental illness by some social workers. Despite a number of highly publicized cases in which communication failures and breakdowns between Social Services and other agencies ended in children's deaths, and the efforts made in the Children Act to integrate child protection responsibilities, only child specialities have really been affected — adult psychiatry and psychology has remained something of a law onto itself (Rouf 1997). But 'although services are arranged into specialities, the lives of our clients are not' (Rouf 1997, p. 23).

Specifically, mental health and Social Services have very different managerial patterns, one 'flatter' than the other. The hierarchy in Social Services departments is more pyramidal, from social worker up through unit manager, child protection co-ordinator, service manager, and senior management. In mental health trusts, the typical 'flat' pattern is simpler: consultant-led teams, trust management, and ultimately the health authority. In Social Services departments, issues travel up the pyramid of responsibility and accountability very quickly; in mental health, by contrast, clinical management decisions remain at the team level until a very high threshold of concern has been reached (Jones 1997). Kathy McAllister's decision to forward her letter to senior personnel might well thus be normal good practice to her, whereas to the mental health team it probably looks inflammatory. Some mental health trusts have brought their managerial arrangements nearer to those of Social Services by appointing a named doctor and nurse to liaise with Social Services — another layer of case management — in an attempt to prevent or resolve conflicts arising in cases like this one.

Interagency tensions and disputes do not, however, arise solely from differences in managerial structures. Deeper philosophical issues about risk and responsibility are at stake, falling into two principal categories:

1 Risk assessment and moral luck.
2 Objects of duty and responsibility.

Risk assessment and moral luck
For understandable reasons, mental health and Social Services are likely to have different attitudes towards risk assessment and risk aversion. To a large extent this incompatibility results from having different objects of concern, of being responsible in the one case for the adult patient and in the other for the vulnerable child. The question of 'protecting whom' — of the proper object of one's professional duty — will be explored further under the next heading. But different attitudes towards risk assessment are not explained solely by different objects of responsibility. There is also the important question of how things can

go wrong, and how they can go wrong in different ways for the two sets of professionals. This is where the issue of moral luck comes in, as it has in other cases.

What counts as 'getting it wrong' in psychiatry? To the extent that the medical model obtains (see Case 3.1, Elizabeth Orton), the answer is 'failing to cure'. It is the possibility of cure which underpins the therapeutic relationship in psychiatry, although as in all areas of medicine — avowedly so in palliative care — the alleviation of suffering might more properly be construed as the goal. However, most clinicians admit that there are some boundaries on the sanctity of the therapeutic relationship, such as patient autonomy or public protection. It is in the name of protecting the public that the General Medical Council guidelines clearly state that there are limits to patient confidentiality, such as the actual duty to report suspected child abuse (GMC 1995, p. 13). It is also clear in law that an abusing parent cannot claim the protection of medical confidentiality — although this applies more to the accident and emergency situation in which a doctor suspects abuse in a child presenting with 'accidental' injuries (Mason and McCall Smith 1991, p. 185). Against that interpretation, the case of A-G v. Guardian (1990) established that there is a public interest in a legally enforceable notion of confidentiality, which requires three elements:

1   Information divulged must have the necessary quality of a confidence.

2   Information must have been given in circumstances imparting an obligation of confidentiality.

3   Unauthorized use of information must be to the detriment of the party who communicated it.

This last condition is the most controversial in Alan's case. Perhaps the clinicians are more concerned with social harm? — the possibility that he will never see his children again if he is deemed a risk to them. Might a strict policy of confidentiality, extending to silence over his discharge date, even harm Alan? — by collusion with his irresponsibility, by excess advocacy, or by failure to get him to confront the possibility he has denied, that he did intend to harm the boys. If, however, we accept that divulging the information is against Alan's best interests (although it is hard to see what clinical harm could be done by releasing his discharge date), then the psychiatrists might argue for maintaining confidentiality on a legal basis. Some clinicians may go further, feeling that there is an actual moral duty to cure which overrides all other ethical considerations, and which enjoins strict confidentiality. This is a paternalistic outlook, and it is not clear that Anya and Paul feel so strongly paternalistic. But it does appear that Alan's clinicians are concerned with preserving the therapeutic relationship from outside 'intrusion', and with avoiding the breakdown of the therapeutic relationship which they feel a breach of confidentiality may provoke. Although they are of course concerned with the boys' welfare too, they have some reason in this case to feel that it is by no means certain that Alan tried to kill his sons.

For Social Services child protection staff, however, 'getting it wrong' means failing to protect vulnerable children. The extreme of 'getting it wrong' would be the boys' deaths. Because that harm is so very great (in itself, not only because it would almost certainly lead to media denunciations), Social Services are unwilling to tolerate even a very small probability of its occurrence. This is a perfectly rational attitude, exemplifying the logic in Pascal's wager (Dickenson 1991, p. 63) — a loss which approaches infinity in its magnitude is so great as to cancel out all probability considerations. No matter how unlikely the harm may be, even the smallest probability of it is intolerable. It is not so much a matter of necessarily believing Tom's account of the swimming pool incident rather than Alan's, as of fearing the consequences of not preferring Tom's account.

Must we simply accept that the two services have differing attitudes towards risk assessment, and 'ne'er the twain shall meet'? To the extent that the law favours one interpretation over the other, that view of risk assessment must be accepted. As Kathy McAllister points out, Social Services child protection staff must be given sufficient information to fulfil their statutory obligations. However, that does not necessarily entail full information-sharing, as she claims: there may be some room for compromise over what information Social Services genuinely needs to know. But there is a significant risk here — withholding information means that one bears full responsibility for an adverse outcome, where sharing information with patients or other agencies might have averted tragedy. Although English law does not recognize the American notion of *informed* consent, and continues to allow a medical standard to determine how much information must be shared (Sidaway v Bethlem RHG 1985), it is against doctors' own interest in avoiding remorse to be the sole 'owners' of crucial information.

Objects of duty and responsibility

To whom do you owe a duty? We have already looked briefly at the notion of the goals of medicine — cure or alleviation of suffering. The duty of care in medicine, including psychiatry, is primarily to the individual patient, but the doctor has wider moral responsibilities which are recognized in guidelines on confidentiality (for example, a duty to the public). But what about duties to 'significant others'? Might Paul and Anya be said to have a duty to Alan's children as well? Could that duty be even more pressing than their duty to protect Alan's best interests? — perhaps because children are more vulnerable than adult patients. That seems an unpromising line of argument: particular children might be less vulnerable than extremely ill psychiatric patients. The extent of duty cannot hinge on ready-reckoning the extent of vulnerability: we might not know the extent of vulnerability until later, if things did indeed go dreadfully wrong.

In a contractual interpretation of medicine, the doctor–patient relationship would be primary because a sort of contract had been put into effect between those two parties when the patient sought care. The duties specified by such a contract might include complying with treatment and providing necessary information on the part of the patient, and provision of the best available service and honouring of patients' reasonable wishes on the part of the doctor. But although contractual models are increasingly influential in public policy (Davis *et al.* 1997), they are not the legal basis of health care — at least not in the National Health Service, where there is no actual contract between patient and doctor.

Contract is a useful metaphor in ethics — whatever its merits or demerits in law — for recognizing others as active agents, rather than passive objects of concern, and indeed one of us has argued for such a Hegelian approach to contract elsewhere (Dickenson 1997). But in this case there does not seem to be a great deal of mileage in a contractual approach. It will not bridge the abyss between mental health and Social Services, only widen it, if the psychiatrists insist that their 'contract' is with Alan and Alan alone, regardless of the danger to his children, Social Services' statutory responsibility. Alan's wife, Valerie, will be left out of the equation altogether. We might not want to say that the clinicians have a duty to Valerie, but she feels badly let down by them.

If the clinician's duties are construed too extensively, however, we encounter what Thomas Nagel terms 'the problem of excess objectivity'. It is important to amplify our concern beyond the doctor–patient dyad, to take the wider world into account — and this the contractual model fails to do. Yet the opposite risk is to make the clinician responsible for too much and, ironically, to erase his or sense of moral efficacy. Once we expand beyond the doctor–patient relationship, and include the wider world in calculations of moral duty, we may be so overwhelmed by everything which we are obliged to take into account that we can see no point in acting at all.

> Once people are seen as being parts of the world, there seems no way to assign responsibility to them for what they do. Everything about them, including finally their actions themselves, seems to blend in with the surroundings over which they have no control. (Nagel 1986, p. 120)

This is the problem of excess objectivity. Nagel's nearest thing to a solution is 'a kind of reconciliation between the objective standpoint and the inner perspective of agency which reduces the radical detachment produced by initial contemplation of ourselves as creatures in the world'. Specifically in relation to the problem of moral luck and responsibility, he suggests the maxim: 'Since we can't act in light of everything about ourselves, the best we can do is to try to live in a way that wouldn't have to be revised in light of anything more that could be known about us.' (Nagel 1986, p. 121)

How can this be applied to Alan's case? Anya and Paul cannot act in light of everything that could be known about Alan's future risk to his sons, but they can try to ensure that they will not regret their actions if the unexpected occurs. It appears that the unexpected, to them, would be for Tom's version of events to have been the correct one; for Alan to discharge himself prematurely, with no improvement; for Social Services to be unable to act because they have not been told the discharge date and Valerie does not notify them; and for the boys to die in an 'accident' of Alan's contriving. If that worst case occurred, Anya and Paul would not be responsible for the boys' death, but they would be responsible for a certain kind of professional arrogance in thinking they could ignore the worst-case scenario.

Practitioner commentary (CASE 7.1)

Dr Gwen Adshead Consultant Psychotherapist, Broadmoor Hospital and Honorary Senior Lecturer, Department of Forensic Psychiatry, St George's Hospital Medical School

This case raises a large number of issues for me as a forensic psychiatrist with, perhaps unusually for those working in this area, a training in psychotherapy. The Department of Health's (1991) document, *Working Together*, makes it a matter of good practice to liaise closely with Social Services in matters of child protection. At the same time though, the Royal College of Psychiatrists' (1996) document, *The Duties of a Consultant Psychiatrist*, state that a consultant's first duty is to their patient. So there is considerable room for uncertainty in the clinical management of cases like Alan Masterson's. I will consider five issues which strike me as central.

1 Dangerousness and hospitalization
The first issue is the underlying rationale for admitting Alan Masterson to hospital because he has done something dangerous (allegedly). This itself supposes a model in which a mental disorder (however defined) gives rise to behaviour which is dangerous to others, the response to which is therefore to address the supposed disorder rather than to control the behaviour.

This model further supposes that if the disorder is treated/cured effectively, the potentially risky behaviour will be reduced or abolished. But the links between mental disorder and risky behaviour are often unclear (Monahan and Steadman 1994; Wallace *et al.* 1998). Mental illness itself is rarely like a disease with discrete boundaries of 'illness and wellness'; rather, mental disorders tend to be more like disabilities with acute or chronic exacerbations. The patient is thus much more like someone living with a disability than someone who has say, pneumonia, from which he or she recovers.

2 The limitations of consequentialism in psychiatry

The second issue (which is related to the first) is the limits of consequentialist argument in situations like this in which there are competing duties. Consequentialist argument inevitably leads to an emphasis on 'evidence', which is often lacking in psychiatric settings. In this case, for example, what evidence do we have that breaches of confidentiality will lead to a 'shattering' of trust, especially if Alan Masterson is informed of the breach? Alan Masterson *may* well be angry with his clinician, but he may *not* be; possible predictions about Alan Masterson's future mental state in response to a breach of confidentiality must be even harder than most risk assessments. Because there is a lack of the type of crucial evidence which makes consequentialist arguments appropriate to pursue, consequentialism in psychiatry falls back on evaluative statements dressed up to look like clinical ones, such as, in this case, 'surely it would be better if…'.

In psychiatry, the limits of consequentialism are closely linked to the difficulties of risk assessment (itself a type of consequentialism). Alan Masterson's case illustrates how psychiatrists may have to select evidence and end up taking adversarial positions. For example, the narrative talks about psychiatrists being on 'Alan Masterson's side'; but even to perceive the situation in terms of 'having sides' is already to have signed up to a particular set of expectations. The narrative suggests that the psychiatrist is not certain that Alan Masterson tried to kill his sons; but there is an equally plausible account of these events in which it is just as certain that Alan Masterson *did* try to kill them.

There is a link between these two first issues in what we take 'cure' to mean. In medicine, we normally interpret it as using medical means to make someone better. Alan Masterson, however, appears to be admitted to hospital only in response to dangerous behaviour, rather than because of any pathological change in mood or other psychological needs. Might it not be more honest to concentrate simply on making him safe, rather than concentrating on his mental state which allegedly has some connection with his risky behaviour?

3 Continuing uncertainties over the duty to disclose

There is certainly other mental health law which is relevant to the duty to disclose. The Tarasoff case, for example, which mandates doctors in the USA to warn and to protect individuals who may be at risk from their patients, is not currently law in the UK but may well end up being so[1].

In the UK we have three relevant cases:

1 *Palmer* v *Tees Health Authority* (1998), in which a court found that doctors did not have a duty to prevent harm to unidentifiable individuals (and by extension suggested there might be the possibility of a duty of care to named and identifiable individuals, just as some states have found in relation to *Tarasoff*).

2 *Clunis* v *Camden and Islington Health Authority* (1988), which found that the health authority were not liable for Mr Clunis' behaviour, but might have been if he had been legally insane (that is, if he did not know what he was doing or he did not know he was wrong).

3 *W* v *Egdell* (1990). In this case the Court of Appeal found that a doctor *may* disclose confidential information where there is a risk to the public, and indeed *may* have a *duty* to do so in some cases.

Overall, the legal approach seems to be that doctors in the situation described in this case may disclose confidential information without breaching their duty of care. However, there is still no mandate to do so. The Clunis decision suggests that as Alan Masterson became more ill, the duty to protect him from being violent to others might increase.

4 Consent and disclosure

The issues of consent in this case show just how difficult consent is in psychiatry. The Sidaway (1985) case (noted in the narrative) refers to consent to *treatment*, and the doctor's duty to disclose relevant *information about treatment decisions* to patients. It is not about confidentiality, unless one is arguing that disclosure of information might be seen as part of an overall treatment plan. In certain forensic psychiatric circumstances, issues of disclosure are relevant to treatment (for example, of sex offenders). However, in this case there is a tension between the doctor's duty to obtain consent from Alan Masterson for treatment, Alan Masterson's consent to any disclosure by doctors, and the doctor's own professional duty to disclose information to third parties. It is important to separate these out.

5 Ethics and relationships

This case might look very different if Alan Masterson were seen as a nodal point in a network of relations and not as an isolated individual (Agich 1993; Attanucci 1988; Adshead, in press). In this model of relationship ethics:

1 duties to ill persons such as Alan Masterson might include some degree of duty to their carers and their dependants;

2 we might understand Alan Masterson's capacity to be autonomous as including a capacity to relate to others who are part of his network and who make up part of his social identity;

3 the psychiatrist would then have a duty to restore Alan Masterson's capacity to relate to his sons and his wife;

4 input from both Alan Masterson's wife and their sons would be relevant here, not in an adversarial way, but as information relevant to understanding how Alan Masterson relates to other important people in his life;

5 the fact that Alan Masterson's wife, or their children, are afraid of him, has to be considered a matter of *his* (Alan Masterson's) *own* health.

This last point in particular, and the impact of relationship ethics generally, is a further and important aspect of the many ways in which mental health ethics are different from and considerably more difficult than the ethics of physical medicine.

References (CASE 7.1)

A-G v Guardian Newspaper Ltd (No. 2) [1990] 1 AC 109.

Adshead, G. (forthcoming) A different voice in psychiatric ethics. In *Healthcare Ethics and Human Values* (ed. Fulford, K.W.M., Dickenson, D., and Murray, T.H.). Oxford, Blackwell Science.

Agich, G.J. (1993) *Autonomy and Long-Term Care*. Oxford, Oxford University Press.

Attanucci, J. (1988) In whose terms: a new perspective on self, identify and relationship. In *Mapping the Moral Domain* (ed. Gilligan, C., Ward J., and Taylor, J.). Cambridge (Mass.), Harvard University Press.

Clunis v. Camden and Islington Health Authority (1988) 2 WLR 902.

Davis, G., Sullivan, B., and Yeatman, A. (1997) *The New Contractualism?* Melbourne, Macmillan Education Australia.

Department of Health (1991). *Working Together under the Children Act 1989*. London, HMSO.

Dickenson, D. (1991) *Moral Luck in Medical Ethics and Practical Politics* (1st edn). Gower, Avebury Press. (2nd edn (forthcoming), published as *Risk and Luck in Medical Ethics*. Cambridge, Polity Press.)

Dickenson, D. (1997) *Property, Women and Politics: Subjects or Objects?* Cambridge, Polity Press.

General Medical Council (1995) *Guidelines on Confidentiality.* London, GMC.

Mason, J.K. and McCall Smith, R.A. (1991) *Law and Medical Ethics.* London, Butterworths.

Monahan, J. and Steadman, H. (1994) *Violence and Mental Disorder: Developments in Risk Assessment.* Chicago, University of Chicago Press.

Nagel, T. (1986) *The View from Nowhere.* Oxford, Oxford University Press.

Palmer v. Tees Health Authority and Another (1998) Court of Appeal. *Times* Law Report, 1 June 1998.

Rouf, K. (1997) Child protection issues within the mental health setting: a forgotten problem. *Clinical Psychology Forum,* **99**:23–7.

Royal College of Psychiatrists (1996) *The Responsibilities of Consultant Psychiatrists. Council Report No. 51.* London, Royal College of Psychiatrists.

Sidaway v Bethlem RHG (1985) 1 All ER 643.

Tarasoff v The Regents of the University of California (1974) 118 *California Reporter* 129, 529, P2d 553.

W v Egdell (1990) 1 All ER 835.

Wallace, C., Mullen, C., Burgess, P., Palmer, S., Ruschena, D., and Braune, C. (1998) Serious criminal offending and mental disorder. *British Journal of Psychiatry,* **172**: 477–84.

CASE 7.2

Philip Caversham — sense, nonsense, and supervision registers

Synopsis A man in his early forties, with a history of indecent assaults and a diagnosis of paranoid schizophrenia, is reluctant to continue attending out-patient follow-up or to co-operate with any form of continued supervision. He could be placed on the Supervision Register without his knowledge but (a) it is not clear that in practice this would give greater control and hence reduce the risk of re-offending and (b) it could alienate Philip, if he found out, thus actually increasing the risk of re-offending.

Key dilemma Should Philip be put on the Supervision Register?

Main topics Ethical issues arising from uncertainties of risk assessment.

Other topics Moral luck; supervision registers; dangerousness; community care; criminal law; responsibility; consent to treatment.

Philip Caversham, now in his early forties, was cautioned for an indecent exposure involving a schoolgirl when he was twenty-eight. Since then he has served a period of probation and a prison sentence, both for indecent assault. He has had lifelong psychosexual problems: his marriage was never consummated, and his wife divorced him after his prison sentence. The first psychiatric assessment only took place some years after he had begun to offend, while he was in prison. He was diagnosed as suffering from paranoid schizophrenia and was treated with injected antipsychotic drugs. However, he does not accept this diagnosis; instead he claims that his ordeal in prison accounts for his psychiatric problems. His sense of grievance against the psychiatric profession is considerable, and he categorically denies that there is anything wrong with him.

Since his release two years ago, Philip has committed no further offences and has had no hospital admissions. He used to attend a psychiatric out-patient clinic erratically, but accepted merely the very minimum level of medication by injection, fearing that the drugs were poisonous. It seems that he only attended the clinic because he dreaded being sectioned or imprisoned. His behaviour in the clinic was always very eccentric: he stared around the room while talking, casting the occasional darting glance at the interviewer before looking hurriedly away in a manner suggesting delusions of thought interference — although he rejected any such interpretation with outrage. He would terminate any attempt at interview abruptly, usually with cutting remarks about the skills and training of his clinicians, Nick Fox and Margaret Shanley. Nick and Margaret felt that only an increased dosage would protect him in the long term from psychotic relapse, but Philip was very hostile to any such suggestions. He refused to participate in any care planning or assessment.

About ten months ago, when interviewed in the presence of Parvadi Mehta, a second-year clinical medical student, Philip became extremely agitated. He stared at her pointedly, shouting that the girls he assaulted had 'asked for it'. This was the first time he had spoken of his offences; in the past he always refused to discuss them. A month later, in an interview designed to assess his risk of further sexual offending, he spoke out angrily in a similar vein about 'slags'. After that Philip disappeared from follow-up altogether, but sent a coherent letter, claiming that he had been misunderstood in both interviews. He was willing to return for follow-up only on condition that there was no further insulting talk of delusions or psychosis. Nor was he willing to accept any more drugs, he stipulated. Anyone the 'shrinks' think well enough to live in 'the so-called community', he remarked tartly, was well enough to refuse drugs. His sexuality had been channelled into art, he claimed; recently he gave an exhibition of his amateur paintings — proof, he said, that he was flourishing without the psychiatrists' interference. But whereas he told the clinical team that he painted landscapes, they know that he is actually primarily interested in female nudes.

The clinicians' preferred management would be to increase Philip's medication, see him more often, refer him to a forensic psychiatrist to get a risk estimate for re-offending, and finally, place him on the hospital Supervision Register. They are concerned about the two violent outbursts, and fear that Philip's condition is declining rather than improving, as he insists it is. But if they call him in to discuss these courses of action, Philip is likely to break off even the minimal contact he now has. Placing him on the Supervision Register, unlike the other three courses, could be done without his knowledge or co-operation. But given that there are no new resources available, what would it achieve? Perhaps it would only stigmatize Philip without offering him any extra help.

Nick and Margaret have considered whether it will improve Philip's compliance with long-term management to keep the Supervision Register in reserve as a threat, along the lines of section (which he does seem to respect). This they find preferable to the harder approach which they could actually take under aftercare legislation — conveying Philip to a treatment centre without his consent. On the other hand, if Philip were to find out that he had been placed on the Supervision Register behind his back, it might only increase his hostility to the doctors. Ironically, by placing him on the Supervision Register, Nick and Margaret feel that they would lose the last shreds of their ability to supervise him.

Philip and his clinicians, Nick and Margaret, are at odds over the correct interpretation of his behaviour, and thereby over his future dangerousness. Whose version should prevail? It is the risk of harm to others which gives the clinicians' version greater potential legitimacy. They cannot just take Philip at his word, given his history of offending. Equally, however, they cannot be certain that he will offend again, and indeed he offers a coherent if not entirely plausible argument about why he is unlikely to do so. So the problem boils down to assessing the risk, which in turn dictates what treatment, if any, should be imposed, with or without Philip's consent.

But can *any* compulsory treatment be justified if Philip is deemed well enough to live in the community? It is advances in psychopharmacology which enable borderline cases to manage out of hospital, one might reply (Lindley 1986, pp. 157–8), and therefore the question is misguided. Philip would not be out in the community without the drugs; it is back-to-front, 'Alice-in-Wonderland' reasoning to infer his right to refuse medication from the fact of his being in the community, as he does. The disagreement in this case cannot be solved so easily.

Like the case of Tom Benbow (Case 3.2), the example of Philip Caversham also illustrates the particular ethical problems surrounding risk assessment in long-term psychiatric management. How much intervention can be justified by future risk of harm? — to himself in Tom's case, to others in Philip's. An initial means of gaining some purchase on the question of risk assessment in Philip's case might be the notion of significant harm in child protection legislation: in England and Wales, for example, in the Children Act 1989. Evidence that harm has occurred in the past is not enough, unless it points to significant likelihood of harm continuing into the future (White *et al.* 1990, p. 102). (The notion of significant risk is also enshrined in paragraph 3.72 of the Department of Health's 1994 *Draft Guide to Arrangements for Inter-Agency Working for the Care and Protection of Severely Mentally Ill People.*) Do Philip's actions point, then, to significant likelihood of future harm? His self-justification in terms of channelling his sexuality into art sounds rather specious, and there may well be danger to the models he paints or to the schoolgirls he passes. But because these risks are only probabilities for a statistical aggregate, we cannot yet say for certain that any particular girl or woman is in danger. Here the parallel with child protection breaks down: typically the child on the 'at risk' register is at risk from known adults.

It is axiomatic that someone who may be dangerous but has not actually committed any crime cannot normally be detained preventively under the criminal law. Under mental health legislation the situation is different, but even so, there are time limits which even the most risk-averse clinician must respect. For example, compulsory admissions for assessment under Section 2 of the Mental Health Act 1983 may not extend beyond 28 days and cannot be renewed. An emergency admission under Section 4 of the 1983 Act (or Section 24 of the Scottish Act) is only valid for 72 hours. Under Section 3 of the 1983 Act, the patient may be detained for treatment for up to six months, renewable only if specified conditions are met.

Although service user groups have queried how effective these limits are in practice, when boundaries are absent — as in long-term care — the justification for compulsory treatment becomes more obviously problematic, and the informed consent of the patient particularly critical. Indeed, community care can be seen as an attempt to escape from preventive detention, and as a more just system for those with mental illness (Chadwick and Levitt 1995). Nevertheless, long-term management, as under the Supervision Register, raises particular problems, compared to the expressly limited time-frame of treatment under Sections 2 or 3 of the Mental Health Act 1983, because there is simply more uncertainty about prospective benefit (Dickenson 1997). This is the issue in Philip's case as well.

The Supervision Register was introduced for England and Wales in 1994 in response to the Ritchie Report on Christopher Clunis, a patient with schizo-phrenia who killed a stranger while being cared for in the 'community'. It was intended to provide heightened vigilance over ex-patients considered to be at risk of serious violence, suicide, or significant self-neglect. The register was fol-lowed by a new Aftercare under Supervision Order passed by Parliament in 1995 under the Mental Health (Patients in the Community) Act. This autho-rizes the allocation of a named supervisor (usually a community psychiatric nurse) and a community RMO. A power of 'arrest' (according to the mental health charity MIND) is given by the provision in the Aftercare under Supervision Order that the ex-patient can be 'conveyed' to a safe place, such as residential or day-care provision, without his or her consent.

Many clinicians — like Nick and Margaret — find this power disturbing and unwelcome. There is also considerable scepticism amongst practitioners about whether the purpose of the Supervision Register is to benefit the patient following discharge, or to ensure that a key worker is identified and made formally responsible for the ex-patient's behaviour. The Royal College of Psychiatrists expressed 'strong concerns' about the DOH guidelines for the introduction of supervision registers. As an article in the *BMJ* put it, psychiatrists are put

> in an untenable position subject to a duty of care over a 'patient' who probably does not want to see them and who may actively evade them. It may or may not be reasonably possible to know whether the patient is actually dangerous...but the duty of care may extend as long as the patient is on the register. (Harrison and Bartlett 1994, p. 552)

This could have been written to describe Philip's case.

Supervision registers and Aftercare Under Supervision Orders are a halfway house which lack the frank paternalism of drug treatment orders or early recall orders, but they are also less than satisfactory to autonomy-minded psychia-trists, ethicists, and lawyers. Some critics even argue that long-term patients' rights would actually be better served by community treatment orders incor-porating due process — much as it may be fairer to have appeals against invol-untary committal go to normal legal institutions, as in Scotland. There is no requirement under the supervision order legislation to inform patients that their names have been placed on the register, and no process of appeal, although there is a built-in process of review every six months. However, it might be argued that supervised discharge does respect autonomy insofar as it allows patients who would otherwise be hospitalized to live in the community.

The example of Philip Caversham is a case about risk assessment, in building up a diagnosis and treatment plan, and about what might happen if that process of evaluation goes wrong. That is, if things turn out badly, who bears the responsibility? If no further treatment is imposed on Philip except his self-imposed art 'therapy', he may well re-offend — and then what? In the USA, practitioners have still been found civilly liable for releasing patients who have since harmed others. (For example, Semler *v* Psychiatric Institute of Washington (1976); Durflinger *v* Artiles (1983) P 2d.) But apart from the fear of legal liability, there is also an important paradox about ethical responsibility — the issue of moral luck (Williams 1981; Nagel 1976; Dickenson 1991).

We generally hold people morally responsible only for that which was within their control, but in practice we regard actions as right and wrong partly according to what happens as a result of the moral agent's decision. Yet this notion of personal responsibility as dependent on luck in outcomes seems to threaten the agent's ethical integrity: 'While one can be lucky in one's business, in one's married life, and in one's health, one cannot, so it is commonly assumed, be subject to luck as far as one's moral worth is concerned.' (Statman 1994, p. 1). In particular, the concepts of professional responsibility and justification for one's diagnostic and treatment decisions seem radically undermined by moral luck.

'Moral' or 'ethical' feels incompatible with 'luck' for clinicians, who are likely to be blamed for irresponsible or unprofessional behaviour if they get treatment decisions wrong — and, even more importantly, to blame themselves too. If Nick and Margaret decide not to exercise their powers to place Philip on the Supervision Register or to convey him to a treatment centre, and another girl is assaulted, will they reproach themselves? There seems to be something deeply wrong with the prospect of the clinicians shrugging such an assault off as just bad luck. Yet in another sense, what Philip decides to do is beyond their control: he would be the agent who commits the crime. And long-term management in the community gives the practitioner less control over the patient, compared with the ward situation.

Is the psychiatrist who decides not to take out a Supervision Order or to place a possibly dangerous person on the Supervision Register morally at fault if that person harms someone, or merely unlucky? What would be the appropriate reaction for the clinician who 'gets it wrong?' Perhaps a more subtle typology of blame and self-criticism is called for. Bernard Williams, who first developed the notion of moral luck, suggests that we can distinguish between failure of the agent's 'project' and his or her own failure. The sentiment of 'agent-regret', which applies to the latter kind of failure, is felt specifically about the agent's past actions, rather than about external states which have gone wrong. As a concomitant, it carries along with it the desire to atone in some way for the wrong which has been committed.

It does seem excessive, however, to ask that Nick and Margaret should feel that they have failed personally if Philip commits another assault, and should want to atone. Agent-regret seems a certain route to guilt, burn-out, and disillusionment among the most conscientious clinicians. It also implies a kind of hubris or fatal arrogance: only an all-seeing divine judge could know everything that bears on a decision and always give the right weight to it. Yet Williams is right, we think, to dismiss as 'very importantly wrong' the view that we can always avoid self-criticism if we have considered all available information carefully before making the decision and have done everything possible to avoid the unfortunate outcome (Williams 1994, p. 256). Such a perspective involves an unhealthy distance from one's own actions and a failure to distinguish ethical dilemmas from ordinary practical rationality (prudential decisions such as what car to buy).

We will return to the paradox of moral luck in other case studies, where it will be analysed from other angles: for example, in the case of Gilbert Ryan (Case 8.1), a wandering patient who is a risk to himself. For now, let us return to what moral luck implies about risk and consent in cases such as Philip's, where the clinicians' assessment differs from that of the patient. A focus on ill luck in outcomes concentrates the mind wonderfully: although the most obvious way in which things could turn out badly would be for Philip to re-offend, there are actually two ways in which things could turn out badly in this particular case. Philip's therapeutic outcome could be worsened, the clinicians feel, if they place him on the Supervision Register without his consent.

Consent seems to us the key to the dilemmas of moral luck. If a procedure turns out badly, the normally competent physician cannot be held ethically at fault if he has obtained informed consent. In general, the effect of informed consent, as one of us has argued elsewhere (Dickenson 1991), is to transfer responsibility for ill luck in outcomes from the doctor to the patient. On the surface, the question may appear to be who has authority to give consent; but in relation to long-term consequences, the question is who bears responsibility if something goes wrong.

If Nick and Margaret bypass the consent procedures — as the supervision register legislation may well tempt them to do — then they bear the responsibility for any worsening in Philip's condition, against their expectations of therapeutic success. This may appear to put the clinicians in a cleft stick: damned if they seek Philip's consent to being put on the Supervision Register and he absconds altogether; damned if they don't and he finds out they have acted behind his back, destroying what little therapeutic alliance has been constructed. Of the two possible adverse outcomes — and it is important to recognize that both are possible — the second should actually occasion more self-blame in the clinicians than the first. The first is Philip's choice, not Nick and Margaret's.

Practitioner commentary (CASE 7.2)

Dominic Beer Senior Lecturer (Guy's, King's, St Thomas', and Institute of Psychiatry) and Honorary Consultant Psychiatrist in Challenging Behaviour and Intensive Care Psychiatry, Oxleas NHS Trust (approved under Section 12(2) Mental Health Act 1983).

This case exemplifies a number of key issues confronted by mental health professionals working in the fields of general and forensic psychiatry. It shows that many of the old chestnuts are as hot as ever! How does one weigh up issues of patient autonomy against the protection of others? Allied to this — what does the professional do when the patient's capacity for autonomy is compromised by illness? The professional's 'duty of care' may 'trump' autonomy, even when the duty to protect others from the patient is not considered to be an issue.

In this brief commentary I want to pick up three issues. First, how risk assessment, with all its inherent difficulties, might proceed in practice. Second, how the new Supervised Discharge Aftercare Orders would help in practice with a case like Philip Caversham's. Third, how the new Mental Health Act for England and Wales would help, if as proposed, it includes a tribunal to deal with issues of compulsory treatment.

For the clinician looking after Philip Caversham, the first priority is to complete a formal risk assessment. The adage 'past behaviour predicts future behaviour' is highly pertinent; the Initial Police Risk Assessment for Sex Offenders uses such data (Grubin, 1998). From the criminal history, one point is scored for each of the following: index offence has sexual element; pre-convictions include offence with sexual element; index conviction includes non-sexual assault; person has been convicted on at least four separate occasions.

If we count Philip's last conviction for indecent assault as the index offence, then he scores 2. This puts him in the medium-risk category for re-offending (1 point low; 2–3 medium; 4+ high). If at least two of the following aggravating factors are present, then the risk is increased one level:

- Any contact offences with male victim.

- Any sex offence with a stranger victim.

- Never married or lived with lover for two years.

- Ever taken into local authority residential care.

- Substance abuse problem (more than recreational).

It is unclear from the history available if Philip scores two on these factors, but since he is already a medium risk on actuarial grounds, the clinician is sufficiently alerted to be concerned.

The next step for the clinician is to assess what might make the risk in the case greater or smaller. This requires a thorough assessment of Philip's psychiatric, psychological, and social functioning. It is doubtful whether this can be done as an out-patient, given his non-engagement with services. If he is unwilling to be admitted voluntarily, then an assessment for admission under the Mental Health Act should be arranged. The rationale for this is that there is evidence that he has delusions of thought interference: his behaviour is eccentric; he refuses to take medication; there are other worrying factors such as painting nude women; and he refuses to engage in discussion of previous offences. A Section 3 Order, under the Mental Health Act (allowing admission to a hospital for treatment), can be applied for once it is clear that (1) he is suffering from a mental disorder, and (2) that he needs to be treated in hospital.

Once he is in hospital, then further risk assessment can be performed by a forensic psychiatrist and psychologist. Let us suppose that the assessment shows that he is indeed psychotic, but that his sexual fantasies and aspirations are not directly linked to his mental illness. It also reveals that his current sexual interests include young women and adolescent girls and that his previous offences had only failed to proceed to rape because he was fortuitously interrupted. The assessment shows that his psychosis acts as a disinhibitor, because his grandiose beliefs make him more likely to fulfil his sexual needs.

It is clear that, given this risk assessment, merely placing a patient like Philip on the Supervision Register will achieve very little (Hindler 1999). In fact, it is likely that the Department of Health will permit health authorities to withdraw a patient from the Register if a risk assessment has been performed as part of the Care Programme Approach (Department of Health, 1999). One of the possible reasons for this is because Supervised Discharge Aftercare has been introduced (Section 25a, Mental Health Act 1983 in England and Wales). Supervised Discharge Aftercare Orders give the health authority the power to make a patient who has been under a Treatment Order subject to certain conditions on discharge from hospital (for example, to be resident at a specific place, to allow access to a supervisor, to attend at specified places and times for medical treatment, occupation, education, or training).

This brings me to my second point — how a Supervised Discharge Aftercare Order would help in a case like Philip Caversham's. These are being increasingly used in mental health practice (Pinfold *et al.* 1999). In the first place, the criteria for a Supervised Discharge Aftercare Order are different from those for being placed on the Supervision Register. They are:

1 The patient suffers from mental disorder.

2 There would be a substantial risk of serious harm if he were not to receive the aftercare services.

3 His being subject to a Supervised Discharge Aftercare Order is likely to ensure that he receives aftercare services.

Unlike the Supervision Register, the patient can appeal against this section of the Mental Health Act. This is clearly a key difference from the patient's point of view and one which might improve compliance. A more important difference from the Supervision Register, however, which is more likely to increase compliance, is that resources are attached to the Supervised Discharge because the Supervisor is unlikely to agree to supervise the patient in the absence of such resources. In this case, residence at a staffed hostel and attendance at out-patients, at a day centre, and at group therapy for sex offenders may be stipulated.

Although drug treatment cannot be enforced under a Supervised Discharge Aftercare Order, in practice, if medication is refused then the patient can be assessed for admission under Section 2 of the Mental Health Act. The Mental Health Act Commission's *Threshold for Admission and the Relapsing Patient* (1998) states that 'A patient may be admitted under Section 2, despite the absence of signs of mental disorder if the patient's health has begun to deteriorate and that there are signs of relapse, ie it is clear that the disorder is beginning to manifest itself in the familiar way'.

While Supervised Discharge Aftercare Orders are, in my view, a considerable advance on the Supervision Register for cases like Philip Caversham's, the fundamental problem with 'compulsory treatment' still remains for the physician — that of combining a therapeutic role with the role of custodian. My third point, then, is that Philip Caversham's case reinforces the importance of current proposals to include, in the new Mental Health Act for England and Wales, a tribunal system for deciding issues of compulsory treatment. The current draft of the new Act provides for the possibility that a tribunal will be able to make the decision to compulsorily admit a patient. If this becomes law it will allow patients and clinicians alike to feel that their therapeutic relationship has not been so adversely affected by the process of 'sectioning'.

Arrangements of this kind, in which a tribunal is responsible for compulsory admissions and treatment, would have the further salutary consequence of relieving psychiatrists of the impossible responsibility they currently bear for the behaviour of their patients. In the UK, public attitudes, which are constantly 'hyped' by the media, are of blaming the doctor when 'something goes wrong' and one of their patients commits a crime. The new arrangements will bring us more into line with European practice (for example, van Lysebetten and Igodt 2000). Our European colleagues find it hard to understand how mental health professionals in Britain have allowed themselves to get into this situation.

References (CASE 7.2)

Chadwick, R. and Levitt, M. (1995) 'The ethics of community health care.' Paper presented at the Riverside Mental Health Trust, 30 January.

Department of Health (1994) *Draft Guide to Arrangements for Inter-Agency Working for the Care and Protection of Severely Mentally Ill People.* London, DoH.

Department of Health (1999) *Modernising the Care Programme Approach — a Policy Booklet.* London, DoH.

Dickenson, D. (1991) *Moral Luck in Medical Ethics and Practical Politics* (1st edn). Aldershot, Gower Publishers. (2nd edn (forthcoming), published as *Risk and Luck in Medical Ethics.* Cambridge, Polity Press.)

Dickenson, D. (1997) Ethical issues in long-term psychiatric care. *Journal of Medical Ethics,* **23/5**:300–4.

Durflinger v. Artiles (1983) 673 P 2d.

Grubin, D. (1998) *Sex Offending Against Children: Understanding the Risk.* Home Office Policing and Reducing Crime Unit, Research Development and Statistics Directorate.

Harrison, G. and Bartlett, P. (1994) Supervision registers for mentally ill people: medicolegal issues seem likely to dominate decisions by clinicians. *BMJ,* **309**:591–2.

Hindler, C. (1999) The supervision register: 19 months after its introduction. *Psychiatric Bulletin,* **23**:15–19.

Lindley, R. (1986) *Autonomy.* Houndmills, Macmillan.

Mental Health Act Commission (1998) *The Threshold for Admission and the Relapsing Patient.* Nottingham, Mental Health Act Commission.

Nagel, T. (1976, reprinted 1979). Moral luck. In *Mortal Questions* (Nagel, T.) Cambridge, Cambridge University Press.

Pinfold, V., Bindman, J., Friedl, K., Beck, A., and Thornicroft, G. (1999) Supervised discharge orders in England: compulsory care in the community. *Psychiatric Bulletin,* **23**:199–203.

Semler v. Psychiatric Institute of Washington DC (1976) 538 F 2d 121.

Statman, D. (1994) Introduction to *Moral Luck* (ed. Statman, D.). State University of
New York.

van Lysebetten, T. and Igodt, P. (2000) Compulsory psychiatric admission: a comparison of English and Belgian legislation. *Psychiatric Bulletin*, 24:66–8.

White, R., Carr, P., and Lowe, N. (1990) *A Guide to the Children Act 1989*. London,
Butterworths.

Williams, B. (1981) *Moral Luck*. Cambridge, Cambridge University Press.

Williams, B. (1994) Postscript to *Moral Luck* (ed. Statman, D.), pp. 251–8. State
University of New York.

Reading Guide

This Reading Guide covers some of the ethical aspects of the prediction of dangerous behaviour. A particularly problematic area is confidentiality and we
include a separate section on that topic. As we indicated in the introduction to
this chapter, this is an area in which the uncertainties that are endemic to psychiatric practice are perhaps most critical ethically. Hence the third section of
this Reading Guide is on 'moral luck'.

Predicting dangerous behaviour (ethical aspects)

Recent reviews of the now very large literature on the prediction of dangerousness include Hazel Kempshall and Jackie Pritchard's *Good Practice in Risk
Assessment* (1997) and Anthony Maden's 'Risk assessment and management in
psychiatry' (1998). The Royal College of Psychiatrists' *Management of
Imminent Violence: Clinical Practice Guidelines* (1998) includes extensive bib-
liographies. Ethical aspects of risk assessment have been relatively neglected. In
Psychiatric Ethics (Bloch *et al.* 1999), George Szmukler reviews the issues in
community care (Chapter 17), and Roger Reele and Paul Chodoff consider the
role of a 'dangerousness criterion' for involuntary hospitalization (Chapter 20).

The ethics of the use of Supervision Registers in community care is discussed by Donna Dickenson (1997). Although not concerned with psychiatry,
Kenneth Calman's article 'Cancer: science and society and the communication of risk' (1996) covers important aspects of the relationship between evidence on risk and public attitudes. The gross public stigmatization of people
with mental disorders in respect of dangerousness is explored by Pamela
Taylor and John Gunn in 'Homicides by people with mental illness: myth
and reality' (1999).

The *Bulletin* of The Royal College of Psychiatrists publishes brief articles
reporting psychiatrists' actual experience of implementing arrangements for
'care and control' in the community: for example, Milton (1998), Knight *et al.*

(1998), and Mohan *et al.* (1998) on supervised discharge; Lowe–Ponsford *et al.* (1998), Vaughan (1998), and Hindler (1999) on Supervision Registers; and Wallace and Ball (1998) on the Care Programme Approach. These articles are particularly helpful in grounding ethical discussion on reality. They indicate, for example, the key role of resources (see Reading Guide to Chapter 8).

Confidentiality

Most of the large textbooks on medical ethics include sections on confidentiality: Chapter 17 of Gillon's *Philosophical Medical Ethics* (1986) or Chapter 7 of Beauchamp and Childress' *Principles of Biomedical Ethics* (1989) are both excellent starting points. Confidentiality in medical records is covered in detail in Chapter 2 of the BMA's *Medical Ethics Today* (1993). The BMA issued new guidelines in 1999 on *Confidentiality and Disclosure of Health Information*. The importance of being aware of different perspectives in this area is illustrated by Weiss' (1982) article on the expectations of patients, physicians, and medical students.

The ethical aspects of confidentiality specifically in psychiatry are reviewed by David Joseph and Joseph Orek in Chapter 7 of *Psychiatric Ethics* (Bloch *et al.* 1999). This includes a discussion of the issues raised by potentially dangerous behaviour. Confidentiality is also a growing issue in relation to publication. A valuable review of the practical, ethical, and legal aspects of confidentiality in respect of case reports is provided by the article by Wilkinson and colleagues, 'Case reports and confidentiality: opinion is sought, medical and legal' (1995). The Royal College of Psychiatrists have recently reviewed the issues raised by confidentiality in all areas of psychiatry, including research. Their report is forthcoming. A recent edited collection explaining all aspects of confidentiality in mental health is Chris Cordess' *Confidentiality and Mental Health* (2000).

The concept of significant harm, as used in the Children Act 1989, is also of interest: evidence that harm has occurred in the past or is occurring at present is not enough, unless it points to significant likelihood of harm occurring in the future. See Richard White *et al.*'s *A Guide to the Children Act 1989* (1990).

Moral luck

The nub of the moral luck debate is set out in essays by Thomas Nagel, 'Moral luck,' in *Mortal Questions* (1979) and Bernard Williams, *Moral Luck*, in the volume of the same name (1981). Further development of the concept and application to medical ethics can be found in Donna Dickenson's *Moral Luck in Medical Ethics and Practical Politics* (1991) and the considerably extended second edition, *Risk and Luck in Medical Ethics* (forthcoming).

Reading Guide: references

Beauchamp, T.L. and Childress, J.F. (1989; 4th edn 1994) *Principles of Biomedical Ethics*. Oxford, Oxford University Press.

Bloch, S., Chodoff, P., and Green S.A. (1999) *Psychiatric Ethics* (3rd edn; 1st edn 1981). Oxford, Oxford University Press.

BMA (1993) *Mental Ethics Today: Its Practice and Philosophy*. London, BMA.

BMA (1999) *Confidentiality and Disclosure of Health Information*. London, BMA.

Calman, K.C. (1996) Cancer: science and society and the communication of risk. *BMJ*, **313**:799–802.

Cordess, C. (2000) *Confidentiality and Mental Health*. London, Jessica Kingsley Publishers.

Dickenson, D. (1991) *Moral Luck in Medical Ethics and Practical Politics* (1st edn). Aldershot, Gower Publishers. (2nd edn (forthcoming), published as *Risk and Luck in Medical Ethics*. Cambridge, Polity Press.)

Dickenson, D. (1997) Ethical issues in long-term psychiatric care. *Journal of Medical Ethics*, **23/5**:300–4.

Gillon, R. (1985) *Philosophical Medical Ethics*. Chichester (England), John Wiley and Sons.

Hindler, C. (1999) The supervision register: 19 months after its introduction. *Psychiatric Bulletin*, **23**:15–19.

Kemshall, H. and Pritchard, J. (ed.) (1997) *Good Practice in Risk Assessment II: Key Themes for Protection, Rights and Responsibilities*. London, Jessica Kingsley Publishers.

Knight, A., Mumford, D., and Nichol, B. (1998) Supervised discharge order: the first year in the South and West Region. *Psychiatric Bulletin*, **22**:418–20.

Lowe–Ponsford, F. L., Wolfson, P., and Lindesay, J. (1998) Consultant psychiatrists' views on the supervision register. *Psychiatric Bulletin*, **22**:409–11.

Maden, A. (1998) Risk assessment and management in psychiatry. *CPD Psychiatry* (Rila Publications), **1/1**:8–11.

Milton, J. (1998) Section 17 of the Mental Health Act. *Psychiatric Bulletin*, **22**:415–18.

Mohan, D., Thompson, C., and Mullee, M.A. (1998) Preliminary evaluation of supervised discharge order in the South and West Region. *Psychiatric Bulletin*, **22**:421–3.

Nagel, T. (1976, reprinted 1979). Moral luck. In *Mortal Questions* (Nagel, T.) Cambridge, Cambridge University Press.

Royal College of Psychiatrists Research Unit (1998) *Management of Imminent Violence: Clinical Practice Guidelines to Support Mental Health Services*. London, Royal College of Psychiatrists.

Taylor, P. J. and Gunn, J. (1999) Homicides by people with mental illness: myth and reality. *British Journal of Psychiatry*, **174**:9–14.

Vaughan, P.J. (1998) Supervision register in practice. *Psychiatric Bulletin*, **22**:412–15.

Wallace, J. and Ball, C. J. (1998) Use of the Care Programme Approach register by an inner-city old age psychiatry team. *Psychiatric Bulletin*, 22:489–91.

Weiss, B.D. (1982) Confidentiality in expectations of patients, physicians, and medical students. *JAMA*, 247(19):2695–7.

White, R., Carr, P., and Lowe, N. (1990) *A Guide to the Children Act 1989*. London, Butterworths.

Wilkinson, G. *et al*. (1995) Case reports and confidentiality: opinion is sought, medical and legal. *British Journal of Psychiatry*, 166:555–8.

Williams, B. (1981) *Moral Luck*. Cambridge, Cambridge University Press.

CHAPTER 8

Teamwork and the organization of services

Multidisciplinary teamwork, including users as well as providers, is the key to successfully working through the ethical issues explored in preceding chapters. This in turn depends on good communication skills

Issues of teamwork, although not separated out as such, have been woven through many of the ethical dilemmas raised in earlier chapters. The different models of disorder represented by different members of multidisciplinary teams were important in coming to a balance between moral and medical conceptions of mental disorder in Chapter 3; in Chapter 4, the different value perspectives of team members as well as of users and carers were crucial to diagnosis; these perspectives were important, too, in the discussion of aetiology in Chapter 5, in coming to an understanding of the meanings (as well as to explanations of the causes) of mental disorder; the skills base of the multidisciplinary team was important to treatment in Chapter 6 generally, but also to the management of involuntary treatment discussed in Chapter 2; and shared decision making was essential to the problems of risk management discussed in Chapter 7.

Where a multidisciplinary team works well, problems in all these areas are readily tackled, if not always easily resolved. Too often, though, what happens in practice is that different professional groups find themselves in competition or even in open conflict. In this chapter we explore some of the ethical issues specific to multidisciplinary teamwork, in one case where the professionals involved were in open conflict, in a second where they co-operated.

Case 8.1 concerns Gilbert Ryan, an elderly man with moderate dementia and a tendency to wander off, but who was otherwise well cared for by his loving but disabled son. The option of tagging was raised as a way of making it possible for him to stay with his son, but discussion of this was blocked *ex cathedra* by a local Social Services policy.

Case 8.2, Sam Mason, illustrates the continuing problems of community treatment which is blocked by the primary carer (in this case the patient's father). Although not finally resolving the problem, co-operation between agencies was effective in 'damage limitation'.

These two cases illustrate a range of wider ethical issues raised by community care. Thus Gilbert Ryan's story (Case 8.1) graphically illustrates how resource issues underpin and determine every aspect of community care. This in turn is an aspect of the wider question of the extent to which what is ethical is determined by what is practical. As the American bioethicist George Agich has shown in a detailed discussion of ethical issues in the care of people with long-term illnesses, autonomy is an empty concept without the physical as well as psychological resources required to make our choices meaningful (Agich 1993). Jim Birley (in Chapter 11) makes a similar point in his comments on the dire state of many people with long-term mental illnesses in some of the territories of the former USSR. Gilbert Ryan reminds us that our options in community care in the UK are largely determined, less dramatically but no less decisively, by our resources.

The counterpart to resources is needs. Gilbert Ryan's story also reminds us that professionals may have a very distorted understanding of the needs of those with long-term mental disorders. Modern methods of needs assessment aim to take into account the views of users as well as providers of services. Some of these methods have actually been devised by users (Avon Mental Health 1996). The Oxford psychiatrist Max Marshall (1994) has shown that earlier, provider-only based methods of assessment were based on a misconception of the very concept of need. But it is important to be aware that this shift to 'patient autonomy' — to a recognition of the importance of the values of users in needs assessment — is a recent development in mental health. There is still a tendency to slip back to a 'doctor knows best' or, as in Gilbert Ryan's case, a 'social worker knows best' perspective. Gilbert Ryan's story, and indeed that of his learning-disabled son, shows that even where a long-term mental disorder involves cognitive impairment, a balanced approach to the assessment of need, reflecting the perspectives of users and carers as well as of different members of the multidisciplinary team, is essential to good clinical care.

Sam Mason's story (Case 8.2) leads into a discussion of the role of legal options other than the Mental Health Act for providing care and control (for example, Guardianship Orders and the Children Act). However, it also illustrates the limitations of the individual-centred approach of the law, the mechanisms of rights, principles, and so on, in the context of community care. What is needed, we argue, as a counterbalance to this approach, is an ethic which is itself less individualistic and more communitarian. We discuss two possibilities — 'relationship ethics' and the 'ethics of care'. This is a growth area in medical ethics and we include relevant recent publications in the Reading Guide at the end of this chapter. But Sam Mason's case offers a warning note. For it reminds

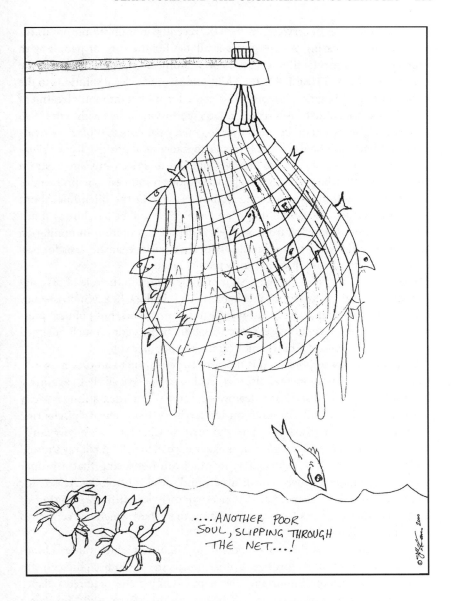

us that, *contra* the ethics of care and relationship ethics, relationships may be harmful as well as helpful, and carers may be intrusive as well as supportive, when it comes to young people's choices.

A common factor in Gilbert Ryan's and Sam Mason's stories is the need to balance care and control. This is at the heart of many of our most pressing problems in community care, not only at the level of teamwork but also in the overall organization of services. In the UK, recently announced proposals for substantially increasing the resources available for the care of people with severe long-term mental illnesses are to be welcomed. On the other hand, the review of the Mental Health Act 1983 looks set to opt for legal solutions to the problem of providing greater control — some form of community treatment order is a likely candidate. Aftercare Under Supervision Orders within the 1995 Act already give psychiatrists the power to convey patients to a place of treatment. But what will be the effect if this is upgraded to a positive legal obligation? Will psychiatrists find themselves obliged to search out and restrain patients? Will they be given responsibility without resources? The problem of responsibility without resources is already present in the dilemmas about Supervision Orders (discussed in the last chapter). It will be a sad irony if just as medical ethics is moving from a largely individual to more communitarian ethic, we should find ourselves saddled with a narrowly legalistic basis for balancing care with control in community mental health.

Whatever form it takes though, a shift of some degree in the role of psychiatry towards social control seems inevitable, at least in the UK. Psychiatrists may believe that their primary responsibility is to their patients, but political pressures and public perceptions seem set to saddle them with a much enlarged responsibility to society. Control, not care, is the popular vote.

Psychiatrists may respond to this defensively, retreating to an ever narrower scientific conception of mental disorder. Such a response is likely to aggravate the problems of interdisciplinary teamwork, for it will harden attitudes, deify ideologies, and intensify competition for territory. An exclusively scientific conception of mental disorder, we have argued (in Chapter 3), is anyway mistaken in principle; even if it were not, as experience in the USSR plainly showed (Fulford *et al.* 1993), it is incapable in practice of ensuring that a proper balance is maintained between medical care and social control. One reason for this, as we noted in Chapter 3, is that a narrowly scientific conception of mental disorder excludes from consideration the values which are central to maintaining this balance.

We are brought back then to a model of psychiatry in which values, alongside facts, are central. According to this model, the multidisciplinary team will be an increasingly important ally in maintaining the required balance as the pressures on psychiatry to shift from care to control build up. For a well-functioning multidisciplinary team, reflecting as it does different value perspectives, can help to bring a balance of values to clinical decision making. The importance of this was transparent in the diagnostic problem in Case 4.3, Simon Greer — the problem of whether Simon Greer was suffering from schizophrenia (and hence in principle subject to psychiatric control as well as care) or going through a religious experience. Here, as we noted, the multidisciplinary team can play a key role in coming to a balanced view over the value judgements on which the DSM's Criterion B for schizophrenia depends.

Similar value judgements were implicit, however, in the concepts of rationality and responsibility embedded in the diagnostic judgements in the other cases in Chapter 4, and in the wider moral and political judgements by which, in Chapter 3, mental distress and disorder were identified as pathological in the first place. Value judgements have also been important in the meanings which were central to the aetiological assessments in Chapter 5, in the outcome preferences governing issues of autonomy of treatment choice in Chapter 6, and in the utilities by which risk and dangerousness (as opposed to mere probabilities) were assessed in Chapter 7. Now, finally, in this chapter, values are central to the different perceptions of need on which the definition of adequate resources and hence an ethically sound community care provision depend. And it is only within an ethically sound community care service that ethically sound community control is possible, even in principle.

This leads us to a final point about the central place of teamwork, including users as well as providers, in mental health care. To make this point we need to take two steps back — the first, to the promissory note we left at the end of Chapter 4 about the importance of definition, and the second, to the discussion of the role of law in Chapter 2. Thus, the value of law, as we noted in Chapter 2, is that it provides clear criteria which set limits to what is acceptable in mental health care. This is part of its appeal, particularly in a discipline like mental health in which diversity and uncertainty are the norm. It is for similar reasons, as we indicated in Chapter 4, that clear psychopathological criteria, as incorporated into classifications like the DSM, are attractive to psychiatrists.

The practical utility of clear criteria, however, in disciplines such as law and psychiatry, has led to a widespread assumption that explicit definitions are a *sine qua non* for clear thinking. 'Define your terms' is the clarion call in psychiatry no less than in law! Yet the message of the cases described in this book has been that many of our deepest dilemmas in psychiatry turn on concepts which have stubbornly resisted definition: the concept of 'need', for example, in this chapter; the concept of 'risk' in Chapter 7; a whole range of deep metaphysical concepts (freedom, personal identity, and so on) underpinning dilemmas of treatment in Chapter 6; 'meaning' and 'cause' in Chapter 5; 'rationality', 'autonomy', and 'capacity', together with some of our core psychopathological concepts such as 'delusion', in Chapter 4; and, by no means least, in Chapter 3, the very concept of 'mental disorder' itself.

The difficulties of definition presented by concepts such as these reflect the fact, spelled out in Chapter 1, that psychiatry is conceptually as well as empirically difficult. The difficulties, though, have been taken by many, not least in psychiatry itself, as an indication that compared with other areas of medicine, psychiatry is a muddled discipline. It is important, therefore, to recognize that clear definition, notwithstanding its success with concepts such as schizophrenia, is the exception rather than the rule. The rule, indeed, is that in general we are actually much better at *using* concepts than at *defining* them.

You can see this in a general way by noting how little help you get from dictionary definitions in trying to understand the meaning of an unfamiliar word. This should not come as a surprise, since we learn the meanings of concepts primarily through shared use in a social context (as we grow up) rather than from dictionaries. But if you doubt that people are better at using concepts than at defining them, try defining 'time'. This is a standard philosophical example of a concept which we are so good at using (we use it all the time, *sic!*) that we fail to notice that we are unable to define it[1].

A medical example of a concept which is easier to use than to define is the concept of physical illness. Unlike the concept of mental illness, physical illness is not problematic in use. That is to say, in psychiatry, as we have seen (particularly in Chapters 3 and 4), there are often problems about whether a given mental condition is or is not a genuine mental illness. (It is these problems which have led to the whole psychiatry v. antipsychiatry debate about the validity of the concept of mental illness.) But in physical medicine, while there are problems aplenty of *differential* diagnosis (of what particular *kind* of illness someone is suffering from), there are few problems about whether a given physical condition is or is not a genuine physical illness. Correspondingly, therefore, while there has been debate about the meaning of physical illness, it has been widely assumed that physical illness is relatively transparent in meaning compared with mental illness. Nothing could be further from the truth! As one of us has shown elsewhere (Fulford 1989, Chapter 1), the psychiatry v. antipsychiatry debate about *mental* illness actually turns on unrecognized difficulties about the meaning of *physical* illness.

That a concept is difficult to define is, therefore, no indication that it is invalid, still less that those using it are muddled. This has a number of important implications, theoretical and practical (Fulford 1990). One theoretical implication has to do with how we understand psychiatric science. Much of the stigma attached to psychiatrists and their patients alike arises from the assumption that the difficulty we have with the meanings of our core concepts is a mark of a primitive or underdeveloped science. From this flows marginalization, lack of resources, and many other practical consequences crucial to good practice in mental health. Hence we, users and providers together, should fight back. Instead of accepting a 'Cinderella' role to the medical scientific model, we should recognize that in this respect, psychiatry is closer to theoretical physics than biology. In theoretical physics, like psychiatry, many of the *key* scientific problems are conceptual (including the concept of time) as well as empirical[2]. Therefore the conceptual problems with which we are concerned in psychiatry — from the disputed nature of mental disorder onwards — are the marks not of a muddled science but of a science at the cutting edge of understanding.

A practical implication of recognizing that psychiatry is conceptually difficult (rather than muddled) has to do with the organization of services (Fulford 1998). This brings us back to the crucial role of the multidisciplinary team. Where we have difficulties with the meaning of a concept (as we have with the meaning of 'mental disorder' and the family of related concepts we have encountered in the cases in this book), we should look as much to the processes by which the concepts in question are *used* as to the criteria by which they are defined. Criteria, to reiterate, are important. They are not enough, however. We must be concerned also with the processes by which we, as *users* of the relevant concepts, come to a shared understanding of their meanings. But in mental health, we are *all* users of mental health concepts, service users (the term is doubly apposite!) as well as service providers, and among service providers, not just psychiatrists, but social workers, community psychiatric nurses, psychologists, managers — indeed, all those working in multidisciplinary teams.

In mental health, then, 'shared use in a social context' means, literally, the multidisciplinary team, including users as well as providers of services. We noted the important role of the multidisciplinary team in Case 4.3 (Simon Greer), in providing a variety of perspectives which could be crucial in coming to a balance of values. Recognizing that we are better at using concepts than at defining them takes this role a step further, to the full range of difficult concepts (including rationality and responsibility) implicit in psychiatric diagnosis. This throws the onus of good practice firmly back on us all, users as well as providers, to develop the communication skills on which good practice crucially depends. This in turn means that it is, above all, in the multidisciplinary team that the practice skills model outlined in Chapter 2 — bringing together communication skills with a philosophically enriched bioethics — is essential to good practice in mental health.

References

Agich, G. J. (1993) *Autonomy and Long-Term Care*. Oxford, Oxford University Press.

Avon Mental Health (1996) *The Avon Mental Health Measure: A User-centred Approach to Assessing Need*. London, MIND Publications.

Bridgman, P.W. (1927) *The Logic of Modern Physics*. New York, Macmillan.

Fulford, K.W.M. (1989, reprinted 1995; 2nd edn, forthcoming) *Moral Theory and Medical Practice*. Cambridge, Cambridge University Press.

Fulford, K.W.M. (1990) Philosophy and medicine: the Oxford connection. *British Journal of Psychiatry*, **157**:111–15.

Fulford, K.W.M. (1998) Replacing the Mental Health Act 1983? How to change the game without losing the baby with the bath water or shooting ourselves in the foot. *Psychiatric Bulletin*, 22:666–70.

Fulford, K.W.M., Smirnoff, A.Y.U., and Snow, E. (1993) Concepts of disease and the abuse of psychiatry in the USSR. *British Journal of Psychiatry*, 162:801–10.

Kendell, R.E. (1975) *The Role of Diagnosis in Psychiatry*. Oxford, Blackwell Scientific Publications.

Marshall, M. (1994) How should we measure need? Concept and practice in the development of a standardised assessment schedule. *Philosophy, Psychiatry, and Psychology*, 1/1:27–36. (Commentaries by Crisp, R. and Morgan, J., 37–40)

CASE 8.1

Gilbert Ryan — tracking and tagging

Synopsis A 79-year-old man, with moderately severe Alzheimer's disease, is admitted to hospital after being knocked over by a car whilst wandering the streets in the early hours of the morning. He has always been a keen walker. He lives with his learning-disabled son, who is devoted to him. Tagging is discussed with him as an alternative to staying in hospital (there being no Social Services nursing home placement available), but he is unable (or unwilling) to consent.

Key dilemma Should he be discharged home, with a tag, at least for a trial period? Or is this merely endorsing inadequate resources for care/supervision?

Main topics Resources; use and misuse of technology; clinicians' responsibility for risk.

Other topics Principlism; duty of care; consent; advance directives; guardianship; Supervision Orders; moral luck; Kant; negligence; doctrine of double effect.

Gilbert Ryan, a 79-year-old widower, lives with his learning-disabled son Stephen in sheltered housing. He has mild to moderate Alzheimer's disease, with very poor short-term memory. His language abilities are reasonably well preserved, as is his mobility. Always very active as a younger man, Gilbert still enjoys 'getting out and about', as he puts it: 'got to get some air'.

The difficulty is that now his 'getting out and about' has got out of control. Until recently, the problems were confined to Gilbert's uncertainty over which of the sheltered housing flats was his own, when he came back from walks with his dog Barney. This was not too serious: Stephen, who is very attached to Gilbert, was usually waiting at the gate to fetch his father back home. But now Gilbert has taken to wandering in the very early hours of the morning, when Stephen is still asleep. Gilbert normally wakes around

3.00 a.m., but sometimes rises several times during the night, at unpredictable hours.

A number of times Gilbert was found by the milkman, near the entrance to the flats. But two months ago, in January, things took a sudden turn for the worse. After going missing for an entire day, Gilbert was located unconscious, a mile away, in a ditch with the dog — the victim of a hit-and-run motorist. Luckily Barney's body heat was detected by the search team, using a heat detector. Gilbert's own body temperature had fallen so low as to be undetectable.

Fortunately there were no serious injuries. Gilbert recovered in hospital and was then admitted informally as an emergency case to a psychogeriatric unit. His sleep patterns have become more settled with mild night-time sedation, and a urinary infection, which might have caused his restlessness, is now under control. At first he desperately wanted to return home to Stephen, but after ten days, he is now less keen to leave the ward. However, he does not want his mobility impaired by sedative drugs (to which he is peculiarly sensitive): getting out and about is still his major preoccupation.

Gilbert's consultant, Hassan Shah, has called a case conference to discuss the risk management issues. Gilbert is very hesitant when crossing the road, in observations of his traffic assessment. When he does start to cross, he is unable to react to drivers. Hassan is not at all happy about releasing Gilbert to return home. But if the risks of a trial at home are considered acceptable by the case conference, he would like to stipulate that a tracking device should be part of the care package. He has tried to talk about tracking to Gilbert during his intervals of competence, but has not succeeded in getting a meaningful consent. Whether this is due to Gilbert's inability to remember and understand the options, or to outright opposition, seems unclear. Stephen does not understand the idea of tracking, but he is enthusiastic about it because then he can have 'Dad home'.

Jane Vargos, a senior social worker who is 'Approved' under the Mental Health Act to deal with compulsory admission of at-risk patients, warns that Social Services locally are very opposed to tagging and tracking. She might be subject to disciplinary action if she approved the use of any electronic device of this kind. An additional difficulty is that Social Services do not have any money to fund placement of patients in nursing homes, except on a strictly one-to-one basis. This means that in-patient psychogeriatric units, often needed as part of the emergency management of patients who wander, will be increasingly less able to respond to such emergencies because their beds will be blocked by patients awaiting placement in nursing homes. The implications are that patients with wandering problems will increasingly be

> managed in the community, with the increased exposure to risk that this necessarily entails.

How much should what is 'ethical' be determined by what is practical? 'Ought implies can', in Kant's famous formulation. To have an ethical obligation, one must be in a position to carry out the obligation. Instead, Hassan Shah and his team are in a very difficult position — a cleft stick, in fact. The case conference cannot approve tagging or tracking Gilbert without putting Jane Vargos at risk of disciplinary action, since Social Services policy is strictly anti-tagging. On the other hand, they cannot bank on the ready availability of the in-patient psycho-geriatric unit as part of Gilbert's care plan, because Social Services policy on nursing home placements has created a bed-blocking problem in the unit. The effect as the clinicians see it is that psychiatric services must decide whether they will be party to countenancing increased risk because of scarce resources.

Yet because clinicians owe a duty of care to the individual patient, generalized resource considerations cannot be allowed to dominate altogether. That sort of excuse feels profoundly unethical to most doctors, and might also be negligent in law. The courts have generally been reluctant to intervene in resource alloca-tion questions, viewing them instead as a political matter for Parliament (Wilsher *v* Essex AHA (1986)). However, the principle is not absolute: for example, in Knight *v* Home Office (1990) the court warned that staffing short-ages could not be a 'complete defence' against a charge of negligence in failing to prevent a prisoner from hanging himself. Whether a reasonable level of care has been provided cannot ignore the question of whether unreasonable risks have been taken, although the standard is more lenient in health care law than in tort (Montgomery 1997, p. 181). So would discharging Gilbert with a track-ing device infringe that duty of care? What's wrong with the proposal?

There is no denying that the idea of tracking is uncomfortable. For many, this kind of electronic dog-lead seems to dehumanize the patient. Harry Cayton, President of the Alzheimer's Disease Society, warned in an editorial in the society's newsletter: 'Time to get out your "Living Will" and write on it in large letters, "I want to be allowed to wander. I need to take risks. I'm a person, not a dement." '

But even a person whose competence is not in doubt is not permitted to take any and all risks — not if their risk-taking poses unnecessary, intolerable harm to others. This is what motorway speed limits are about. The difference here is that Gilbert primarily poses a risk to himself: he is the one likely to be knocked over, perhaps killed this time, if his wandering is not monitored. But according to the view we have put forward in other studies, such as the case of Ida Harbottle (Case 6.2), the right to risk self-harm is rarely unqualified—because other people usually get hurt too, although perhaps in less obvious ways. In this case, Stephen will be shattered if anything happens to his father. More broadly, 'the wandering old man who gets knocked down in the road has inflicted harm on the driver as well as himself' (Oppenheimer 1991, p. 369). Even the hit-and-run driver may have had a conscience, which must now be troubled.

In contrast to Harry Cayton's view, one might want to argue that tracking and tagging devices are a rare example of a new form of technology which actually poses no moral dilemma. If Gilbert can be sent home with a tracking device, his autonomy seems to be reconciled with his best interests and with the clinicians' duty of beneficence (doing good). He has more freedom than he would in the psychogeriatric ward, and is less at risk of institutionalization. Arguably, unless the monitoring becomes so zealous that Gilbert has little or no freedom of movement, it even enhances his autonomy, rather than diminishing it, as Cayton implies. But if Gilbert gets into trouble again, he can be located before serious harm occurs: so the principle of '*primum non nocere*' ('first do no harm') is also served. (We need to be careful here: the principle 'first do no harm' refers to harm done by doctors, strictly speaking. In Gilbert's case the harm which we want to prevent would be done by careless motorists, icy roads, or inadequate lighting. It is probably better to stay within the cautious bounds of maintaining that at least no direct iatrogenic harm is done by tracking or tagging, in the purely physical sense.)

Stephen's interests are also best honoured by allowing Gilbert to return home with a tracking device. One might argue that this way Stephen does not bear sole responsibility for monitoring his father, and he gets to enjoy Gilbert's company and assistance. So rather than having to balance Gilbert's right to wander against Stephen's needs, tracking appears to allow both equal weight. This is an advantage in institutional contexts as well as in community care. Tracking devices for demented patients allow ward doors to be unlocked, so that non-demented patients can benefit; they allow all patients to move around at will, freeing clinicians from the difficult burden of trying to balance the rights of one group against the safety of the other. Of course, clinicians must remain sensitive to the issue of whom the tracking device is really for. The by-product of other people's interests must be just that: Gilbert's interests come first. But conflict of interests may be avoidable.

On the face of it then, fitting Gilbert with a tracking device preserves the principles of autonomy, beneficence, and non-maleficence (first do no harm). But we keep coming back to problems about resources and distributive justice — the fourth of the principles used in the common framework (Beauchamp and Childress 1994). Abuses of justice are all too possible. For example, although tracking is very resource-intensive, there is the real possibility that tagging might be used to excess, as a substitute for proper supervision. That could be an excuse for cutting staffing levels, reducing the available resources still further and raising the legal problems about negligence and risk.

And what if the device isn't foolproof? Suppose a failure of the device leaves Gilbert lying in a ditch again, when he could be safe in hospital. Wouldn't the clinicians be responsible if they relied too heavily on tracking as a substitute for proper supervision? That raises not only pragmatic issues, but also issues about moral luck, which we first encountered in the case of Philip Caversham (Case 7.2).

Normally, as we have argued before in this book and elsewhere (Dickenson 1991), it is the giving of informed consent to treatment which transfers responsibility for ill-luck in outcomes from doctor to patient. This is only true within the limits of negligence, of course: I cannot be said to consent freely to an operation if the only surgeon in town is habitually drunk during half his operations, and I have no other hope but the operation. We have discussed the negligence issues in connection with tracking and tagging — the danger that these devices might be used as a substitute for proper supervision, and the law's warning that resource shortage cannot be a complete defence against charges of inadequate supervision. What we have not yet covered, however, is the issue of consent. If Gilbert does not give a consent which Hassan Shah regards as satisfactory, is it impermissible to fit him with a tracking device? Contrariwise, if he does consent, can he be said to have taken responsibility for any future ill-luck in outcomes? — including the worst-case scenario in which the device malfunctions, leaving him dead in a ditch.

There is no doctrine of proxy or substituted consent in English law, in contrast to many American jurisdictions (for example, In Re Quinlan (1976) and In Re Jobes (1987)). This means that no one else can give consent on Gilbert's behalf — including Stephen (even if he were capable of fully understanding what tracking involves). In the absence of a new judicial forum to settle treatment decisions for incompetent patients — such as have been mooted by the Law Commission (Law Commission 1995) — no one else can make the decision for Gilbert. Guardianship and Supervision Orders seem less relevant, since the issue is not requiring Gilbert to attend for treatment or to reside in a specified place (the objectives of these orders). So it does not appear that Social Services (under a Guardianship Order) or the trust (under a Supervision Order) can take the decision about tracking or tagging on Gilbert's behalf. But there are very real doubts about whether Gilbert is competent to consent to the tracking device.

Of course, even a moderately demented patient like Gilbert could express his refusal of consent, once the tracking device is fitted, by tearing it off. More passively, he could refuse to put it on when he changes his clothes. But if he simply forgets, is that refusal of consent? Is it sufficient to say that we won't track or tag patients who positively refuse to wear the device, but will feel free to track any others? Then tracking becomes the default option. This may not be an actual battery (as is physical touching without adequately informed consent), but it is clearly undesirable. There is also a risk that Gilbert will be given a choice between sedatives (to which he is clearly opposed) and tracking, and that he will choose tracking as the 'least worst' option — but not altogether freely.

What if the team makes it clear that tracking will only be done on a trial basis? Perhaps then the requirement of Gilbert's consent is not so important? Legally this is not clear, but ethically it may feel more comfortable. The use of trials of treatment has been suggested as a management strategy for demented patients with life-threatening illness (Reilly *et al.* 1994). One advantage lies in the hope that if doctors have to obtain periodic renewal of consent from a patient with fluctuating competence, the odds are that they will 'strike lucky' at some point or other, catching the patient on a competent day later, if not sooner. The difficulty lies in knowing what would constitute the conditions under which the trial could be stopped altogether (what counts as success?) and in specifying who has the power to stop the trial (ultimately only the patient?). At an earlier stage of Gilbert's dementia, it might have been appropriate to ask him what he would want done if he started wandering. This could have been noted in his management plan — although it would probably not be considered an advance directive in legal terms (Cayton is mistaken in thinking that it could be). But if Gilbert gives a clear refusal of tracking on that hypothetical 'good day' when he fluctuates into competence, then the trial has to be stopped.

It does seem as if pragmatic and ethical issues are too deeply intertwined in this case for comfort. Even if tracking and tagging turned out to be ethically praiseworthy, how could we be sure that the decision to fit Gilbert with a tracking device was being done purely for reasons of autonomy, non-maleficence, and beneficence, rather than to solve the resource dilemma? There is a serious risk of hypocrisy here.

In fact, a complete care plan involving tracking, with other forms of support allowing Gilbert to continue living at home, might not turn out to be cheap at all. This is how we would know whether we had chosen the tracking option for the right 'ethical' reasons rather than the wrong 'pragmatic' ones. If such a programme of management were actually revealed to be more expensive than in-patient care, the clinician who had chosen it only to save resources would be disappointed — even if it also turned out to enhance Gilbert's autonomy and protect his clinical best interests. This parallels the doctrine of double effect, which allows doctors to relieve pain (the good effect) even if they are aware that there is an increased risk that the patient will succumb to morphine overdose (the bad effect). The usual charge against the doctrine of double effect is hypocrisy — but if the doctor is not disappointed if pain is relieved although the patient does not die, then she or he genuinely intended the good effect only.

Practitioner commentary (CASE 8.1)

Dr Catherine Oppenheimer Consultant in the Psychiatry of Old Age, Warneford Hospital, Oxford

Gilbert Ryan's case raises a number of issues of which anyone working in a psychogeriatric team will be all too aware. There is no single right way to deal with these issues (Oppenheimer, 1999) but I want to highlight some aspects, to which a different approach, or at any rate a different emphasis, may be relevant.

First, there is the key dilemma about where Gilbert Ryan's care should be based. As described in the case history, this amounts to 'live at home with electronic devices' v. 'nursing home care'. A third possibility would be 'live at home with humans supervising you'. This might mean care assistants visiting in the day and/or night sitters at night. The choice of supervision and the type of care input would vary according to individual decisions about 'expense', or the perceived 'oppressiveness' of supervision, and so forth. For example, provision of night sitters is an extremely expensive resource and Social Services would therefore probably not be able to agree to it. They might, though, provide someone to *call in* during the night. Policies and practice vary widely in this area, but in my view one would only consider putting Gilbert Ryan in a nursing home if he had reached the stage of needing considerable personal care (dressing, attention to hygiene, and so on). A concern about his safety would not be enough by itself to justify this.

The option of 'receiving care at home' raises an interesting issue about consent, by the way. We rarely ask patients for 'fully informed consent' to carers visiting them, even though we do pay attention to their refusal to allow it.

A second issue relevant to this case concerns the distinction between 'tagging' and 'tracking'. These are very different practically, and the ethical issues arising from them are not the same. 'Tagging' is shorthand for those devices which issue a warning signal when a person has crossed a boundary, such as going out of the door of a house — like the devices which tell you that a garment has been shoplifted. Something similar is used when prisoners on parole are 'tagged'. But tagging gives you *no* clues as to where the person has gone. Hence the only advantage of tagging in a case like Gilbert Ryan's is that the carers get an early warning of the fact that he has gone.

A third issue is the extent to which Gilbert Ryan's own needs and concerns have been explored. The psychiatrist in this case is clearly very concerned and 'involved', but it is important to understand the needs to which Gilbert Ryan was responding when he 'wandered'. If he wanted fresh air and exercise, I would try to maximize his opportunities for these during the day in the hope of reducing his drive to wander at night. (If feasible, Stephen could be encouraged to walk with him, for example.) If it was sleeplessness which was driving Gilbert to wander, it would be very reasonable to arrange exercise *and* medication in a regular daily regime to help him sleep at night. If it was the desire for company, I would try to meet that need in the daytime. Respecting Gilbert's autonomy does not necessarily mean trying to facilitate what he *says* he wants to do, without further enquiry — it means trying to understand more deeply what he wants. That is one of the key purposes of an assessment on a psychogeriatric ward.

Finally, I am concerned by the apparent conflict of purposes between Social Services and the psychiatric team in Gilbert Ryan's story. If there had been a more positive working relationship in this case, then a Guardianship Order, which provides a legal framework for legitimizing *any* element in an agreed care plan (including the use of electronic devices), might well have been relevant. Similarly, on the question of resources, there is no necessity for conflict between the two services. Social Services *do* have to safeguard the way they use resources, just as we do in psychiatry, in the interests of their clients as a whole; but they also should (and normally *do*) balance this against the welfare of particular individuals in particular cases. This case is a good example of the need for Health and Social Services to work together to devise the best plan for each individual client or patient, rather than defensively 'hiding behind policy'. In many areas, Health and Social Services enjoy good working relationships. Gilbert Ryan's case shows just how vital this is to good clinical care.

References (CASE 8.1)

Beauchamp, T.L. and Childress, J.F. (1994) *Principles of Biomedical Ethics* (4th edn). Oxford, Oxford University Press.

Dickenson, D. (1991) *Moral Luck in Medical Ethics and Practical Politics* (1st edn). Aldershot, Gower Publishers. (2nd edn, forthcoming, published as *Risk and Luck in Medical Ethics*. Cambridge, Polity Press.)

Knight *v* Home Office (1990) 3 All ER 237.

Law Commission (1995) *Mental Incapacity. Report no. 231*. London, HMSO.

Montgomery, J. (1997). *Health Care Law*. Oxford, Oxford University Press.

Oppenheimer, C. (1991) Ethics and psychogeriatrics. In *Psychiatric Ethics* (2nd edn) (ed. Bloch, S. and Chodoff, P.), pp. 365–90. Oxford, Oxford University Press.

Oppenheimer, C. (1999) Ethical problems in old age psychiatry. In *Psychiatric Ethics* (3rd edn) (ed. Bloch, S., Chodoff, P., and Green, S.A.). Oxford, Oxford University Press.

Re Jobes (1987) 108 NJ 394.

Re Quinlan (1976) 70 NJ 10.

Reilly, R.B., Teasdale, T.A., and McCullough, L.B. (1994) Projecting patients' preferences from living wills: an invalid strategy for management of dementia with life-
threatening illness. *Journal of the American Geriatric Society,* **42**:997–1003.

Wilsher v. Essex AHA (1986) 3 All ER 801, 834.

CASE 8.2
Sam Mason — the breakdown of a therapeutic alliance

Synopsis A 15-year-old youth, schooled at home by his father after divorce, suffers repeated psychotic breakdowns. His father insists that there is nothing wrong with him and refuses to co-operate with treatment.

Key dilemma Should he be removed from his father?

Main topics Legal mechanisms for intervention and their ethical basis; the family's role.

Other topics Communitarian ethics (advantages and disadvantages); therapeutic alliance; expressed preference and best interests; consent to treatment (children and young people); family; autonomy; paternalism; confidentiality; relationship; Brody; Callahan.

Sam Mason, aged 15, is a thin, withdrawn youth — the youngest of three children: originally there were four, but a younger sibling died in infancy. The death of the youngest child eventually broke up the marriage. Sam's father, Gerald, seems to have reacted to these two blows by concentrating all his efforts and affection on Sam. On the divorce, a residence order was made in the father's favour, consistent with Sam's own preferences; Sam's mother, Abby, lives about four hours distant with her second husband and two stepchildren. Gerald is a strong believer in home schooling, but now that his older sisters have left home, Sam has little companionship.

Several months ago, the psychiatric services for Sam's area were contacted directly by Abby, who wanted him to be seen by a psychiatrist — but without Gerald knowing. According to Abby, Sam was becoming more and more preoccupied and reclusive, refusing to see his mother and stepfather. Jenny Reed, the child and adolescent psychiatrist, was afraid she might just be drawn into a dispute between Sam's parents, so her instinct was to proceed cautiously. But she did contact Sam's GP, who agreed that it might be a good idea for him to be seen. A referral was arranged on rather vague grounds of 'general age-specific assessment'. Gerald appeared content to co-operate, perhaps under the impression that this was part of the 'bargain' for being allowed to educate Sam at home.

When Jenny saw Sam, she found that he was indeed detached and pre-occupied, posturing and muttering to himself. He revealed that he had received 'personal communications' from a gangsta rapper, via the radio, but added that this had stopped a few months ago. A presumptive diagnosis of schizophrenia was made, and after lengthy discussion of the alternatives, Sam agreed to a period of admission for assessment. Dr Reed telephoned Gerald to tell him of what she believed to be Sam's voluntary agreement.

Gerald was furious at being duped, as he saw it, and at psychiatric services' unwelcome intrusion into his family business. 'Nanny state gone mad,' he fumed. 'There's nothing wrong with Sam. You lot are all in it together, aren't you? Did the school put you up to this? Schooling at home produces weirdos, that's the message, is it?' When Gerald asked Jenny who had suggested that Sam should be assessed, she had no option but to tell him that it was his ex-wife, which did not improve matters. In turn, Sam now refused to be admitted or to have any treatment. Dr Reed telephoned Abby, who, as someone with parental responsibility, might give consent to compulsory admission; but while Abby was concerned, she would not support that course. Although in law one parent's consent is sufficient in cases of disagreement, Abby was unwilling to 'go it alone'. It seemed best for the GP, Nigel Raynsford, to try to maintain contact, since Gerald flatly refused to let Sam have anything further to do with psychiatric services. And perhaps it was better to wait and see — after all, the diagnosis of schizophrenia was not firm.

Four months later Nigel phoned to ask Jenny to make an emergency home visit, as Gerald and Sam had now refused any further contact with the GP's surgery. Jenny arrived on a freezing January morning to find Sam standing naked in the garden, maintaining a fixed and unnatural posture, including a 'schnautzkrampf' or 'pig's snout' posture of the mouth. He was completely uncommunicative. Gerald, in tears, was trying to urge him indoors.

Sam was admitted under section, over Gerald's objections. He improved in hospital, but whenever Gerald visited, he did his best to dissuade Sam from taking his medication or attending OT. Sometimes Abby visited too, but her visits rarely coincided with Jenny's times on the ward. Gerald, on the other hand, seemed to be there all the time, complaining about Sam's treatment and urging him to appeal against his section — which he did. After a lengthy hearing at which Gerald gave extensive 'evidence', the appeal was dismissed. Sam was placed on depot medication and given increasingly extended periods of leave in order to acclimatize him for eventual discharge with visits by the community psychiatric nurse.

Over the next few months, with Sam back at home and the section still in place, the therapeutic alliance broke down still further, Jenny and her team felt. Appointments with the community psychiatric nurse were postponed or cancelled, so that the intervals between injections began to lengthen ominously. If the nurse called, Sam was never at home — even if an appointment had been arranged. On the rare occasions when he could be seen, Sam did appear relatively well. He had obtained a part-time job, at his father's urging, and seemed less withdrawn. Apparently he had also begun visiting his mother again. Another appeal was launched, but before a result could be announced, the psychiatric team decided to cancel the section order.

A year after Sam's first admission, Abby again phoned Jenny to say that she was concerned. She had heard from a friend of Sam's that he had lost his part-time job. Apparently he had not told Gerald, but pretended to go 'out to work' at the usual hours. Abby had not said anything to Gerald, but she was becoming increasingly worried: she had not heard from Sam for six weeks, and there was never any answer when she phoned.

Jenny paid another home visit. This time she found Sam lying naked in bed, again in a semi-catatonic state. Finally he began talking, admitting that he felt depressed and that he had lately taken to standing on the edge of the top floor of a multi-storey car park. He was readmitted under section for several months and then agreed to be transferred to a hostel when discharged. But the day he was transferred, Gerald turned up at the hostel, and Sam went home with him. The only concession which could be extracted from Sam and Gerald was a promise to allow visits by the community psychiatric nurse.

Now, according to the nurse, Sam appears to be having another psychotic relapse, but is actively refusing either hostel or hospital placement. The clinicians have considered the possibility of a specific issue order and/or a new residence order under the Children Act, requiring him to live with his mother and attend for depot medication. But Abby is reluctant to take Sam on: there is always tension between him and her two teenage stepchildren, and she is also rather hurt that he has broken off contact so often. Gerald remains adamant that there is nothing wrong with the boy. Sam has told the nurse that he doesn't want any further treatment because he doesn't want to upset his father.

This is a case about the rightful domain of the family. As part of a general backlash against the excesses of the earlier individualistic, autonomy-worshipping tendency in medical ethics (Callahan 1996), some medical ethicists have argued that the rights and needs of the family should count more in decision making (for example, Lindemann Nelson and Lindemann Nelson 1995). Yet in this case, a perfectly well-meaning family threatens to drive its youngest member to suicide, perhaps, ironically, because the father fears the loss of another child so deeply.

When the therapeutic alliance with the father breaks down, the professionals in Sam's case feel helpless. This suggests that reports of the 'death' of the family have been greatly exaggerated: even in 'broken' form, it can still wield considerable power, if only negatively. Yet it is also powerless in this case to achieve its positive goals — nurturance and protection. The overwhelming sense which comes from this case study is that no one in the family feels they can do anything: Abby is afraid to take Sam in because her stepchildren object; Sam will do nothing to help himself because he is afraid of upsetting his father; Gerald weeps at his son's condition, even though he insists that there is nothing wrong with the boy.

Another dynamic which we must watch out for involves the 'sick role'. To the extent that patients accept the 'sick role', it is usually said that they become more dependent on the institution — less autonomous, in fact. We could equally well argue that to the extent that Sam accepts his 'sick role', he actually becomes less dependent on the psychiatric team and more dependent on his father. Once again, his autonomy needs upholding, but it is hard to see how to break that dynamic. If psychiatrists intervene and section him, he becomes more passive and institutionalized; if he obeys his father's preferences instead, he becomes less and less likely to achieve any sort of break from his family.

What we witness then, is a tragic impasse, particularly poignant because of the tremendous damage already done to Sam by his severe, early-onset catatonic schizophrenic illness. Despite his high level of dependence on his family, 'life with father' is doing Sam no good at all. To some extent Sam seems aware of this when he is separated from his home environment, for then he does cooperate with treatment plans. Yet he has chosen to live with Gerald, and clearly feels something for his father: he is not a mere victim, nor is Gerald an unfeeling bully. How can we recognize and respect these feelings without despairing acceptance of the situation to which they have given rise? It is not enough to assert Sam's 'rights' when Sam himself is more concerned about not upsetting his father. Ironically, telling Sam he must assert his rights to treatment, for the sake of his own best interests, would be paternalistic. Rights and autonomy are more often seen as opposed to best interests and beneficence, and paternalism is associated with the latter.

What action can be taken against the negative power of the family, and how? Use of the Mental Health Act has not proved productive so far. With a long-term, early-onset mental illness such as Sam's, Jenny is unhappy about ongoing hospitalization, and indeed every section order is appealed. But when she arranged discharge to a hostel, her long-term care plan for Sam was 'subverted' by Gerald.

If Sam were to be treated under the common law, rather than under the Mental Health Act, he could be compelled to accept treatment, provided that one of his parents gave consent. As Montgomery states, citing Section 2(7) of the Children Act 1989, 'It is now clear that parents may act independently, and the approval of one will be sufficient, even if there is a disagreement.' (Montgomery 1997, p. 292) In Re W (1992), an anorexic girl of Sam's age was held to be unable to reject force-feeding so long as someone with parental responsibility consented (in W's case, the local authority, as she was in their care). In an earlier case, Re R (1991), it had been held that a young person with fluctuating lucidity could not be considered competent to reject treatment to which someone with parental responsibility had consented. The case of W went one step further: even a fully competent young person cannot refuse treatment in English law. Legal commentary (for example, Kennedy 1992) at the time of the R decision suggested that R's right of refusal could have been better upheld under the Mental Health Act. The courts have been reluctant to use this legislation with young people for fear of lifelong stigmatization, as they perceive it. But as Howard Brody points out in *The Healer's Power*, the power to label is also the power to excuse the sufferer and to mobilize social resources on his behalf (Brody 1992).

There are various possible legal remedies as alternatives to the Mental Health Act. Section 8 under the Children Act 1989 can direct specific steps, and in Sam's case it appears that a residence order is already in force under this section. A further 'specific issue' order could specify that Abby and Gerald must consult with each other over the future course of Sam's mental illness — although it is debatable how productive that will be, when Gerald does not recognize that Sam has an illness.

Aftercare Under Supervision procedures under the Mental Health (Patients in the Community) Act of 1995 might provide an alternative remedy, requiring Sam to reside at a specific address and attend for treatment. Supervised discharge also gives professionals legal power to 'take and convey' patients to these named places, although many psychiatrists are very reluctant to use these powers, as the case of Philip Caversham (Case 7.2) showed. In any event, there is no actual power to treat or to detain the patient for treatment.

Guardianship procedures under the Mental Health Act may also require a patient to reside in a specified place and attend for treatment, or give access to a doctor or other specified person to enter the patient's residence. It would be better for Sam, of course, if that specific place were with the parent who does not oppose treatment, since with guardianship there is no sanction for noncompliance with conditions. (Guardianship does not provide powers of compulsory treatment, although the position differs between England and Scotland: see R. *v* Hallstrom 1986.) Perhaps Abby's stepchildren might accept

Sam's living with them more readily if an actual order were in force? That might bring the seriousness of the situation home to them, and give Abby some 'ammunition'. But there is no reason to think that Gerald will be any happier about this than he is about treatment under section — probably less so, since it deprives him of Sam's company.

Critics of autonomy as the be-all and end-all of medical ethics are right to emphasize that we are caught up in a web of relationship — that 'no man is an island'. In Sam's case, simply insisting on either his right to refuse treatment or his right to accept treatment regardless of his father's preferences is largely an academic exercise. Any long-term treatment plan that ignores his feeling for Gerald simply won't work. Waiting until Sam turns eighteen is an equally irrelevant strategy: Gerald's influence over him will not automatically cease on his eighteenth birthday. In fact, Gerald's hold is so strong that the clinicians seem to think in terms of the therapeutic relationship having broken down when Gerald says so.

But Gerald is not the patient. It is even doubtful whether he is part of the wider category of the therapeutic alliance. He is not interested in Sam's therapy; nor is he the therapists' ally in any sense. Rather, he is interested only in frustrating the treatment plan. The obvious inference is that he is in some sort of denial, but that may be too crass. Perhaps he has reasons for his hostility: when Jenny decided to follow Abby's request that the reason for the initial assessment should be kept secret from Gerald, perhaps she was already ruling Gerald out of the therapeutic alliance. Although she feared being drawn in on the side of one parent rather than another, her action did just that. Rather than accepting the dynamic of confrontation and secrecy, it might have been better to have tried to work with both parents from the beginning. Instead, Gerald has alternated between getting too much attention and too little from the psychiatric team, and Sam's confidentiality has not really been respected either.

The key point, none the less, is that it would be contradictory to respect Gerald's wishes out of an ethic which emphasizes relationship, because relationship appears to be the last thing Gerald wants for Sam. Or rather, he cannot see beyond his own longings for his relationship with the boy, to the stark facts of Sam's illness and the pressing realities of his needs. He is the male version of what has wryly been called a 'smother-mother': not the stereotypical unconcerned father, but an overly concerned though deeply diligent one. By allowing Gerald so much power in the 'therapeutic alliance', the clinicians are also depriving themselves of what Howard Brody identifies as the particular potency of the therapeutic relationship to heal. He believes that the physician–patient relationship should itself be treated as a vital therapeutic tool, especially in primary care, which can promote a mode of relating to each other which encourages full participation and recognizes the patient's importance in defining and identifying the nature of his illness and the aims of treatment.

Advocates of the ethic of care (those who most emphasize relationship) fail to recognize, however, that relationship can be a bad thing (Gordon 1996; Noddings 1984). It comes with an ideological freight of 'goodness' which we need to question, just as intensely as communitarians and ethicists of care interrogate autonomy. Daniel Callahan, for example, favours what he calls a 'vital institution' principle as a counterweight to autonomy, offsetting the harmful effects of individual choice on key societal institutions such as the family. When vital institutions are threatened by too much deference to individual autonomy, we ought not to defer to autonomy, he argues. 'Overrun with claims of autonomy, we are losing the moral commons in medicine. Nothing seems more important than to try to regain it.' (Callahan 1996, p. 42) Elsewhere in this casebook we, too, have been sceptical of autonomy and cognisant of relationship. But we need to remember an older truth, which feminists recognized long before they became enamoured of the ethic of care: families also stifle individuals, abuse them, and do them harm — even when they most intend their good.

Practitioner commentary (CASE 8.2)

Dr D.M. Foreman Consultant/Senior Lecturer in Child and Adolescent Psychiatry, Keele University

This case is presented as one where there is a possible conflict between the child's and the parent's rights in the treatment of a schizophrenic youngster, and the limitations of the law in resolving it. This commentary will take an opposing view, proposing instead that the ethical dilemmas described here result from how these rights have been claimed. Some of the events described in this case occurred before the Children Act 1989 was implemented in 1991. We will see that many of the concerns identified here have been incorporated into that legislation.

It is said that accidents happen, but disasters take careful planning. Gerald's outburst at having been duped followed his discovery of the information not given by Sam's GP and child and adolescent psychiatrist at their first contact. Distorting information for therapeutic reasons is only acceptable in rare circumstances of persistent resistance (Foreman 1990) or dangerous parental behaviour (Foreman and Farsides 1993) — conditions not apparent here. This principle was clearly incorporated in the Children Act's first guidelines on working with parents in difficult circumstances (Home Office *et al.*

1991). This case is a good example of one where any therapeutic advantages of withholding information turn out to be more apparent than real.

How we talk about our patients is as important as what we say, as it is the 'how' that determines the language-game that we wish to play (Wittgenstein 1999). The patient and family are described here as if they were simply recipients of therapy, who are able to do no more than comply or interfere with what is offered. The fundamental principle of respect for a patient's autonomy (Beauchamp and Childress 1994) implies that patients are active participants in the treatment process. The role of parents as custodians of their offspring's autonomy has recently been explicated (Foreman 1999), showing it is appropriate that the parents represent different points of view to the clinicians. The language used does not allow the possibility of such behaviour in the parents, so it is not possible for the clinicians to compose a treatment programme that could include the parents' concerns. The parents, indeed, would have good reason to avoid services that, from *their* perspective, not only fail to attend to their concerns but even blame them (the parents) when further difficulties arise.

Irrespective of whose fault it is, the overriding issue when any caretaking relationship breaks down is the child's welfare. This again is enshrined in the Children Act. However, current case law allows a child to be treated against his or her wishes up to the age of 18 without legal constraint, irrespective of the views of the parents (Kennedy and Grubb 1994). Also, the Children Act cannot guarantee that a child lives with a particular parent in these circumstances. The psychiatric service would first have to show that any order was better than none, and the court is also required by law to take the child's ascertainable views and wishes into account under the 'welfare checklist'. Finally, the Children Act allows a child to refuse a psychiatric examination. Thus, though the Section was allowed to lapse, the Mental Health Act offers the best current protection for a child's rights while under psychiatric treatment, as the case study points out.

We can now see that this case is not about 'the rightful domain of the family'. Instead, it shows how principles need to be correctly *specified* and *balanced* (Beauchamp and Childress 1994) before they can start to influence real clinical situations. We see Gerald taking the child to the doctors without difficulty at first, the doctors attempting to engage first one, then the other parent, and Gerald initially agreeing to co-operate with the doctors. So all the parties understood the importance of a therapeutic alliance involving both the patient and all the patient's caretakers. In this particular case, there were two problems with specification, both relating to respect for autonomy. The initial absence of full and clear information limited the family's opportunities to express their positions except through defiance. Also, the language used conflated the differing roles of caretaker, present or absent parent, and patient — all were treated similarly, as reluctant recipients of medical instruction. In the end, Gerald ended up being cast as a patient himself.

The story ended with the psychiatrists attempting to place Sam in a hostel, despite extended family networks being valuable for a good outcome (for example, Birchwood *et al.* 1992), while the family continued to undermine the psychiatrists' equally important attempts to give appropriate medication. This shows the impact of the problem with balancing in this case: the desire to do good overrode the need to minimize harm, despite these principles being equivalent (Beauchamp and Childress 1994).

It might have been the case that Gerald would have been equally intransigent had more ethical approaches been followed. In that case, the arguments just presented would be the same, with Gerald demonstrating clear lack of respect for Sam's autonomy. Being a custodian for your child's autonomy makes the luxury of unreasonable conduct unethical as well (Foreman 1999).

This case exemplifies the importance of ethical care in planning case management in clinically difficult cases. If, even unintentionally, the ethical dimensions of treatment plans are not specifically included, then the plan is likely to fail, while everyone blames each other for the debacle.

References (CASE 8.2)

Beauchamp, T. and Childress, J. (1994) *Principles of Biomedical Ethics* (4th edn). Oxford, Oxford University Press.

Birchwood, M., Cochrane, R., Macmillan, F., *et al.* (1992) The influence of ethinicity and family structure on relapse in first episode schizophrenia. *British Journal of Psychiatry*, **161**:783–90).

Brody, H. (1992) *The Healer's Power*. New Haven, Yale University Press.

Callahan, D. (1996) Can the moral commons survive autonomy? *Hastings Center Report*, vol. 26, no. 6, pp. 41–7.

Children Act (1989). London, HMSO.

Department of Health (1991). *Working Together under the Children Act 1989*. London, HMSO.

Foreman, D.M. (1990) The ethical use of paradoxical interventions in psychotherapy. *Journal of Medical Ethics*, **16**(4):200–5.

Foreman, D.M. (1999) The family rule: a framework for obtaining consent for medical interventions from children. *Journal of Medical Ethics*, **25**:491–6.

Foreman, D.M. and Farsides, C. (1993) Ethical use of covert videoing techniques in detecting Munchausen syndrome by proxy [see comments]. *BMJ*, **307**:611–13.

Kennedy, I. (1992) Consent to treatment: the capable person. In *Doctors, Patients and the Law* (ed. Dyer, C.), pp. 58–62. Oxford, Blackwell.

Kennedy, I. and Grubb, A. (1994) *Medical Law: Text with Materials*. London, Butterworths.

Lindemann Nelson, H. and Lindemann Nelson, J. (1995) *The Patient in the Family: The Ethics of Medicine and Families*. London, Routledge.

Montgomery, J. (1997) *Health Care Law*. Oxford, Oxford University Press.

R. *v* Hallstrom, *ex parte* W (No. 2) (1986), 2 All ER 306.

Re R (1991) 4 All ER 177.

Re W (1992) 4 All ER 627.

Wittgenstein, L. (1999) *Philosophical Investigations* (2nd edn) (trans. Anscombe, G.E.M. and Rhees, R.). Oxford, Blackwell.

Reading Guide

Given the importance of multidisciplinary teams in mental health, there is surprisingly little literature on the ethics of teamwork as such. Chapter 11, on 'Inter-Professional Relations', of the BMA's *Medical Ethics Today* (1993) is a helpful review of the issues. In this Reading Guide we cover two areas that are critical to good teamwork: (1) professional ethics and the role of codes, and (2) resources.

Professional ethics and the role of codes

Excellent introductions to these two areas aimed specifically at psychiatry are Allen Dyer's 'Psychiatry as a profession' and Sidney Bloch and Russell Porgiter's 'Codes of ethics in psychiatry' (Chapters 5 and 6 respectively of Bloch *et al.*'s *Psychiatric Ethics*, 1999). Ruth Chadwick's edited collection *Ethics and the Professions* (1995) gives a good overview. The ethical connections between codes of practice, concepts of disorder and the practice skills required for good clinical care in psychiatry are explored by K.W.M. Fulford and S. Bloch in *Codes, Concepts and Clinical Practice Skills* (forthcoming). The ethics of teamwork between professionals and voluntary organisations is explored in Chris Heginbotham's *Return to Community* (1999).

Resource issues

A comprehensive discussion of the ethical and legal issues raised by rationing of health care resources is Chapter 12, 'Rationing and allocation of health care resources', in the BMA's *Medical Ethics Today* (1993). Relevant medical codes of practice include the GMC's *Good Medical Practice* (1995) and the World Medical Association's *Declaration of Lisbon on the Rights of the Patient* (updated

1995). These emphasize the importance of acting in the best interests of one's patient, yet also having regard to resource issues.

The two main approaches to ethical analysis of the proper basis of resource allocation are 'QALY theory' and 'needs theories'. Both have generated large literatures. Illustrative discussions of QALY theory include Alan Williams (1995), Michael Loughlin (1996), and John Harris (1991). A critical account, directly relevant to psychiatry, is Roger Crisp's (1994) 'Quality of life and health care'. The most influential recent 'needs theory' of justice is John Rawls' *A Theory of Justice* (1972), a version of which is developed particularly for the health care context in Norman Daniels' *Just Healthcare* (1985).

Much of the literature assumes that what people actually want and need is largely self-evident. For a review of evidence to the contrary, see the medical sociologist Ray Fitzpatrick's chapter in *Essential Practice in Patient-Centred Care* (1996), edited by Fulford *et al.,* and the commentary by the philosopher Martyn Evans (1996). The practical importance of attending to what people want is brought out by Max Marshall's work in developing a modified 'needs for care' assessment schedule (1994) for use with the long-term mentally ill.

There has been relatively little bioethical discussion of these issues in the context of primary care, most of the literature being concerned with 'high-tech' medicine. For a valuable overview directly relevant to psychiatry, see Tony Hope and Catherine Oppenheimer's chapter in Robyn Jacoby and Catherine Oppenheimer, *Psychiatry in the Elderly* (2nd edition, forthcoming). An application of resource and justice debates in philosophy to everyday clinical practice can be found in the chapter on allocation of scarce health care resources in Parker and Dickenson, *The Cambridge Workbook in Medical Ethics* (2000).

The question of whether efficiency is a value-laden concept is considered by Dickenson in 'Is efficiency ethical? Resource issues in health care' (1995), and the related question of whether prioritization by evidence-based medicine can enable us to avoid political and ethical questions about justice in 'Can medical criteria settle priority-setting debates? The need for ethical analysis' (1999).

Reading Guide: references

Bloch, S., Chodoff, P., and Green S.A. (1999) *Psychiatric Ethics* (3rd edn). Oxford, Oxford University Press.

BMA (1993) *Medical Ethics Today: Its Practice and Philosophy.* London, BMA.

Chadwick, R. (ed.) (1995) *Ethics and the Professions.* Aldershot (England), Avebury Press.

Crisp, R. (1994) Quality of life and health care. In *Medicine and Moral Reasoning* (ed. Fulford, K.W.M., Gillett, G., and Soskice, J.M.), Chapter 13. Cambridge, Cambridge University Press.

Daniels, N. (1985) *Just Health Care*. Cambridge, Cambridge University Press.

Dickenson, D. (1995) Is efficiency ethical? Resource issues in health care. In *Introducing Applied Ethics* (ed. Almond, B.) Oxford, Blackwell.

Dickenson, D. (1999) Can medical criteria settle priority-setting debates? The need for ethical analysis. *Health Care Analysis*, 7:1–7.

Evans, M. (1996) Commentary on Fitzpatrick, R. 'Patient-centred approaches to the evaluation of healthcare'. In *Essential Practice in Patient-Centred Care* (ed. Fulford, K.W.M., Ersser, S., and Hope, T.), pp. 240–3. Oxford, Blackwell Science.

Fitzpatrick, R. (1996) Patient-centred approaches to the evaluation of healthcare. In *Essential Practice in Patient-Centred Care* (ed. Fulford, K.W.M., Ersser, S., and Hope, T.), Chapter 15. Oxford, Blackwell Science.

Fulford, K.W.M. and Bloch, S. (forthcoming). Psychiatric ethics: codes, concepts and clinical practice skills. In *New Oxford Textbook of Psychiatry* (ed. Gelder, M., Andreasen, N., and Lopez–Ibor, J.), Chapter 17. Oxford, Oxford University Press.

GMC (1995) *Good Medical Practice*. London, GMC.

Harris, J. (1991) Unprincipled QALYs: a response to Cubbon. *Journal of Medical Ethics*, 17:185–8.

Heginbotham, C. (1990) *Return to Community: the Voluntary Ethics and Community Care*. London, Bedford Square Press.

Hope, T. and Oppenheimer, C. (1997) Ethics and the psychiatry of old age. In *Psychiatry in the Elderly* (2nd edn) (ed. Jacoby, R. and Oppenheimer, C.). Oxford, Oxford University Press.

Gordon, S. (ed.) (1996) *Care, Autonomy and Justice: Feminism and the Ethic of Care*. Boulder, Co, Westview Press.

Loughlin M. (1996) Rationing, barbarity and the economist's perspective. *Health Care Analysis*, 4: 146–56.

Marshall, M. (1994) How should we measure need? Concept and practice in the development of a standardised assessment schedule. *Philosophy, Psychiatry, and Psychology*, 1/1:27–36. (Commentaries by Crisp, R. and Morgan, J., 37–40)

Noddings, N. (1984) *Caring: A Feminine Approach to Ethics and Moral Education*. Berkeley, University of California Press.

Parker, M. and Dickenson, D. (2000) *The Cambridge Workbook in Medical Ethics*. Cambridge, Cambridge University Press.

Rawls, R. (1972) *A Theory of Justice*. Oxford, Oxford University Press.

Williams, A. (1995), Economics, QALYs and medical ethics — a health economist's perspective. *Health Care Analysis*, 3(3):221–6.

World Medical Association (September/October 1981; updated September 1995) *Declaration of Lisbon on the Rights of the Patient*. WMA.

SECTION THREE

Teaching and research

Putting theory into practice: a sample teaching seminar

One of the general themes running through the cases described in Chapters 3–8 of this book has been the extent to which legitimately different ethical perspectives may bear on clinical problems in psychiatry. We have reflected this in the open nature of our discussions of these cases. Thus we have not prescribed ethical 'solutions' but, rather, have highlighted the issues, indicated relevant guidance, and reviewed alternative strategies. Those committed to a particular ideological point of view may find this approach unsatisfactory. It is important that such points of view are respected in psychiatry: there must be room for an Islamic ethic, a Christian ethic, a humanist ethic, and so on. But if there is an ethic guiding this book, it is of valuing diversity, of making room for individual perspectives within a framework of mutual respect. Everyone has their ethical sticking points, of course. And for a profession to function effectively, its members must agree clear ground rules: this is one reason why professional codes are important (Fulford and Bloch, forthcoming). All the same, as one of us has argued elsewhere, good practice in psychiatry depends ultimately on 'extending the limits of tolerance' (Fulford 1996).

But what does this mean in practice? In becoming conscious of the extent of the ethical difficulties in psychiatry, how do we avoid an ethical counterpart of the obsessional's *folie de doute*; in recognizing the open nature of these difficulties, their essential rather than merely contingent uncertainty, how do we avoid ethical paralysis? How, in a word, do we convert theory into practice?

Putting theory into practice is the task of this chapter, which focuses on 'teaching' as the main conduit (apart from practice itself) through which all theory, whether scientific or ethical, is converted into practice. We will be looking, first, at three ways of incorporating case materials into teaching psychiatric ethics. We will then outline in rather more detail an approach based on clinical problem solving. Finally, we will illustrate how this approach can draw on the materials in this book by revisiting one of our cases (Case 3.1, Elizabeth Orton) in the context of a teaching seminar.

A couple of preliminary points are important. First, the model of teaching we have in mind is not that of a one-off, 'life event' at medical school, but of lifelong learning. Hence the ideas we set out in this chapter are as applicable to continuing professional development seminars as to undergraduate clinical training. Second, if teaching is to be an *effective* conduit from theory to practice, we need to bear in mind the distinction between 'learning' and 'doing', introduced at the end of Chapter 2.

You will recall that the moral philosopher R.M. Hare distinguished two levels of ethical reasoning — level 1 being the level of immediate decision making in the hurly-burly of day-to-day clinical care; level 2 being the level of reflection on practice. In terms of this distinction, the approach set out in this chapter is at level 2. It is an approach to ethical reasoning which can be adopted in the more reflective circumstances of, say, a clinical case conference or a research ethics committee. In this chapter then, we are still not *quite* at the clinical 'coalface'. But as Hare argued, it is the lessons we learn at level 2, in reflecting *on* practice, which are crucial to the way we react at level 1, *in* practice.

Using case material in teaching psychiatric ethics

Teaching and learning styles vary widely and teaching methods in psychiatric ethics should be correspondingly flexible. So far as the use of case material is concerned, we can distinguish three main approaches.

1 **Use of cases in issue-based teaching** The use of cases to illustrate key ethical issues is the approach adopted in the sister volume to this book — Bloch, Chodoff, and Green's *Psychiatric Ethics* (1999). For example, in their Chapter 24 on 'Teaching psychiatric ethics', the American psychiatrists Robert Michels and Kevin Kelly focus on the issue of sexual relations between psychiatrists and their patients. This is an important issue: the current public preoccupation (at least in Britain and America) surrounding sexual ethics makes it a matter of central concern for any profession's ethical identity. And as Michels and Kelly argue, it also illustrates many of the most pressing ethical concerns specifically for psychiatry, arising, in particular, from the unequal power relations between professional and patient in the area of mental health.

   A danger with issue-based teaching, however, is that it tends sometimes to be driven by high-profile and not necessarily representative problems. In medicine, the big issue for sexual ethics is sexual relations between patients and professionals. As Michels and Kelly show, this may be an issue for psychiatry too. But the problems faced by the therapist in our Case 5.2, Francesca Gindro, remind us — if reminder were needed — how subtle are the ramifications of sexuality in psychiatry. Hence, even in a well-defined area like sexual ethics, there is a risk that issue-based teaching may artificially restrict the kind of cases selected.

2 **Case vignettes** Brief case examples have a number of uses in ethics teaching. They are particularly helpful in bringing ethical issues to life for those with limited clinical experience — medical students, for example, or those from non-medical disciplines, such as law and philosophy. In Chapter 2 we showed how a case vignette questionnaire can be used with experienced psychiatrists to raise awareness of ethical issues by contrasting what we *think* we do and what we actually *do*! Yet another use of the brief vignette is to raise the question — what additional information would you need in order to decide what to do? However, the power of the brief vignette, to quickly focus attention on issues, is also its limitation. For the brief vignette, by definition, lacks the substantive narrative detail on which the clinical decisions we take in everyday practice depend.

3 **Building on case histories** It is the importance of narrative detail in tying theory to practice which is behind our use of long case histories in this book. As we emphasized in the Preface, our aims are first and foremost practical. These practical aims, filtered through the details of the case histories described in preceding chapters, have taken us into areas of deep philosophical theory. There is no contradiction here. As we argued in Chapter 1, deep philosophical theory is an essential complement to good practice in psychiatry. Equally, philosophical theory without the narrative detail of clinical case histories is empty. But bring theory and practice together, in a problem-solving approach to ethics teaching, and, as we anticipate in Chapter 2, ethical reasoning emerges as an essential practice skill.

In the remainder of this chapter then, it is practical decision making, and the specific role in this of ethical reasoning, with which we will be concerned. In contrast to the open style of our discussions in earlier chapters, we make a number of specific and concrete suggestions about how a problem-solving seminar in psychiatric ethics could be run. Our intention though is not to suggest that this is how such seminars *should* be run! Still less should the further discussion of Case 3.1 given later in this chapter be considered definitive. Our aim in providing concrete examples is rather to illustrate how the cases and commentaries given in Chapters 3–8 can be used to stimulate discussion and open up debate.

The clinical problem-solving approach

Our general approach then, is that of ethical reasoning as a clinical practice skill. Problem solving in clinical ethics can be thought of as involving four stages:

1 clarifying the problem

2 getting a deeper understanding of it

3 formulating a response

4 follow up.

These stages are the same as for more technical aspects of clinical problem solving: Stage 1 (clarifying the problem) is a diagnostic stage; Stage 2 (deeper understanding) is that of drawing on background theory; Stage 3 (responding) is the stage of developing a management plan; and Stage 4 (follow up) is literally, follow up. This mirroring by ethics of the technical aspects of clinical problem solving is integral to the practice skills approach. Practice skills are the skills required for the successful application of technical knowledge and skills to clinical problems (Hope *et al.* 1996). Hence as a key practice skill, ethical reasoning is wound inextricably into the clinical process.

The four stages of the clinical problem-solving process will form the core of any practice skills seminar in psychiatric ethics. For the teaching to be effective though, the seminar should always begin with a carefully planned introduction which contextualizes the cases to be considered and sets out the key learning objectives. Similarly, it should end with a 'debriefing' session which includes a clear resumé and summary of the 'take-away' messages. Expert commentary, from someone experienced in the relevant clinical area, is also especially helpful at this stage. Effective teaching also depends on what happens before and after the seminar. Thorough preliminary planning is of course essential, but so too are strategies for reinforcing learning after the seminar is over. Overall, therefore, the seminar can be thought of as involving the following key elements:

- **Preliminary planning**
- **Introduction:** including
  Title/topic
  Plan of the seminar
  Contextualization
- **Clinical problem solving**[1]: this occupies the main part of the seminar and covers

  Stage 1 — clarifying the problem
  Introduction of the case
  Extracting ethical issues from the case
  Defining the core problem(s)

  Stage 2 — deepening understanding
  Review of the issues raised by the core problem(s), drawing on the discussions in Chapters 3–8 of this book and other materials (from bioethics, law, ethical codes, and so on)

Stage 3 — formulating a response

Theoretical material introduced in Stage 2 is applied to the core problem(s)

Stage 4 – follow up

Possible outcomes are reviewed

- **Debriefing:** the themes of the seminar are drawn together and summarized. This includes
Expert commentary (where available)
Key learning points
Any questions

- **On-going learning:** this depends on
Guide to further reading
Subsequent seminars (with cross-referencing of topics)
Integration with clinical experience

In practice, the stages of a seminar often overlap and interact. Also, the time taken for each will vary greatly. However, the most common fault in all teaching is that we fail to leave sufficient time for the later stages of the seminar, in particular debriefing. A rough guide is to allow a *full quarter* of the time available for Stage 4 (outcomes) and debriefing. Thus, in a two-hour seminar, approximately *30 minutes* should be given to introducing the case and clarifying the problem (that is, everything up to the end of Stage 1); *30 minutes* for Stage 2 (deepening understanding); *30 minutes* for Stage 3 (formulating a response); and *30 minutes* for Stage 4 (outcome) and debriefing. The time plan and summary of a two-hour seminar is given in Table 9.1.

The stages of a clinical problem-solving seminar

We will now go through each of these stages in more detail before illustrating how they might be worked through in a seminar based on our Case 3.1 (Elizabeth Orton).

Preliminary planning

Much of the work of any teaching is completed before the teaching itself gets going! Estimates vary, but for a new session you can expect to spend at least four hours' preparation for every hour of teaching. Even with a session you have taken before, preliminary planning is essential. This should cover the following.

Definition of the aims of the seminar

A common fault in ethics teaching is attempting to cover too much. One way to focus a seminar is by reference to the four general aims of ethics teaching

Table 9.1 Clinical problem solving in psychiatric ethics: an example of a 2-hour seminar plan

Preliminary planning	Define aims, identify cases, background reading, etc.	
	START OF SEMINAR	Time in mins (approx)
Introduction		10
(MAIN AIM – to start from where the group is 'at')		
Title	Descriptive title of the core problems to be discussed	
Topic/plan	Brief description of the core problem and seminar plan	
Contextualization:	Relate to the group's own experience	
Clinical problem solving		
Stage 1 ~ clarifying the problem		20
(MAIN AIM — to increase awareness)		
Small groups	Discussion of the case	
Questions to consider	1) What ethical difficulties are there? Do a problem list.	
	2) What is/are the core problem(s)?	
Plenary	Discussion of the two questions	
Stage 2 ~ deepening understanding		30
(MAIN AIM — to increase knowledge)		
Lecture presentation	Discursive review of the core problem(s), drawing on relevant ethical discussions in literature (including chapters in this book), guidelines, codes of practice; legal points; communication issues; etc.	
Plenary	Questions and discussion	
Stage 3 ~ formulating a response		30
(MAIN AIMS — (a) to change attitudes (i.e. by looking at the problem from different points of view) and (b) to improve reasoning skills)		
Small groups	Discuss:	
	1) how the literature bears directly on the core problem, and hence	
	2) how to formulate an action plan	
Plenary	Discussion of proposed action plans	
	Note: focus is on ethical reasoning — i.e. principles, casuistry, perspectives; deontology; consequentialism; analytic ethics — all as part of clinical problem solving	
Stage 4 ~ outcome and follow up		10
(MAIN AIM — to develop 'reflective practice')		
Plenary	Review possible outcomes	
Debriefing		20
(MAIN AIM — to fix key points)		
Commentary	By practitioner with relevant experience (may be integrated into above stages)	
Key points/questions	Summary of 'learning points' (by reference to seminar aims)	
	END OF SEMINAR	2 hrs total
Ongoing learning		
(MAIN AIM – to reinforce learning)		
Further reading	Focused guide to further reading as take-away handout	
Subsequent seminars	Cross-refer between seminars	

This table illustrates on way in which the cases and discussions given in Chapters 3–8 of this book may be incorporated into seminar teaching aimed at improving clinical problem-solving skills. Seminars may of course vary enormously in style and content, but should always incorporate the four key stages of:

1 clarification of the problem;
2 deepening understanding;
3 formulating a response; and
4 outcome and follow up.

They reflect the stages of all clinical problem solving and hence allow ethical and technical aspects of a case to be woven together in an integrated approach to the development of good 'practice skills'. (See also text.)

outlined in Chapter 2 — *awareness, attitudes, knowledge,* and *thinking skills.* Table 9.1 shows how the seminar aims are related to the four stages of the clinical problem-solving process; the main aims of each part of the seminar are shown. Obviously there is considerably more overlap than we have indicated: ethical reasoning, for example, is often important at Stage 1 (clarifying the problem) as well as at Stage 3 (formulating a response); similarly, the different models of disorder will be spelled out at Stage 2 (from the literature) as well as emerging from the process of clarifying the problem (at Stage 1). Table 9.1 also indicates the aims of other stages of the seminar, in particular the importance of take-away materials and cross-referencing of seminars for reinforcing the learning process.

A time plan

In ethics teaching there is constant tension between the need for clear educational objectives and the importance of an open, interactive style which encourages participants to develop their own thinking skills. Clear objectives can be secured through explicit aims, but an interactive style requires a clear structure to the seminar. A good way to achieve this is by setting out a time plan, with the main stages and points to be covered, in a one-sheet summary. This gives a series of benchmarks against which to maintain progress. Approximate times for the main stages of the seminar are shown in Table 9.1.

Introduction

The initial scene setting and contextualization of a case are crucial to the educational process. Scene setting includes obvious (but often neglected) organizational details: making sure that you have case histories of appropriate length and well-structured reading lists; and checking that equipment (for example, the overhead projector) is working. Introducing co-teachers or visiting speakers and giving their backgrounds are also important. It is often helpful to put up on a blackboard or whiteboard the 'game plan' of the seminar (that is, the title and the main stages). This can be referred to initially and then used to keep everyone on track.

The aims of the seminar are also sometimes put up in 'hard copy'. However, this can have the effect of closing down discussion too early. Hence it may be better to introduce the aims briefly and then return to them at the end of the seminar in the form of a summary of the key learning points.

Contextualization involves anything which helps the participants to pinpoint where they are 'at'. Particularly with a new or mixed group, it is important to make sure that the problem to be discussed is carefully related to their own experience. One way to do this is with an initial 'buzz' group: members of the group are asked to work in pairs for, say, five minutes, to think of examples from their own experience of the problems to be tackled; these are then shared in a question-and-answer session with the group as a whole. The examples produced in this way are often very rich and may indeed be used as the basis for the rest of the seminar. Using a set-piece case history, on the other hand, makes it is easier to be sure that the key issues will be covered. The two approaches can be combined, of course. Beginning with a set case, for example, one can build in time for participants to suggest applications from their own practice. Or they could be sent the set case in advance and asked to think of similar problems they have encountered.

Clinical problem solving

We are now ready to start the clinical problem solving proper. This will occupy most of the seminar, starting with Stage 1, clarifying the problem.

1) Clarifying the problem

At this stage, the presenting problem is made explicit and we try to clarify its elements. Cases described in the literature are often idealized (much of the literature on medical ethics still deals in abstractions and general principles). In practice, ethical aspects of clinical problems are as complex and multifaceted as technical aspects. Hence an important problem-solving skill is to be able to recognize the ethical problems for what they are, to disentangle them, to make them explicit. A second problem-solving skill is prioritizing. It is helpful to do a problem list, but the problems are not usually all equally pressing, and there is often a core problem on which the practical difficulties turn.

2) Deepening understanding

Having made the problems explicit, the next step is to get a deeper understanding of them. The first step here is understanding what *kind* of problem you are dealing with. Although clinical cases are highly individual, most ethical problems fall into a limited number of general kinds: there is a taxonomy! Identifying the *kind* of problem you are dealing with allows you to tap into all the relevant literature, guidelines, legal principles, and so on.

The topics covered will vary, of course. But we have prefaced each of our discussions with topic lists so that they can be easily cross-referenced. Thus, following the areas covered in the discussion of Elizabeth Orton's case in Chapter 3 would include dual role issues, autonomy, confidentiality, iatrogenic harm, and risk. But the core issues all centre around the concept of mental illness and how this drives the balance between treatment and social control. Thus, deepening understanding of these issues could draw in material from Case 3.2 on values in psychiatric diagnosis, or perhaps aspects of autonomy and rationality from Chapter 4. But the objective at this stage is to get across the 'knowledge' component of the seminar.

3) Formulating a response

Having clarified the core problem, understood its general nature, and read up on relevant literature, the next stage is to formulate a response in the circumstances *of the particular case*. This is the stage at which the thinking skills of bioethics and philosophy are particularly relevant. For example, a case involving involuntary treatment will have led (at Stage 2) to the now very large literature *on* this topic. This literature includes, as in Chapter 2, applications of the 'four principles' — though of course it covers much else besides! But insofar as you are employing the principles approach, at Stage 3 you will be thinking *for yourself* about the balancing of these principles in the particular case.

Other methods of ethical reasoning may be helpful in formulating a response. As we describe in Chapter 2, case-based reasoning (casuistry) and perspectives are frequently important, as are recent approaches such as narrative ethics and virtue ethics. But also significant may be conceptual analytical skills (if the case turns critically on whether someone is genuinely ill — for example as in Chapter 3) or the general philosophical ethical approaches of deontology and/or consequentialism (for example, utilitarianism). These specifically ethical ways of approaching a problem, moreover, will need to be combined in the clinical context both with generic thinking skills (see Table 1.1, Chapter 1) and with communication and other clinical skills.

4) Outcome and follow up

It may seem odd to include this stage in ethical problem solving. However, it directly reflects our strongly clinical approach. As a branch of philosophy, ethics has been reflective and abstract. This is its strength; it allows us to stand back and analyse a problem. Even consequentialist ethical theories (such as utilitarianism) are primarily concerned with guiding choices by reference to *anticipated* outcomes. It is really only 'moral luck' ethical theorists who have given actual outcomes an ethically central place. But as an aspect of practice skills, monitoring how things actually turn out ethically is vital. It is vital clinically: we should always review how a case is progressing. It is also vital for skills development: it is only by reviewing how things work out that we are able to monitor our own performance. There is a need generally for more research on the outcome of ethical review, for example in the functioning of research ethics committees (see Chapter 10).

Debriefing

In the final part of the seminar it is important to find ways of pulling together and integrating what has been learnt. The key learning points should always be summarized against the original seminar aims. It may be helpful to spend some time asking the group what they have learned from the seminar. If it is a clinical group, this can be extended to thinking about where they might find ideas from the seminar helpful in their day-to-day practice. Finally, an expert commentary — either at this stage in a seminar or as the case evolves — is an excellent way of pulling the issues together and picking up points which may have been missed.

Ongoing learning

Reinforcement is the key to successful learning. Ideally, this should be by reference to seminar materials in the context of everyday clinical work. Sometimes 'ethics' teachers are also clinical supervisors. Where they are not, it is often helpful to ask a seminar class to bring examples from their own clinical work to later seminars.

Other ways of reinforcing learning include:

- *Guides to further reading*. We have structured the guides to further reading at the end of each chapter to cover, as far as possible, relevant topic areas. Extended reading guides, if offered as take-away handouts, should distinguish key readings and optional extras.

- *Cross-referencing between seminars*. The interconnected nature of the topics covered by psychiatric ethics makes it easy to cross-refer between seminars. This is a powerful way of reinforcing learning, especially if combined with occasional questions to see whether students have followed up on materials from the guides to further reading!

Example of a clinical problem-solving seminar

In the remaining section of this chapter we illustrate the clinical problem-solving approach, building on the first case history and discussion in Chapter 3, Elizabeth Orton.

Preliminary planning

Elizabeth Orton's story illustrated some of the ethical problems arising from overuse of the concept of mental illness. As we noted in Chapter 3, problems of this kind are becoming increasingly common for multidisciplinary teams working in community-based programmes. However, the origins of these problems, which lie in differences between team members in their 'models of disorder', are not well recognized. Hence it is particularly important, before launching into the seminar proper, to think how the case should be presented. Thus we start with defining the *aims* of the seminar thus:

- **Awareness:** of different models of disorder (conceptual), their influence on clinical decision making (communication), and their ethical as well as scientific significance (ethics).

- **Attitudes:** greater tolerance of different approaches, as between professionals and patients and within multidisciplinary teams (communication).

- **Knowledge:** of (1) specific models (conceptual); (2) dual role issues (ethics, law); and (3) bias in psychiatric assessment (communication).

- **Thinking skills:** use of three main methods of ethical reasoning.

The time plan is as shown in Table 9.1

Introduction

The introduction to the seminar includes:

- **Title/topic** — 'To treat or not to treat?'
- **Reference to the 'game plan'** (on the board; see the following box)

To treat or not to treat?

Plan of seminar
Introduction
Case history
=> Problem
Background literature
Action plan
Outcome
Conclusions

- **Contextualization** — brief question-and-answer session to locate the topic in the group's own experience.

Clinical problem solving

Stage 1 — clarifying the problem

The case to be worked on is now introduced. A brief introductory synopsis is usually helpful. Participants should each have a copy of the case to read and 'mark up'. They are then asked to discuss it in small groups with specific questions to answer. Thus:

Synopsis: A psychiatrist is asked by Social Services to see a woman (Elizabeth Orton) who in his opinion is not mentally ill. If he refuses, Elizabeth's baby (Anthony) will be taken away and put 'in care'. Elizabeth says she does not want her baby, but her husband (Tim) says he does, and Elizabeth wants to keep their marriage intact.

Questions: Imagine yourself as the doctor here, Dr Isaacs. Like most real-life cases, Elizabeth's story raises a number of issues — some explicit, others implicit. Start by brainstorming these issues, thinking as widely as you can and writing down a checklist of problems. Include issues which you think could be there, behind the explicit story as it were, as well as those which are openly presented. Then, as a second stage, review your list in order of priority, and try to extract a core problem.

Case history (as distributed to each member of the class): Elizabeth Orton is a thirty-five-year old solicitor with a ten-month-old baby, Anthony. She has a congenital hip malformation which has required numerous surgical procedures and sometimes confinement to a wheelchair, although at present her mobility is quite good. Anthony's delivery, however, was by Caesarean section, and afterwards Elizabeth suffered some postnatal depression. Although there are now no clinical signs of depression, she continues to insist that she does not want the baby. Her fifty-year-old husband, Tim, who is semi-retired, does most of the child care outside the hours when Anthony attends a day nursery, but recently he was away for six nights. During that time Elizabeth telephoned her health visitor for help, upset because she had shaken the baby.

The health visitor alerted Social Services, who (together with the police) have the statutory responsibility for investigating cases of suspected child abuse, and the child protection machinery was set in motion. Anthony was placed on the Child Protection Register. When Anthony is not at his day nursery, Tim or another designated person must be with the baby; Elizabeth is no longer allowed to care for him on her own. She has also been required by Social Services to agree to see a psychiatrist. If she does not accept psychiatric treatment, she has been told that Anthony may well be taken into care — to which Tim is deeply opposed.

Elizabeth insists that she is perfectly willing to have the baby taken away from the home, but that she fears her marriage would not survive. In a way she would be happier if the baby could be adopted immediately: what she dreads is the social embarrassment, her husband's grief, and the uncertainty of the child's long-term future if a series of short-term fostering placements are arranged. So she is co-operating very minimally with the requirement of psychiatric treatment, which she calls 'emotional blackmail.' At the most recent interagency child protection case conference, however, it was decided to keep Anthony at home, on the 'at-risk' register, and to continue the requirement of psychiatric care for Elizabeth, in the hope that she will develop more 'normal' maternal feelings.

The consultant psychiatrist treating Elizabeth, Daniel Isaacs, feels caught in an extremely awkward position. He has developed a reasonably good therapeutic relationship with Elizabeth because, he thinks, she feels he is the only one who is concentrating on her rather than on the baby. He does not actually believe that Elizabeth has any form of mental illness. Although his opinion was sought at the case conference, he thought that this finding was not very welcome. In addition, he had doubts about whether he should have revealed confidential clinical information about Elizabeth in that setting. (Elizabeth and Tim were also invited to attend, but chose not to.) Dr Isaacs also got himself into hot water by pointing out that in his experience, fathers who posed a threat of violence to their children were not usually asked to seek psychiatric treatment, so long as the mother was there to protect the child. 'Probably not', he was told, 'although the child would still be on the 'at-risk' register. But could we please concentrate on the child's best interests, and leave gender politics out of this?'

Plenary discussion

After working on the case in pairs, a problem list is developed on the board through feedback from the class as a whole. The topics that may come up include those covered in our discussion in Chapter 3, but seminar groups are often very sharp at identifying novel ethical aspects of a case. This stage of shared feedback and discussion is crucial for raising awareness — one of the key objectives in ethics education.

A checklist of problems for Elizabeth Orton's case:

1 consent (Elizabeth is attending under duress);

2 confidentiality (Dr Isaacs could be asked to reveal information);

3 the blurred boundary between Dr Isaacs' responsibility to protect 'society' and to act in the interests of his patient;

4 the role of diagnosis (gender bias in the 'norms' applied; and the psychiatrist, as an 'expert', colluding in this);

5   the concept of 'mental illness' (as defining the proper role of the psychiatrist);

6   clinical responsibility and legal obligations (for example, the potential conflict between Dr Isaacs' role as a psychiatrist and his responsibilities under
the Children Act);

7   the effect of her disability in Elizabeth's perceived and real situation; and so
on.

How these problems are now put in order of priority may vary considerably.
It is important in discussing different suggestions to bring out that the problems are inter-related; hence in focusing on one problem, the discussion could
move in a number of directions. However, a key step towards developing some
form of action plan is to extract the essence of the problem.

The core problem for Dr Isaacs: the boundary between psychiatric treatment
and social control.

Stage 2 — deepening understanding
At this stage in the seminar it is often helpful to move to a more discursive style
of presentation. There will be a number of points to cover. The participants will
have worked hard on the problems and should be ready to sit back for a bit and
take on board some ideas and information. It is important to keep the exchange
of ideas going, but the style can switch to more of a lecture.

Materials covered at Stage 2: these could include:
1   high-profile cases of abuse (USSR, Japan) but also endemic/sporadic cases
in all areas;
2   the influence of culture/gender in diagnosis;
3   sociological/firsthand literature (patients themselves) regarding abusive
coercion;
4   the variety of models of mental disorder;
5   the polarity between medical and agent-centred models;
6   the importance of finding a balance between these extremes; and
7   the role of different perspectives (of patients, of carers, and of different
members of the multidisciplinary team) in achieving this balance.

Stage 3 – formulating a response
The group now has to do some work again! Working in their pairs, they are
given two tasks:
1   to apply the materials from Stage 2 to the core problem.
2   to develop an action plan.

Questions for the group: We have covered a lot of material. We now need to
think about two questions. (1) In what ways does this material help Dr Isaacs,

in particular by giving a deeper understanding of what lies behind his feeling of being caught in the role of 'policeman in the guise of doctor'? (2) What would one do in practice? Write down your answer to question 1. Then, working in your groups, use one or more of the methods of ethical reasoning to work out and write down a brief action plan.

Response to question 1: the aim of this first task is to reinforce learning — a common problem with teaching in this area is that general theoretical points are not applied carefully to particular situations. The literature covered in Stage 2 is all relevant in principle, but there are a number of points that will apply particularly strongly to the core practical dilemma.

Points from the literature for Dr Isaacs: the literature helps Dr Isaacs in at least three ways —

1 It provides a clear endorsement of his concerns. This is crucial practically in a situation in which one person is being pressured by others to act against their instincts. The literature shows time and again that the situation is indeed 'unsatisfactory'...this is no mere nicety of clinical sensitivity...still less 'playing with words' (ill or not ill)...nor is it a problem only of totalitarian regimes...psychiatry is coercive, often without recognizing it, and goes beyond its clinical brief into social control all too readily...Dr Isaacs is right to be alert to all this — and especially where a state agency, motivated by strongly held values (the child's best interest) has relatively wide powers. So the literature empowers Dr Isaacs to take a stand.

2 It gives him a way of framing or giving shape to his concerns (that is, in terms of the balance between medical and agent-centred models of mental disorder). Elizabeth Orton is being compelled into medical 'treatment'; Dr Isaacs sees her not as a patient but as an agent who is responsible for and has a right to her own choices.

3 It identifies some of the specific factors which contribute to this balance. Thus an important factor driving the medical/agent balance in this case is gender bias: the 'problem' is 'the mother who rejects her child'. The literature is full of examples of gender bias driving psychiatric assessment.

Response to question 2: for this task, the three methods of ethical reasoning outlined in Chapter 2 are often helpful. The principles approach was used in the discussion of the case in Chapter 3 (in relation to issues of autonomy). So this approach has already helped to define the problem. Other methods of ethical reasoning are often helpful in developing an action plan.

Developing an action plan for Dr Isaacs

Casuistic reasoning is helpful in thinking about the balance between agent-centred medical models of Elizabeth Orton's 'disorder'. For example, if she were depressed, Dr Isaacs would probably have fewer reservations about treating her (and this reminds us that it is important clinically to monitor her mental state); similarly, if she had not asked for help at all (from the health visitor) he would probably feel that he definitely should not be involved. (This in turn triggers the question of whether Elizabeth really is as unambiguously 'blackmailed' as she says. She did ask for help after all. She is not wholly against seeing Dr Isaacs.)

Perhaps a key here, though, is perspectives. After all, Dr Isaacs might think: I have been looking at this from my point of view as a compromised professional! But what is Elizabeth Orton's perspective? What are her real concerns? Also, yes of course, what about Tim, her husband? Why did neither of them feel they could come to the meeting? Social Services' perspective, too, could be critical: they feel very strongly about the child protection issue. This is not strictly my (Dr Isaacs') concern, but it will help no one, least of all Elizabeth Orton, if she ends up battering her baby.

Communication issues will obviously be important also. We (those at the case conference meeting) need time to think this through, rather than taking up entrenched positions, in order to understand each other's points of view.

The plan

Rather than confronting the child protection meeting with a refusal, or merely acquiescing to an unacceptable role, Dr Isaacs decides to ask the chair, the Social Services line manager, Jim Jones (note that he gets a name now, he becomes a real person) to take his concerns seriously and to give a few minutes to discussing his precise role. After all, the basis of Elizabeth's referral had never been made clear; psychiatrists are always being accused of 'medicalizing' life's problems; and anyway, if Elizabeth felt 'blackmailed' this would not ultimately help her baby, Anthony.

Stage 4 — outcome and follow-up

Either in whole-class discussion or a further brief 'buzz' group session, the group now thinks about the likely outcome of this course of action. Obviously things could go a number of ways, but the point of including this as a distinct stage of ethical reasoning is to reinforce the importance of monitoring outcomes. It is helpful to break this stage down into immediate and longer-term outcomes.

A possible immediate outcome: Jim Jones (who in fact was a member of MIND) immediately agreed to Dr Isaacs' proposal and apologized for appearing to discount his assessment of Elizabeth's mental state. They then agreed a joint plan. Dr Isaacs would offer Elizabeth two further appointments specifically to clarify whether from her point of view, there were reasons for her to continue seeing him; he would offer to see Tim as well. The social worker responsible would also make clear at her next visit that Tim, as well as Elizabeth, could be offered help. There would be a further meeting if Elizabeth still appeared to feel 'blackmailed', but a firm decision had to be in place one way or another before Tim's next period away.

A possible longer-term outcome: At her next appointment, Dr Isaacs explained to Elizabeth that he would be happy to go on seeing her provided she saw this as helpful, and they agreed on two further meetings before coming to a decision. This led to Elizabeth being able to talk about her own feelings more fully. She had wanted a baby, but then felt trapped as soon as Anthony was born. This was why she had been 'rejecting', but, far from telling anyone (least of all Tim), she felt she must be 'going mad'. This fear intensified when she found herself shaking Anthony — hence her 'cry for help'. But being referred to a psychiatrist then seemed to underscore her worst fears for her sanity.

Elizabeth now recognized that she needed help — not necessarily to accept Anthony but at least to resolve her conflicting feelings. She decided she wanted to go on seeing Dr Isaacs, not specifically as a psychiatrist, but as someone whom she felt she could trust. Also, his opinion that she was not mentally ill was important for her battered self-esteem. Tim welcomed the offer of seeing someone for himself. He had felt excluded and also very hurt. He was very concerned for Anthony if Elizabeth was still negative as he grew up.

Debriefing

Expert commentary: Where possible, it is helpful to have an 'expert' from the relevant clinical field involved in the seminar. The practitioner commentaries accompanying the cases in this book illustrate the range of additional material this can bring in.

Key learning points from this case

1 **Awareness:** of the importance of models of disorder. The ethical problems centred around the different models of disorder held by Dr Isaacs (Elizabeth Orton is distressed but not ill) and Social Services (Elizabeth Orton is mentally ill); this difference was in turn driven by unacknowledged differences of values (Dr Isaacs' responsibility to his 'patient'; Social Services' concern for child protection).

2 **Attitudes:** whether we took sides initially with Dr Isaacs or Social Services, we have seen that both had genuine concerns. Similarly, we now understand Elizabeth Orton's contradictory response to the offer of help. Attitudes of mutual respect and understanding were the key to moving this case forward in a practically effective way.

3 **Knowledge:** we have covered:
  a the different models of disorder (for example, the medical paradigm);
  b the proper use of the Mental Health Act;
  c principles of child protection legislation;
  d empirical work on the causes and outcome of the rejection of babies by their mothers;
  e Tarasoff and Egdell legal cases on confidentiality;
  f consent to treatment;
  g risk; and
  h iatrogenic harm.

4 **Thinking skills:** apparently intractable problems of principle (social control versus treatment) are often resolved in practice on the basis of concrete detail; the relevant detail here was Elizabeth's perspective. The key aspect of this — her fear that she was going mad — had not been recognized because the overwhelming 'value' was the child protection issue. This was behind the view of her as 'mentally ill'; a view that reinforced her fear that she was going mad. Standing on principle (by Dr Isaacs or Social Services) would have been 'legal' but would have deepened the practical problem; at best it would have left Anthony growing up with a mother who resented him. Communication skills and interagency respect were crucial. It was also essential that Dr Isaacs and Jim were both able to pick up on the ethical issues (that is, communication is no good unless you know what to communicate!) This is where the literature, as opposed to merely generic reasoning skills, can be important: the use of casuistic reasoning and perspectives led directly to the practical solution (covering both Elizabeth's concern and Tim's needs).

Ongoing learning

As noted earlier in the chapter, ongoing learning is crucial to ethics teaching. It is supported particularly by a clear guide to further reading, cross-referencing between seminars, and (where possible) integration into clinical practice.

- **Guide to further reading:** In a clinical problem-solving seminar this would cover a subset of the issues in the Reading Guide to Chapter 3, focusing particularly on aspects directly relevant to practice.

- **Cross-referencing seminars:** Relevant cases in Chapters 3–8 include Case 3.2 in Chapter 3 (to compare underuse of the concept of mental illness), Case 4.3 (the importance of values in shaping our conceptions of mental disorder), and Case 7.1 (the range of issues involved in risk management in psychiatry). Both cases in Chapter 8 (on teamwork) are also particularly pertinent.

- **Clinical integration:** Obviously this is only possible where those running the seminars are also involved in clinical training. This is one of the many ways in which team teaching, between an ethicist and someone skilled in the relevant clinical area, can be extremely valuable. In Elizabeth Orton's case, relevant areas of practice of course include social work.

References

Bloch, S., Chodoff, P., and Green S.A. (1999) *Psychiatric Ethics* (3rd edn; 1st edn 1981). Oxford, Oxford University Press.

Fulford, K.W M. (1996) Religion and psychiatry: extending the limits of tolerance. In *Religion and Psychiatry: Context, Consensus and Controversies* (ed. Bhugra, D.), Chapter 1. London, Routledge and Kegan Paul.

Fulford, K.W.M. and Bloch, S. (forthcoming). Psychiatric ethics: codes, concepts and clinical practice skills. In *New Oxford Textbook of Psychiatry* (ed. Gelder, M., Andreasen, N., and Lopez–Ibor, J.), Chapter 17. Oxford, Oxford University Press.

Hope, T., Fulford, K.W.M., and Yates, A. (1996) *Manual of the Oxford Practice Skills Project.* Oxford, Oxford University Press.

Reading Guide

Sources and resources for teaching psychiatric ethics

For introductions to psychiatric ethics, see the Reading Guide to Chapter 2.

The introductory chapter and study guide to Parker and Dickenson, *The Cambridge Medical Ethics Workbook* (2000), includes a comparison of various approaches to reading cases in medical ethics. The workbook as a whole can be used either for teaching, for self-study, or for a combination of the two (which is the method now being developed for the Imperial College School of Medicine MSc in Medical Ethics). A practical manual, including sample seminars, outlines of ethical theory, and a detailed appendix covering literature sources, databases, and courses — all aimed at ethics education in medicine — is *The Oxford Practice Skills Manual* (Hope *et al.* 1996). This method is also described in 'Medical Education: Patients, Principles and Practice Skills' by Hope and Fulford (1993).

Search engines which may be useful for medical ethics include that operated by the Kennedy Center, Bioethicsline; Medline; and Knowledge Finder. There are also on-line discussion groups and list subscriber services such as that run by Feminist Advances in Bioethics. On-line versions of journals such as the *Hastings Center Report* are also useful.

Literature on the effectiveness of medical ethics education is frequently featured in *The Journal of Medical Ethics* and in *Medical Education*. A structured approach to assessing 'ethics' competences in medical students is described by Savulescu *et al.* in 'Evaluating ethics competence in medical education' (1999). Ethics curricula in medical schools are reviewed by John Goldie (2000).

Resources aimed specifically at psychiatry are less readily available. Robert Michels and Kevin Kelly, in Chapter 24 of Bloch *et al.*'s *Psychiatric Ethics* (1999), describe a topic-based approach. The Royal College of Psychiatrists regularly runs ethics teaching workshops as part of its annual meetings.

The four-part process of clinical problem solving, which is at the heart of the approach described here, broadly follows the course of problem-based learning. This is now used extensively in medical schools for general clinical training: see, for example, Holm and Aspergen (1999) or Davis and Harden (1999).

Reading Guide: references

Bloch, S., Chodoff, P., and Green S.A. (1999) *Psychiatric Ethics* (3rd edn; 1st edn 1981). Oxford, Oxford University Press.

Davis, M.H. and Harden, R.M. (1999) Problem-based learning: a practical guide. *Medical Teacher*, 21:130–40.

Goldie, J. (2000) Review of ethics curricula in undergraduate medical education. *Medical Education*, 34:108–19.

Holm, U. and Aspergen, K. (1999) Pedagogical methods and affect tolerance in medical students. *Medical Education*, 33:14–18.

Hope, R.A. and Fulford, K.W.M. (1993) Medical Education: Patients, Principles and Practice Skills. In *Principles of Health Care Ethics* (ed. Gillon, R. and Lloyd, A.), Chapter 59. Chichester (England), John Wiley and Sons.

Hope, T., Fulford, K.W.M., and Yates, A. (1996) *Manual of the Oxford Practice Skills Project*. Oxford, Oxford University Press.

Parker, M. and Dickenson, D. (2000) *The Cambridge Medical Ethics Workbook*. Cambridge, Cambridge University Press.

Savulescu, J., Crisp, R., Fulford, K.W.M., and Hope, T. (1999) Evaluating ethics competence in medical education. *Journal of Medical Ethics*, 25:367–74.

CHAPTER 10

The three Rs of research ethics

Although this book is primarily a clinical casebook, we felt it important to include a brief consideration of research ethics for two reasons. First, the problems raised by ethics of research illustrate and help to draw together many of the issues that are important in clinical ethics. Second, the gap between clinical work and research is narrowing day by day. More and more clinical training schemes include a research component; and those working in ordinary clinical practice are increasingly expected to carry out research projects. These factors, combined with the growing importance of evidence-based practice, mean that even someone who is not directly involved in research, either as a researcher or as a member of a research ethics committee, must be able to assess the quality of a research proposal in its ethical as well as technical aspects.

There is now a considerable literature on research ethics. Besides academic and scholarly papers, there are endless guidelines, regulations, and codes — not to mention evolving case law and legal statutes. Over the last thirty years or so, we have moved from research being de facto subsumed under whatever regulations, tacit or explicit, covered ordinary clinical work, to almost everyone concerned with research feeling it incumbent on them to produce their own set of guidelines. Relevant documents now range from supranational statements of high-level principles, like the World Psychiatric Association's *Declaration of Madrid* (1996), through the codes of practice of professional bodies like The Royal College of Psychiatrists (see the Reading Guide), to the detailed regulations issued by each of the now very large number of local research ethics committees.

We will not be attempting to review this huge literature in this chapter! As with other areas of bioethics, the particular problems raised by research specifically in psychiatry have been relatively neglected. Even so, the literature and regulatory frameworks relevant to psychiatric research within the UK alone are protean. Moreover, there are a number of excellent introductions to research ethics readily available, as we describe in the Reading Guide. These references cover a number of specific topics that we have not attempted to consider here, for example the ethical relevance (or otherwise) of such distinctions as therapeutic versus non-therapeutic research and invasive versus non-invasive protocols.

The aim throughout this chapter will be to provide a framework for ethical thinking which, in reading or writing a research proposal, has *practical* problem solving as its objective. This will undoubtedly lead us into a number of difficult theoretical areas.

As in other chapters, we will be looking at problem solving in research ethics primarily through a case history. However, unlike the clinical cases considered in Chapters 3–8, we will be considering our research ethics case history in a series of stages. These stages correspond to the main stages of thinking through the ethical aspects of a research proposal and are:

1   to decide whether what is proposed is research

2   to consider whether it satisfies the criteria for good practice in research (we will suggest that four principles are helpful here — knowledge, necessity, benefit, and consent)

3   to develop proposals for resolving any problems identified, using casuistic or other methods

4   to follow up.

We will conclude with a brief resumé of the role and functioning of research ethics committees especially in relation to psychiatry.

CASE HISTORY   **The background (initial letter)**

The Director of a large National Health Trust[1] wrote to the Chair of her Local Research Ethics Committee as follows...

Mr L R Smith
Chair
Erehwon Research Ethics Committee

Dear Mr Smith

Re: Primary care mental health evaluation project

Following our conversation before Christmas I am pleased to enclose an outline of the nature and objectives of this project.

Our aim is to compare the cost-effectiveness of two ways of providing mental health services in the community, one based on community mental health teams, the other based on General Practices (family doctor teams). We have approached the Jonsen Centre for Mental Health, who have a well-established reputation for evaluation of mental health services, to assist us in the task of evaluating our preferred model of community-based mental health services alongside a general practice-based model. They have proposed a two-stage study, the first stage involving an audit of mental health needs and how they are being met in the two models, the second stage involving semi-structured interviews of key informants (including users of services). We have obtained financial assistance from West Fenland Health to meet the cost of the project.

I should make it clear that, at this stage, what I am seeking is your opinion as to whether this evaluation of mental health services in Erehwon should be referred to your full Committee for approval. If it is your conclusion it should be, I am assuming you would wish to see copies of the protocols to be used for the 'semi-structured interviews' in the second stage of the project, which have yet to be finalized.

I hope this is helpful. If you do require any further information please do not hesitate to contact me.

Yours sincerely

Christine Ready

Director of Primary Care and Commissioning

Erewhon Health Care

Stage 1 — is this research?

When the need for ethical review of research first began to be acknowledged, there was a vigorous debate about precisely how research should be defined. The main aim of this debate was to distinguish research from ordinary clinical practice. This in turn was motivated by two concerns. First, it was feared that an unduly restrictive approach to clinical work would restrict therapeutic freedom and inhibit innovation. This concern remains with us today, though now more closely associated with the way in which evidence-based guidelines may be allowed to 'trump' individual clinical experience. The second concern was that too broad a definition of research might result in Research Ethics Committees being overwhelmed with applications.

One result of this debate was to mark out a number of distinctions which, although not always capable of being unambiguously drawn, have found their way into the literature on research ethics; the Royal College of Physicians have provided a helpful summary (1996, Section 6). These include therapeutic v. non-therapeutic, and 'unintrusive research'. Part of the importance of these distinctions is to signal different levels of concern about a research proposal. As we will see later, the therapeutic v. non-therapeutic distinction has been invoked in relation to research with people unable to consent. However, there is a growing movement to abandon such distinctions in favour of express assessment of the balance of risks and benefits for all research (the therapeutic v. non-therapeutic distinction may be abandoned in future revisions of such documents as the Declaration of Helsinki).

Measured against these distinctions, the Jonsen Centre proposals seem anodyne. This is clearly signalled in Christine Ready's letter. She emphasizes that she is not actually making an application for ethical review but only requesting an opinion as to whether such a review is necessary. Moreover, she implies that it is only for Stage 2 of the project that the question arises at all, this being the stage at which patients (and others) will be approached for interview. (Note her offer to supply the interview protocols if required.) If the study had been limited to the first stage (an audit), the Research Ethics Committee would not have been approached at all.

Christine Ready's implied distinction between audit and research is consistent with one strand of thought in the research ethics literature. This is to the effect that audit, being 'routine', non-invasive, and therapeutic (in the broad sense of being aimed at identifying best practice for the conditions from which the patients involved in the audit are suffering) is not ethically sensitive. Moreover, as in earlier debates about the distinction between clinical work and research, it is argued that to include audit within the remit of the Research Ethics Committees would both inhibit the proper monitoring and review of services and lead to an overload of the Committees themselves.

There is, though, a central difficulty with this school of thought, reasonable enough as it may seem at first glance — namely that of defining 'audit'. A number of attempts have been made to distinguish audit from research in terms of the procedures involved. As this case illustrates, at best, this approach helps to draw out certain differences of emphasis or degree between audit and some kinds of scientific research, notably research based on laboratory rather than field work.

Similar difficulties were encountered in the debate about the distinction between research and clinical work. The conclusion to which this debate came was that research and clinical work should be distinguished, for purposes of ethical review, not by their respective procedures, but by the *intentions* with which these procedures are carried out. In clinical work, the primary intention is to serve the best interests of one's patients. In research, by contrast, the primary intention is to advance knowledge (though of course with the further intention of benefiting patients). An intentional, rather than procedural distinction, has also been adopted in guidelines from both the

Royal College of Physicians (1996) and The Royal College of Psychiatrists (1990 and forthcoming).

Opinion in the UK is currently swinging towards the view that audit should be included in ethical review: the Association of Local Research Ethics Committees, for example, has come down firmly on this side. More resources may be needed, but ethical review of audit does not have to be resource-intensive. What is required, after all, is review of audit *procedures* or of programmes of evaluation and monitoring, rather than of each and every project. More importantly, though, audit shares with research the key shift of intention — from the best interests of the person who is the subject of the research (or audit) to the intention of advancing knowledge. It is this shift of intention which is at the heart of the greater ethical sensitivity of research and, by extension, of audit. In both cases, the shift implies an inherent conflict of interest and, hence, the need for external monitoring. Moreover, just as ethical review should facilitate good practice rather than inhibit the advance of knowledge, so too should the ethical view of audit. All in all then, returning to Christine Ready's letter, the Chair of the Local Research Ethics Committee, Mr Smith, was in no doubt that both stages of the proposed evaluation should be subject to review, and he wrote requesting full details.

CASE HISTORY (CONTINUED) **The proposals**

The Jonsen Centre proposals began with a brief resumé of the shift in GP referral patterns for mental health problems from hospital specialists (that is, psychiatrists working in in-patient or out-patient settings) to community psychiatric nurses (CPNs) and counsellors. The proposals continued...

> There is evidence that the number of people using mental health services can increase threefold when the service becomes community orientated. The vast majority of this increased demand comes from people with non-severe mental illness. As resources do not increase at the same rate, this puts pressure on Community Mental Health Teams (CMHTs) in terms of the sheer number of referrals and the difficulty they then have prioritizing people with serious mental illness.

Background information then followed on the substantial expenditure proposed by Erehwon Health on community-based mental health services. The core of the Jonsen Centre's evaluation was now introduced...

How then can mental health services have a close working relationship with primary health care without being over-burdened and while still prioritizing people with severe mental illness? Erehwon Health have developed two models of service provision. In one, a CPN is purchased by the Health Agency to serve a consortium of GPs as a member of the Community Mental Health Team; in the other, a CPN is purchased direct by a GP commissioning group and becomes a member of the local Primary Health Care Team.

The Health Agency, the Erehwon NHS Trust, and the GP practices concerned wish to evaluate these two schemes because mental health needs within the practices and the role of a mental health worker within the Primary Health Care Team are currently unknown. In addition, these stakeholders need to know whether policy objectives, such as targeting severe mental illness, are met, and the costs and benefits of this responsive pilot scheme. The Jonsen Centre presents in this paper a range of evaluation options and costs.

Expected benefits

As a result of this evaluation the following key issues will be addressed:

- What are the needs of people with mental health problems attending primary health care?
- What is the role of the CPN working as part of the Primary Health Care Team?
- Do different models of specialist mental health care provision lead to different numbers of referrals from primary health care?
- What mental health services do people referred go on to receive?
- What is the match between people's needs and the resources they receive?
- Are GPs more satisfied with some models of mental health provision than others?
- How do service users view mental health services?
- What are the clinical outcomes for service users?
- How cost-effective are the different models?

Mental health needs in primary health care

The first stage of developing mental health services is an assessment of need. The aim here will be to assess the needs of people using primary health care. To enable a comparison throughout all components of this evaluation, a third GP practice, which will not initially receive the pilot service, will be recruited. The CMHT, psychiatrists, in-patient wards, and day services will be asked to identify all people using mental health services who are under the care of the three practices (total population 42 000). GPs within the practices will then be asked to augment these lists with anybody else who they feel should receive mental health services. Mental health services or GPs, as appropriate, will be asked to rate whether each individual person meets severity criteria as used by the Audit Commission. In addition they will be asked to give socio-demographic details and mental health history, and to complete a Health of the Nation Outcome Scale (HoNOS). A similar needs assessment method has been successfully employed by the Jonsen Centre in a previous study carried out at the secondary level. Estimate three months' work for a full-time junior researcher with support from senior evaluation staff (13 days).

Role of the primary health care and CMHT mental health nurse
On the basis of needs identified, the Jonsen Centre will carry out key informant interviews, for example, with service users, GPs, CPNs, consultant psychiatrists, social workers, trust managers, and purchasers. The results of the needs assessment, key informant interviews, and expertise gained from other evaluations and research will be presented by the Jonsen Centre as advice to a decision-making steering group. Estimate two months' work for a junior researcher plus high level of input from senior staff (10 days).

The proposals then continued with three pages of details of the comparative analyses to be carried out. A final statement was given of The Jonsen Centre's policy on dissemination.

Dissemination
The Jonsen Centre would like to report at regular intervals to a steering group with local purchasers in the lead. An interim written report will be provided after the needs assessment. A final report will be produced after the impact stages. Findings will also be presented to study participants such as the Primary Health Care Teams and CMHT.

Our usual policy is as follows: The Jonsen Centre undertakes work of this nature so as to inform the national mental health field of progressive developments. Publication will therefore be sought by the Jonsen Centre. No individual service user or member of staff will be identifiable in any report or publication, without their express consent. Organizations will be given copies of intended publications in advance so that they may comment.

> The Jonsen Centre takes pride in the quality and independence of its eval-
> uations. Evaluation commissioners should be aware that study findings may
> not be seen as positive by all interested parties.

Stage 2 – is this good research?

Of the three main methods of ethical reasoning — principles, casuistry, and perspectives — principles are particularly helpful in structuring an initial ethical
review of a research proposal. This is true whether one is in the role of proposer or
appraiser (a member of a Local Research Ethics Committee, for example). In
either case, what is most important is often what is left out. What is said may be
important, but what is *not* said — the gaps and contradictions in the proposal —
are often particularly significant ethically. This is not because researchers set out to
deceive themselves or others. It is because the imperatives that drive research push
one to think about a given project from a particular point of view. And as we saw in
Chapter 2, the structured framework provided by the principles approach is
particularly helpful in opening our eyes to aspects of a situation we had neglected.

In relation to research, four principles are helpful in structuring ethical
review[2]:

1 **Knowledge**: the proposed research is likely to produce an increase in knowledge directly or indirectly relevant to patient care.

2 **Necessity**: it is necessary for the research to be carried out with the subjects
   proposed rather than with some less vulnerable group.

3 **Benefits**: the potential benefits arising from the research outweigh any
   inherent risks of harm.

4 **Consent**: research subjects will give valid (that is, free and informed) consent to their participation.

These principles can be applied to research in any area of medicine, but in the
remainder of this section we will apply them to the Jonsen Centre proposals, to
illustrate some of the special problems raised by research in psychiatry and how
these can be overcome.

1 Knowledge

The 'corpus of knowledge' is less well established in psychiatry than in other
areas. As we noted earlier (Chapter 1), this is due to scientific difficulty rather
than scientific inadequacy. All the same, the lack of consensus in psychiatry *is*
problematic.

Against this, psychiatry has the advantage that much of its research is close
to the clinical coalface: the relative lack of mature theories of brain func-

tioning means that the gap between research and clinical practice is much smaller than in, say, biochemical research on neurological disorders. Psychiatry has its theory–practice 'gaps', of course. Genetic research, in particular, leaves a whole series of intervening variables between the data and their practical applications. But the Jonsen Centre proposals fall firmly into the category of research which is directly relevant to practice: it is concerned with the needs of users and the cost-effectiveness of two models for supplying relevant services; its particular focus is those with *severe* mental illness; the design proposed makes the views of users themselves central to the appraisal process.

2 Necessity

This principle, too, presents particular problems for psychiatric research. It implies a rough hierarchy: that *in vitro* preparations be used in preference to animals, that animals be used in preference to healthy subjects, and that healthy subjects be used in preference to patients. But many forms of psychopathology are uniquely human experiences. It is true that there are animal models for some forms of psychopathology (for obsessive-compulsive disorder, for example), but even here the gap between animal model and human counterpart is considerable. (One aspect of this gap is the whole question of the meaning of the phenomena for the individual concerned: see Chapter 5.). Also, when it comes to symptoms like thought insertion, which require such high-level capacities as the ability for self-reflective thinking, animal models are not available even in principle.

The principle of necessity is also relevant as between different groups of patients. For example, in dementia research it is important to work where possible with subjects who still have capacity for consent. Similarly, patients who are being treated under the Mental Health Act or are in prison are generally considered vulnerable groups.

The Jonsen Centre proposals illustrate a rather different point — that notwithstanding the principle of necessity, it is often important in psychiatry actually to involve the most vulnerable groups (that is, those with serious mental illness) to ensure that their voice is heard. What matters here, as with research generally, is the question of intention. Where the intention is to advance knowledge for the benefit of a group of patients as a whole, then we have to be careful not to prejudice those who are least able to protect their own interests. But where it is the interests of the most vulnerable groups that the research is serving, then they have a positive right to be involved. The Jonsen proposals thus illustrate the importance of being clear about the precise objectives of a research proposal — who will benefit, who needs to be protected, and who should be empowered. The danger is that potential research participants are debarred from taking part by a paternalism which would be wholly unacceptable in a clinical context!

3 Benefit

Calculations of the balance of benefits to risk are complicated in psychiatry by both empirical and evaluative factors. Empirical factors include the lack of an agreed 'corpus' of knowledge (already noted). Perhaps even more significant, though, is the diversity of values by which, as we have several times emphasized, psychiatry is characterized. This is important for both sides of the risk–benefit equation: what is an unacceptable risk to one person may be entirely acceptable to another; what is a clear benefit to one person may not be to another.

The Jonsen Centre proposals, insofar as they are confined to gathering information, may appear to present little in the way of risk. This is one reason why audit is often considered not to require ethical review. We will see in a moment that this is an oversimplification. But it is important to be aware just how risk-laden non-invasive techniques like interviewing may be. The standard paradigms of high risk in research are patients being given a new drug or being subjected to an 'experimental' operation. Far less calculable, though, are the effects of being asked a series of probing questions or merely of being 'recruited' into a trial in the first place. Randomization too — the basis of modern research methods — may be a highly adverse experience where subjects feel that they or their relatives have been denied effective treatments (Snowden *et al.* 1997).

Again, the point of emphasizing such hidden risks is not to inhibit research. The Jonsen Centre proposals are clearly aimed at providing key information which will improve the efficiency and delivery of mental health services. But it is essential that all research, and not just obviously 'risky' research, is properly assessed. Too often — in behavioural research (British Psychological Society 1978), in psychotherapeutic research (Holmes and Lindley 1989), and even in social science research (Wing 1999) — what counts as a good or bad outcome is merely taken for granted.

Where values differ, as we found in Chapter 8 in relation to clinical work, there is no 'ready reckoner' way to resolve them. An appropriate range of perspectives should thus be factored into the review process. The Jonsen Centre proposals directly reflect the importance of perspectives in the design of their study: the perspectives of all the relevant parties are represented in the data-gathering process. But this is also important in the ethical review process. In the clinical context, as we noted in Chapter 8, the required range of perspectives is provided by the multidisciplinary team. In research it is provided by a well-balanced Research Ethics Committee.

4 Consent

Both limbs of the consent formula — freedom of choice and information — may be problematic in psychiatric research. We will look at these briefly before applying them to the Jonsen proposals.

Constraints on freedom of choice may be external or internal. External constraints arise from the unequal power relationship between doctors and patients. Pressure to take part in research is rarely overt, but concerns for one's treatment, or inducements, may amount to strong covert pressures. Patients who are being treated on an involuntary basis, and mentally abnormal offenders in prisons or other institutions, are particularly vulnerable in this respect.

Internal constraints on freedom of choice are generated in a number of ways by different kinds of psychopathology: people who are depressed or suffering from long-term schizophrenia are sometimes unduly compliant; obsessive-compulsive disorders may involve a pathological inability to make up one's mind; and patients suffering from psychotic disorders may have aberrant (and often concealed) motivations. A psychotically depressed man, for example, agreed to take part in a research project that involved having some blood taken. He appeared to understand what was being asked of him and to be fully capable of consenting to this procedure. Subsequently, however, it was discovered that his interpretation of the situation had been that he was to be executed. He welcomed this because his profound delusions of guilt led him to believe that he deserved to die and that everyone around him would be better off if he were dead.

Psychopathology may also generate problems for the information limb of the consent formula. Thus, patients with dementia may be unable to retain or recall even quite limited amounts of new information; hypomania involves marked distractability; depression slows information processing; and anxiety may block it altogether.

Furthermore, problems of this kind complicate the general problem in research ethics of how much information is required for consent to be valid. In clinical work, in the UK, a 'prudent doctor' standard (set by the 'Bolam' test: see appendix) still prevails. Even in clinical work, though, law and practice are moving towards a 'prudent patient' test (Brazier and Miola, 2000). In research, this is already the norm (reflecting the more exacting standards arising from the difference of intent between research and clinical work). Thus the Royal College of Physicians suggests that 'any benefits and hazards' must be explained to research subjects. The standard set by The Royal College of Psychiatrists' guidelines is 'important' risks — what is 'important' being a matter for a research ethics committee, which should 'apply commonsense to decide what level of risk would be likely to affect a reasonable person's decision'. This is helpful advice, but only if the committees in question are aware of just how diverse may be the values by which benefits and risks are judged in psychiatry; as we have several times noted in this book, this is very far from being a matter of 'commonsense'.

We can now apply these general principles to the Jonsen proposals. Taking Stage 2 first, which involves interviewing key informants, consent is clearly an issue. Among the key informants will be those suffering from severe mental illness whose capacity to consent may be in question. We return later to the general problem of research with patients unable to consent. But in this case, the general approach recommended by The Royal College of Psychiatrists' guidelines seems apposite. The research participants concerned are living in the community and hence are unlikely to be wholly without the capacity for consent to an interview. Moreover, the aim of the interview, to elicit *their* opinions on the success or otherwise of the local mental health services, is very much in their best interests. To be excluded from the research would indeed be clearly *against* their interests. On the other hand, there is still an issue of power relations (patients may feel the answers they give could prejudice their future care); it is important that the process of consent is carefully geared to the capacities of those concerned. On these issues the LREC felt they needed further information. In particular they wanted to see the patient information sheet and consent form.

Stage 1 of the proposals, however, which Christine Ready had somewhat discounted in her original letter to the Chair of the Research Ethics Committee, in fact appeared *more* problematic to the Committee, involving as it did the release of confidential, and potentially sensitive, information to a third party (the Centre researcher) without consent. It can be argued that this would amount to a clear and potentially serious breach of confidentiality. The Committee asked the Chair to write to the Jonsen Centre for clarification of this part of their proposals. The Chair accordingly wrote...

John Jones
Head of Service Evaluation
The Jonsen Centre for Mental Health

Dear Mr Jones

re: Evaluation of primary mental health care; Project xx

Many thanks for sending me these proposals which were considered by the Erehwon Research Ethics Committee yesterday.

The Committee have asked me to thank you for the clear and detailed information you supplied. They recognize the importance of the project, the need to complete it as soon as possible, and the central place you give to obtaining the views of those with serious mental illnesses.

They have asked for:

1. Further information on the process by which consent will be obtained at Stage 2, including sight of the patient information sheet and consent form.

2. Your comments on the absence of consent for Stage 1. Their concern here is that releasing information to your researcher in the form described could amount to a serious breach of confidentiality.

Yours sincerely

Mr L.R. Smith

Chair, Erehwon Research Ethics Committee

John Jones replied...

Mr L.R. Smith
Chair
Erehwon Research Ethics Committee

Dear Mr Smith

I hope the following notes will provide you with enough information on how we intend to approach service users and store data.

1. Mental health needs in primary care

All primary and secondary services will be asked to identify all people who use, or should be using, mental health services. Names of individuals along with basic socio-demographic details, diagnosis, and professional's Health of the Nation Outcome Scale Rating will be collected. The use of names is essential so that 'doubles' (that is, people who use more than one service) can be identified.

Based on our work elsewhere we would estimate that there will be 5 to 10 people per 1000 population in contact with services. At the top end, there may therefore be 420 people identified, and it would not be feasible to ask each individual for consent to include them in this very limited needs assessment. As soon as all 'doubles' have been identified, all individual identifiers will be stripped from the database.

Raw data will only be available to Jonsen Centre research staff and will only be used for research purposes. The Jonsen Centre is registered under the Data Protection Act. All reports based on this data will be summary in nature and it will not be possible to identify any individual service user. All paper records will be kept in a locked cupboard and only the local researcher will have access. These records will then be transferred to the Jonsen Centre's locked store. Once the needs assessment reports have been accepted all original paper records will be shredded.

2. Role of primary health care and the CMHT mental health nurse

A small number of service users will be approached to participate in a more qualitative semi-structured interview. Consent will be obtained in advance on all occasions. Confidentiality will be assured and no individual will be identified in any report.

Patients will be approached initially through their General Practitioner who will send them the attached information sheet and consent form. If they return the form, an appointment will be made for them with the Jonsen Centre researcher, Rebecca Smith, to be seen at Erehwon Health. The latter have agreed to provide a room for the interviews in which participants can talk freely without fear of being overheard. Rebecca Smith is a former psychiatric social worker and has considerable experience working with people with severe mental illness. The study has been costed to allow her sufficient time to explain the aims of the study to participants and to answer any questions they may have. If they are still happy to proceed she will then continue with the interview.

Our intentions with this study are to provide a feasible way of making the best use of information that is already collected. The only additional data for Stage 1 is the HoNOS, which is set to become part of the Department of Health's minimum data set requirement for all providers. Where users are to be interviewed, in Stage 2, prior consent will be obtained.

Please do get back to me if you require further details.
With best wishes.

Yours sincerely,

John Jones
Head of Service Evaluation
Ref: JJ/JO
Encl: Patient information sheet and consent form

The Jonsen Centre for Mental Health

Evaluation of Mental Health Services' response to needs identified in Primary Care

PATIENT INFORMATION SHEET AND CONSENT FORM

The Jonsen Centre for Mental Health is an independent charity which specializes in developing services and carrying out research into issues around mental health. The Jonsen Centre has been commissioned by Erehwon Health Authority to carry out this piece of research, which focuses on the role of community psychiatric nurses (CPNs) who work in primary health care teams (GP practices) and in the community mental health team.

One way of finding out about the different work and role of CPNs working in primary health care teams and in the community mental health team is to gain the views of people who use these/their services. Your opinions are therefore extremely important in helping to find out how CPNs work in different settings.

The interviews, which will last on average forty minutes, will be conducted by Rebecca Smith, a researcher from the Jonsen Centre, who is based at Coventry Health Authority. The information that you give will only be available to the researcher and a statistician at the Jonsen Centre (who will help in analysing the information) and **nobody** providing your care, including your GP or any health professional, will have access to your answers. You can withdraw from the study at any time and this will not affect the services that you receive. All the information is confidential and will be kept securely. Serial numbers will be allocated to ensure anonymity and confidentiality will be respected at all times. In order to participate in the study please complete the consent form below and return it to your GP.

I agree to participate in the study being conducted by the Jonsen Centre and agree to be interviewed by Rebecca Smith.

Name   ....

Signed   ....

Date   ....

L.R. Smith reviewed all this new information under 'Chair's action'. He felt that the consent procedures proposed for Stage 2 would be acceptable to the Committee. The form made clear in particular:

1 who was doing the research;

2 who had commissioned it;

3 its aims and why the views of participants were important;

4 the name of the researcher;

5 that confidentiality would be ensured (in particular in respect of those on whom the patient depended for services); and

6 that subjects could refuse to take part or withdraw at any time without prejudicing the services they receive.

All the relevant points had therefore been covered. Moreover, the *process* by which consent was to be obtained seemed fine. First, patients would be approached initially through their own GPs. Second, the information sheet was clearly written: some of the language used seemed a little technical (for example, 'serial numbers will be allocated to ensure anonymity'), but the main messages seemed clear. Third, if patients agreed to take part, they would have an opportunity to talk through the project with the researcher, Rebecca Smith, who was experienced in working with people with severe mental illness. Finally, the circumstances in which the interviews would take place (as described in John Jones' letter) were acceptable. Methodologically, there would be some advantage in interviewing patients in the familiar environment of their own homes. But a confidential room at the offices of Erehwon Health should allow patients to talk freely about any problems they had encountered with the services they were receiving.

In relation to Stage 1, however, the further information supplied by John Jones' reinforced his (L.R. Smith's) concerns. It seemed that there really would be a substantial breach of confidentiality, not only for those receiving mental health services but also for those who, in the GP's opinion, 'should be using' them. The problem was clearly recognized by the Jonsen Centre, but, if the research was to go ahead, they considered it essential that information from the GPs should be personally identified in order to avoid double counting. It was not feasible to obtain consent because of the large numbers potentially involved.

Summary assessment

L.R. Smith's conclusions can now be summarized under the four principles of research ethics appraisal (see also Table 10.1).

Table 10.1 Summary assessment of the Jonsen Centre proposals.

Principles of assessment	Features of the proposal	
	Positive	Negative
1 Knowledge	- outcomes directly relevant to patient care - methodologically sound	
2 Necessity	- research subjects appropriate	
3 Benefit	- negligible risk - recruitment to the study is positive - interview non-intrusive - views of those with serious mental illness emphasized	
4 Consent		
Voluntariness	- recruitment is not pressured - location of research appropriate	- Stage 1 involves breach of confidentiality without consent
	- subjects able to withdraw - no prejudice to treatment	
Information	- clearly presented - fully described - two-stage presentation - time for questions	
Capacity	- despite serious mental illness, subjects likely to be competent to consent to these procedures	
5 Other issues		
Remuneration of researchers	- researchers' 'interest' transparent; clear statement of policy on independence	
Compensation	N/A	
Insurance	N/A	

This table sets out in summary form some of the key issues to consider in writing or review-ing a research ethics application. Tables of this kind can never cover all contingencies and each case has to be considered on its merits. However, one advantage of a clear explicit framework is that it highlights the gaps and contradictions that are often crucial in research ethics. Also, the format of positive and negative entries for each item helps to provide a bal-anced assessment. Ethical appraisal should have the aim of facilitating good research rather than merely blocking bad research (see also text).

The Jonsen Centre proposals amounted to an important study which was methodologically sound and likely to produce information directly relevant to patient care (first principle: *knowledge*). It was necessary to work with the groups proposed, in Stage 1 to identify actual and potential needs, and in Stage 2 to ensure that the views of those with serious mental illness were fully represented (second principle: *necessity*). There were few if any risks to weigh against the benefits of the study (third principle: *benefit*). Consent procedures for the interview stage of the study had been carefully thought through. However, this left a problem with the initial data-gathering stage, for which the researchers considered it impractical to obtain consent, but which would involve potentially serious breaches of confidentiality (fourth principle: *consent*).

Stage 3 — action plan

L.R. Smith was now clear that his committee could not approve the Jonsen Centre proposals — important as the research was — in their present form. He could write to John Jones at the Jonsen Centre to this effect, leaving it to him and the commissioning authority, Erehwon Health, either to come up with a revised protocol or to drop their evaluation altogether. Instead, he decided to build on the positive working relationship that had been established to suggest that John Jones might liaise with a member of the Research Ethics Committee who had specialized in mental health research, to see if they could come up with a mutually acceptable plan. This could then be put to the full committee.

In the event, the solution was straightforward, though not without resource implications — an additional step could be introduced into the data-gathering process in Stage 1, whereby the breach of confidentiality could be avoided. The lists of names produced by the GPs would be scrutinized initially by someone from Erehwon Health who was entitled to see them. This 'scrutineer' would be responsible for identifying any 'doubles' and subjects would be labelled only with serial numbers. The Jonsen Centre researcher would then correlate the serial numbers with the information provided about each subject.

Erehwon Health agreed to make the additional resources available and the committee approved the proposal on this basis at its next meeting.

Stage 4 — follow up

Although the revised protocol worked up to a point, a number of difficulties were encountered. First, Erehwon Health found it difficult to provide a scrutineer who could work consistently with the researchers. Hence, there were a number of discontinuities and the Jonsen Centre were not fully satisfied that all doubles had been identified. Second, there was evidence that some 'doubles' were using different names. A single researcher with access to all the relevant information might have been able to identify these. Overall, the Jonsen Centre's conclusion was that the 'blind' method did not work.

On the other hand, there was evidence, particularly from the interviews in the second stage of the research, that a growing number of those with long-term mental health problems were seeking help through advisory groups, such as MIND, or through alternative or complementary services (including local churches and other faiths, counsellors, and psychotherapists). This appeared to be in part because of a growing concern among users about confidentiality. To this extent then, the LREC's original concerns, notwithstanding the method-ological difficulties, were justified.

Most researchers strongly support the principle of ensuring that all research, evaluation, and audit should be considered by local research ethics committees. However, there is a difficult tension to manage. Individual service users' imme-diate interests may be best served by not releasing named information to an organization working on behalf of the health authority. But on the other hand, the health authority has a duty to act in the interest of society and the long-term interests of service users. For the health authority to carry out these oblig-ations they must assess need and evaluate the care provided to meet these needs. To do this effectively, health authorities will require named data. They may of course have the resources to evaluate their own services, but this is not always satisfactory (self-assessment being peculiarly prone to bias).

Social Services already have a duty to find 'best value' by using external agen-cies. Health services may well have to follow suit, particularly if, as is proposed in some parts of the UK, health and Social Services come together into single-provider agencies. Faced with the additional difficulties that this will generate, it will be even more essential that commissioners of research, LRECs, and researchers work together in a positive, problem-solving approach.

The role of the local research ethics committee

Vogue magazine once described a camel somewhat dismissively as a horse designed by a committee. Well, a camel may not be the most elegant of ani-mals, but it is remarkably well adapted to the demands of its environment! Local research ethics committees have a similar functional utility. Properly constituted, they represent a range of perspectives which offer a balanced assessment of the merits and demerits of research involving human subjects[3]. The importance of this, as we noted earlier, goes back to the key difference in intent between research and ordinary clinical work. It is because research is carried out with the intention of advancing knowledge, rather than of serving the best interests of the research subjects, that external scrutiny, independent of the interests of the researchers and those commissioning the research, is essential.

The importance of this principle of independent scrutiny has been illustrated by our case study in this chapter. Christine Ready (who commissioned the research on behalf of Erehwon Health), the local health trust (who were footing the bill), and the Jonsen Centre researchers were all motivated by the urgent need to audit the cost effectiveness of what were perceived as competing models of service provision. Driven by this 'value', either they were, as in Christine Ready's case, unaware of the breach of confidentiality involved in the first stage of the study or, like the researchers, they felt this was unimportant set against the advance in knowledge and hence improved services the study promised. Yet once the study was reviewed by an independent research ethics committee, the importance of confidentiality appeared in a quite different light. Not only that, but through a positive working relationship, the committee were able to facilitate an improved design which avoided the breach of confidentiality. And confidentiality itself eventually emerged as a key consideration for many service users.

The key role of the local research ethics committee in providing a balance of perspectives is also well illustrated by the problems raised by research with people unable to consent. As we noted in earlier chapters, these problems are important in clinical work — acutely so in England and Wales (where there is no legal provision for proxy consent). The thrust of recent case law has been that procedures carried out without the explicit consent of adults who lack the capacity for consent, should either be covered by Statute (as in the Mental Health Act 1983) or be in the best interests of the person concerned (In Re F, 1990; R v Bournewood, 1998). However, the Mental Health Act does not cover research; as we have seen, research differs from clinical work precisely in that it is pursued not in the best interests of the research subjects but with the intention of advancing knowledge. The 'catch-22', moreover, is that in mental health, those without the capacity for consent are those with the most serious disorders and hence those for whom research is most urgently needed.

Various proposals are currently under review for resolving this situation. These proposals, though, all turn on a series of value judgements which will throw the onus of decision back on to research ethics committees. Thus, the MRC guidelines (1998), after reminding us of the urgent need for medical research and our positive ethical obligation to base medical interventions as far as possible on sound evidence, argue that research with patients unable to consent should only be carried out provided a series of safeguards are observed. These include:

1   that the research is into the condition from which the patients concerned are suffering

2   that it is necessary to work with that group rather than with subjects who are able to consent

3   that the study has been approved by a local research ethics committee

4   that the committee has taken independent advice

5 that in the case of therapeutic research, the benefits significantly outweigh the risks

6 that in the case of non-therapeutic research, the risks involved are 'minimal' and that the research is 'not against' the interests of those involved.

These last two safeguards, therefore, involve value judgements — minimal risk; significant benefit; not to mention the ingenious 'not against the interests' of those concerned!

The Law Commission (1995), in advocating a specialized national research ethics committee to cover research with patients unable to consent, would require that committee to make similar value judgements. As in other sections of this book, therefore, issues which at first sight might appear purely 'technical' matters of fact, resolve on closer inspection into hybrid issues involving values as well as facts. The fear, when matters of value are raised, is moral relativism (anything goes). But, as we have repeatedly seen in our earlier cases, the real danger is failing to recognize matters of value for what they are: see, for example, Case 4.3 (Simon Greer); also the abuses of psychiatry in the former USSR (Fulford *et al.* 1993).

Once matters of value are faced squarely, then, as we have further seen, they are at least accessible to ethical reasoning; and where genuine differences of values turn out to be important, a balance of evaluative perspectives can help to avoid the abusive consequences of one value system overriding others. In the clinical context, a balance of perspectives is provided by the different members of a multidisciplinary team (see Chapter 8); in research, it comes from a properly constituted and well-functioning research ethics committee.

Conclusions

In this chapter we have set out a problem-solving approach to research ethics. With hindsight, we can see that this has involved the same four stages as the clinical problem-solving approach outlined in Chapter 9, though with a particular 'spin' arising from the special nature of research.

Thus, *Stage 1,* which involved asking whether the Jonsen Centre proposals amounted to research, corresponds with the stage of *clarifying the problem.* We suggested that the key question here is one of intention — research differs from clinical work in having the intention to advance knowledge rather than to advance the best interests of one's patients. In our case history we saw that this distinction subsumes audit to research for purposes of ethical review.

At *Stage 2,* when we employed four principles geared to the special nature of research (knowledge, necessity, benefit, and consent), we were *deepening our understanding.* In our case history, consent (as the basis for breaching confidentiality) emerged as a key problem. We spent some time on consent because of the special difficulty it raises for research ethics. Since research is carried out with the intention of advancing knowledge, the usual justification for non-consensual treatment (that one is acting in the best interests of the person concerned) does not apply. This led to the central paradox of psychiatric research ethics — that those for whom research is most urgently needed are also those least likely to be competent to consent.

In our case history, though, coming to *Stage 3, problem solving*, we were able to resolve this problem through a small change to the research design. And at *Stage 4, follow up*, we found that although the proposed solution had not been fully implemented, the original issue (confidentiality) had emerged as a major concern for service users.

The key step in our case history — resolving the ethical issue by a change in the research design — reflects the inseparability of ethical and technical aspects of good practice in research. We have focused here mainly on ethical aspects of research methodology, but the title of this chapter, 'The 3 Rs of research ethics' (or the 'reading, writing, and arithmetic' of research ethics), is intended as a reminder of that inseparability.

We have looked, in particular, at research ethics committees and the way in which by providing a balance of evaluative perspectives, they play a vital role in research. This role, moreover, is critical in psychiatry in that the subject is characterized by *diversity* of values. But the operative word here is 'balance'. Some ethicists, and indeed some members of research ethics committees, see their role as that of a moral guardian, protecting vulnerable patients from unscrupulous researchers. There is a clear need for open review in research, as in clinical work, if gross abuses are to be avoided (and Jim Birley will be drawing out this point in the final section of this book). But if research ethics committees are perceived by researchers as a barrier to research, ethical review will be at best adversarial, at worst circumvented. If, on the other hand, the research ethics committee is seen as a partner in the development of good research, everyone, and not least those suffering from mental disorders, will benefit. As the Jonsen Centre case study shows, good communication, in research no less than in clinical work, is inseparable from ethical expertise in the practical problem-solving approach.

References

The British Psychological Society (1978) E*thical Principles for research with human subjects.* London: The British Psychological Society.

Fulford, K.W.M. and Howse, K. (1993) Ethics of research with psychiatric patients: principles, problems and the primary responsibilities of researchers. *Journal of Medical Ethics*, **19**:85–91.

Fulford, K.W.M., Smirnoff, A.Y.U., and Snow, E. (1993) Concepts of disease and the abuse of psychiatry in the USSR. *British Journal of Psychiatry*, **162**:801–10.

Holmes, J. and Lindley, R. (1989). *The Values of Psychotherapy*. Oxford, Oxford University Press.

Law Commission (1995) *Mental Incapacity*. Law Com. No. 231. London, HMSO.

Medical Research Council (1998) *Guidelines for Good Clinical Practice in Clinical Trials*. London, Medical Research Council.

Royal College of Physicians (1996) *Guidelines on the Practice of Ethics Committees in Medical Research Involving Human Subjects* 3rd ed. London, Royal College of Physicians.

The Royal College of Psychiatrists (1990) Guidelines for research ethics committees on psychiatric research involving human subjects. *Psychiatric Bulletin*, **14**:48–61.

The Royal College of Psychiatrists (forthcoming) *Guidelines for researchers and for ethics committees on psychiatric research involving human participants*. London: The Royal College of Psychiatrists.

Snowdon, C., Garcia, J., and Elbourne, D. (1997) Making sense of randomization; responses of parents of critically ill babies to random allocation of treatment in a clinical trial. *Social Science and Medicine*, **45/9**:1337–55.

Wing, J. (1999) Ethics and Psychiatric Research. Ch 22 in Bloch, S., Chodoff, P. and Green, S.A. (eds). *Psychiatric Ethics* (third edition). Oxford: Oxford University Press.

World Psychiatric Association, Geneva (1996) Declaration of Madrid. (Reproduced with a brief commentary in 1999 in *Psychiatric Ethics* (3rd edn) (Bloch, S., Chodoff P., and Green S.A.), Appendix — Codes of Ethics, pp. 511–31. Oxford, Oxford University Press.)

Reading Guide

Research ethics

There is a voluminous literature on the ethics of research generally. A particularly clear and practical introduction is provided by a series of publications from the Royal College of Physicians, in particular *Guidelines on the Practice of Ethics Committees in Medical Research Involving Human Subjects* (1996) and *Research Involving Patients* (1990). Chapter 8 of the BMA's *Medical Ethics Today: Its Practice and Philosophy* (1993) also gives a comprehensive and authoritative review of the issues. *A Decent Proposal: Ethical Review of Clinical Research* by Donald Evans and Martyn Evans (1996) provides a detailed and authoritative introduction to the ethical, legal, and related methodological aspects of clinical research. Parker and Dickenson's *Cambridge Medical Ethics Workbook* (2000) includes a chapter on research ethics which uses a version of the case presented in this book, together with material from a wider European context, including the Helsinki Declaration and the Council of Europe Convention.

A useful introduction to the problems raised specifically by research with psychiatric patients is John Wing's chapter (Chapter 22) in *Psychiatric Ethics* (Bloch *et al.* 1999). The Royal College of Psychiatrists (1990) have produced a clear and most helpful set of guidelines which complement those provided by the Royal College of Physicians. Some of the problems left unresolved by these guidelines are discussed in Fulford and Howse (1993). A new set of guidelines is in preparation by the Royal College of Psychiatrists; other relevant guidelines are listed below.

Kendell (1986) was one of the first to signal the problems raised by the lack of a proper legal framework in the UK for research involving patients whose capacity to consent is impaired. The issue of capacity has recently been comprehensively reviewed by the Law Commission (1995). Their discussion includes a detailed analysis of the potential conflict between the objectives of research (to advance knowledge) and the 'best interests' principle. The Commission has proposed that a special research ethics committee — the Mental Incapacity Research Committee — be established to deal with such cases. The BMA and the Law Society have jointly published a guide to assessing capacity (1995).

It is important to recognize that the process of being involved in research may in itself have positive therapeutic effects: see, for example, Caroll *et al.* (1980) and Ben-Arie *et al.* (1990). Conversely, we should be aware of adverse effects of apparently neutral aspects of research design such as randomization (Snowdon *et al.* 1997).

Reading Guide: references

Ben-Arie, O., Koch, A., Welman, M., and Teggin, A.F. (1990) The effect of research on readmission to a psychiatric hospital. *The British Journal of Psychiatry,* **156**:37–9.

Bloch, S., Chodoff, P., and Green S.A. (1999) *Psychiatric Ethics* (3rd edn; 1st edn 1981). Oxford, Oxford University Press.

BMA (1993) *Medical Ethics Today: Its Practice and Philosophy.* London, BMA.

BMA and The Law Society (1995) *Assessment of Mental Capacity: Guidance for Doctors and Lawyers.* London, BMA.

Carroll, R.S., Miller, A., Ross, B., and Simpson, G.M. (1980) Research as an impetus to improved treatment. *Archives of General Psychiatry,* **37**:377–80.

Evans, D. and Evans, M. (1996) *A Decent Proposal: Ethical Review of Clinical Research.* Chichester (England), John Wiley.

Fulford, K.W.M. and Howse, K. (1993) Ethics of research with psychiatric patients: principles, problems and the primary responsibilities of researchers. *Journal of Medical Ethics,* **19**:85 – 91.

Kendell, R. E. (1986) The Mental Health Act Commission's 'guidelines': a further threat to psychiatric research. *BMJ,* **292**:1249–50.

Law Commission (1995) *Mental Incapacity.* Law Com. No. 231. London, HMSO.

Parker, M. and Dickenson, D. (2000) *The Cambridge Medical Ethics Workbook.* Cambridge, Cambridge University Press.

Snowdon, C., Garcia, J., and Elbourne, D. (1997) Making sense of randomization; responses of parents of critically ill babies to random allocation of treatment in a clinical trial. *Social Science and Medicine,* **45/9**:1337–55.

Wider perspectives

CHAPTER 11

Psychiatric ethics: an international open society

Jim Birley

The basic education of doctors now lays less emphasis on stuffing them with facts (which may rapidly become irrelevant) and much more on teaching them attitudes about themselves, their patients and families, and their colleagues — which they will require to function as 'good doctors' throughout their professional lives. Much of this teaching will come, for better or worse, not from formal occasions but from attitudes displayed or implied by their teachers. Attitudes are, of course, related to skills. A person's attitude to a swimming pool, particularly to its deep end, will be affected by his or her ability to swim. This book is an introduction to the deeper end of ethics, beyond the shallows of autonomy and beneficence, which encourages the reader to develop the skills required to enjoy the experience and to communicate this enjoyment to others.

Even such a personal and private activity as psychiatry is surrounded by a cloud of witnesses — the patient, his or her family, students and staff — and this is becoming more obvious in many of its branches where the work is shared by members of a team. It is becoming increasingly important for psychiatrists to be able to understand and to articulate the ethical framework — its principles and dilemmas — in which they and their patients find themselves.

The authors describe and discuss a series of 'cases', following a sort of 'sonata form'. There is a statement of the main themes; then a development section in which these are discussed in various ethical keys; followed by a return to the original theme (which may have become inverted); and then a coda which distils the main ingredients in a deceptively simple manner and provides some sensible practical guidance and useful references for further reading.

All the cases seem to be very 'real' and describe situations which will be familiar to many psychiatrists. They are an amalgam of real patients and hence do not represent particular individuals. They have the 'extra' reality of being apparently irresolvable — for example, Case 8.2, in which Sam's father seems to be an immovable object in blocking plans for his son's care; or Case 3.2, where Tom Benbow will probably continue to be a nuisance to his neighbours.

Also realistic is the clinical approach by the psychiatric teams. Here, the standard of practice portrayed is very good, although every reader will want to add his or her own gloss. For instance, if the resistance of Sam's father was seen more as heroic than neurotic, he might be more approachable; and there seems to be something rather fishy about Martin's (Case 4.1) 'total isolation'. He drinks and smokes a lot and is not dying of starvation; either he goes out for his supplies or he has a network of suppliers, as housebound people often have, who may be important and unrecognized 'significant others'.

The book provides a rich diet of sophisticated food for ethical thought — and it creates an appetite for more. Indeed there are, inevitably, some issues which have not been considered which I am sure the authors could illuminate. Their focus has been on 'clinical management', but there are also issues covering the management of the 'ethical environment' which doctors, and those for whom they are caring, inhabit.

My views in these matters have been tempered by working in an organization — the Geneva Initiative on Psychiatry — which is helping to improve the ethical and professional standards of psychiatric care in the former Soviet Union. In these countries, under communist rule, particularly in Russia and its republics, medicine had been deliberately downgraded, with its staff employed and controlled by the State through its agents, the local soviet. No independent professional body existed, and no ethical standards were laid down by any licensing authority. There were 'regulations' but, like most regulations, they were generally disregarded. Since 1991, a new Russian Psychiatric Society has been established which has formulated an excellent and detailed ethical code of professional conduct for its members. Like our own Royal Colleges, though, it has no real disciplinary powers, and the rest of the system has not changed while the funding of the health service has deteriorated. The concerns of those in the system are 'existence', rather than 'ethics': enough food, warmth, and sanitation. Yet it is significant that in precisely these adverse circumstances, ethical discussions have been important in changing the attitudes of many psychiatrists: patients, relatives, and staff are treated with more respect, and listened to. Independent psychiatric associations have been set up in other former Soviet countries, and they are gaining power over their education and clinical activity; psychiatric nurses are being trained for the first time; and new mental health legislation has been introduced. It is no accident that the opening lecture at our first (1993) meeting of 'reformers' (which initiated this movement and gave it a flying start) was given by one of the authors of this book, Bill Fulford.

The work of our colleagues in post-Soviet countries has many lessons for us in 'Western' psychiatry. I will briefly discuss four topics — the importance of the physical environment; the need for an 'open society' in health care; supervision registers; and confidentiality.

The quality of the physical environment

For many people, what matters in a hospital is the quality of the general care, cleanliness, food, privacy, access to telephones, and so on. These affect the 'acceptability' of the services. At present, many acute psychiatric wards are over-crowded and frightening places in a poor state of repair. They give a degrading message to both staff and patients. Indeed some patients may have to be admitted compulsorily not because they 'lack insight into their condition' or do not recognize their need to be treated, but because they have only too accurate an insight into the condition of the ward. This creates an unethical situation.

There is not much discussion in this book of this aspect of the ethical issues surrounding compulsory admission. Chapter 2 sets the theoretical issues out clearly and emphasizes the importance of the values of users and carers. Several of the case histories describe the people involved as having been treated on an involuntary basis in the past. But the discussions neglect the importance of the physical environment.

Doctors are perhaps particularly prone to neglecting this aspect of treatment as they spend less time on the wards than do the nurses and the patients, and the public understandably assumes that hospitals provide basic standards of privacy, comfort, and shelter. The present government's 'new money' for psychiatric services has been 'sold' to the public — perhaps on advice from its 'spin doctors' — as meeting the need for it to be protected against supposedly dangerous people, rather than for providing reasonably acceptable services.

Focusing on ethical codes and reasoning applied to a clinical case, while neglecting its physical environment, produces a kind of ethical tunnel vision which would be cured by a very brief visit to an impoverished ward in the former Soviet Union.

Skilled and unskilled care

The 'hotel' aspects of a ward comprise only a small part of the overall picture. Much more important are the attitudes, skills, and numbers of the staff. Are there enough of them, and are they professionally competent? The 'right to treatment' has been superseded by the 'right to high-quality treatment'. Staff now have a professional and ethical duty to keep up to date and review their activities regularly, maintaining their cutting edge on the grinding of the audit cycle. Much of this can best be done as a group activity for all staff, patients, and relatives. But some matters require specific professional and technical attention.

There may come a point when the competence of one or more staff members, at any level, has to be questioned seriously, and acted upon. The recent

Bristol heart surgery tragedy in the UK repeated the history of many of the psychiatric hospital 'scandals' of the 1960s and 1970s (Martin 1984): the 'whistle blowers', often comparative newcomers or junior staff members, were resisted and harassed, and a response came much too late. The bad situation had been recognized but not acted upon, for far too long.

This situation was writ large in the totalitarian regime of the former Soviet Union. But there is also a more subtle parallel with our situation in Western psychiatry in the continuing relative lack of accountability of health service managers. The General Medical Council (GMC), in addition to setting vocational and ethical guidelines, has recently prepared a system for assessing 'competence'. It has powers both to discipline doctors and to remove their license to practice. Corresponding powers for nurses are invested in the United Kingdom Central Council for Nursing, Health Visiting and Midwifery (UKCC). Managers in the NHS, by contrast, have no comparable professional, ethical, or disciplinary body, although the Institute of Health Services Management has provided some general but unenforceable guidelines of good practice. They are thus, technically, in a 'Soviet situation' — controlled by the state through the NHS Executive and with no professional association to train, control, or protect them. The Chief Executive at Bristol was disciplined, and lost his license to practice, but only because he was also a doctor.

All who have considered these matters agree that an overall controlling structure with disciplinary powers is necessary, and that the neglect of the ethical imperative to report and act upon poor care should be punished. However, in practice the most important ingredient, often missing, is an 'open society' at local level where matters can be discussed freely and there are recognized secure channels for reporting concerns. An 'ethically aware' staff will, I believe, make an essential contribution to creating an open society in health care.

Supervision of potentially dangerous patients

This is a topical issue, much in the public mind, as extreme cases such as homicides of strangers by mentally ill persons are given wide news coverage — in spite or because of their rarity (four per year at present: Thornicroft and Goldberg 1998).

Case 7.2 (Philip Caversham) provides an interesting discussion of this problem and the concept of 'moral luck'. How much responsibility can clinicians take for behaviour which they cannot control? The ethical solution proposed is that the responsibility should be shared: the degree of supervision should be negotiated, the patient's agreement should be obtained, and he or she should be fully informed of the 'rules of the game' and the consequences of breaking them. Such procedures are not required at present; a patient can be put on the 'Supervision Register' without obtaining consent.

While ethically commendable and ingenious, such a negotiated agreement would require the consent of the psychiatrist as well. This might not be given. Some genuinely dangerous patients, with a history of violence, are impulsive people with a 'short fuse'. They have not learnt from previous experiences and take an unrealistic view of their own capacity to control themselves. Equally unrealistic may be the views of the clinician who believes he/she can control this type of patient. The 'consent' of the patient may not be 'informed', and the 'competence' of the psychiatrist, with an overstretched clinical team, could be called into question.

The Supervision Register is strongly reminiscent of the infamous 'Register' in the old Soviet Union against which so many of us campaigned. Under its 'rules of the game', the blame for any accident was laid squarely on the shoulders of the psychiatrist, who was punished by fines, demotion, or dismissal according to the severity of the patient's misbehaviour. Had there not been a failure of control in a system specifically designed to control people?

Now a Soviet system is being advocated by our own 'democratic' government. 'Care workers', we read (in *The Observer*, 28 June 1998), 'who allow dangerous mental patients to roam the streets unsupervised will be sacked under plans to shake up the much-criticized "Care in the Community program" .' Also in the same article, we learn that 'Ministers of Health…are planning to rewrite the Mental Health Act to allow professionals to compel patients to continue treatment after they have been released into the community: and they are warning staff that they will be called to account if there are more tragedies such as random killings by the mentally disturbed'. 'It isn't a matter of more training', says a Minister, 'it's a matter of doing the job they are already trained to do'. The Soviet experience gives us a stark warning, if warning were needed, that this is the 'royal road' to demoralized staff, punitive regimes, and, ultimately, a degraded system of health care.

Confidentiality

Related to supervision is another matter which is not much discussed in this excellent book — with whom should we share our information? In the Soviet Union the police had a right of access to the records of all patients on the Register whether dangerous or not. In the UK, patients can now ask to read their notes, which are often presented in 'continuous multidisciplinary' format rather than as a series of separate records from the separate professionals involved in the case. This may make them more useful for immediate consultation, but where should information given in confidence, by relatives for instance, be recorded? Decisions about this raise ethical and practical issues in terms of informed decision making, particularly in the context of 'risk assessment'.

The importance of confidentiality can be overstated if it is used as a means of preventing open criticism of a public service. This is becoming a serious issue in the commercialized NHS, where 'commercial confidentiality', if breached, can in theory lead to punitive damages. The guidance given by the NHS Executive in 1993 on relations with the public and the media discourages 'whistle-blowing', particularly to the Secretary of State or to the media — two pathways which in the past have revealed fearful situations and led to considerable reforms (Birley 1996). Some trusts have equated patient confidentiality with commercial confidentiality. Such actions are not likely to encourage the 'open society' which all are agreed is needed in the NHS.

Conclusions: ethics, clinical governance, and an open society

A regular topic in ethical discourse is whether ethics are 'absolute' or culturally determined. These debates acquire an immediate practical relevance when health workers from one country arrive to 'help' or 'interfere with' the health system of another. There are many international declarations on people's rights to health, and on the duties and behaviour of health professionals, but in certain circumstances they may fade away like morning dew under a scorching sun.

That medicine, and psychiatry in particular, can be corrupted is all too clear from Nazi Germany and the former Soviet Union — although the corruption was quite different in nature and in scale. In the former Soviet Union, the abuse of diagnosis in order to detain dissidents in mental hospitals was practised and defended by only a few powerful leaders of the profession — Academicians with strong connections with the KGB. The rest of psychiatry was not corrupted in this way, but by the corruption acting on the whole of society in the form of control of individual thought and power and the degradation of all the professions. In this system, for over sixty years, most psychiatrists did their best to provide decent care, with very little scientific leadership or originality, in impoverished surroundings. The beginning of the break-up of this totalitarian state was enshrined in the words 'openness' and 'reconstruction'.

As in the former Soviet Union, the NHS is a government-controlled and funded organization. Its control is not 'totalitarian', however, as those working in it have allegiances and support from other organizations representing the staff, the patients, and the public. Attempts at 'reconstruction' of the NHS are regular, expensive, and often ill thought-out events; attempts at 'openness' are fewer, and often made only under protest from the public and those representing patients and carers. But reconstruction without openness is unlikely to work. It often smacks of the five-year plans so familiar to the Soviet public. All large organizations — governmental, commercial, or professional — are inclined to resist openness. But the need for more openness is becoming increasingly clear.

It is connected with the claims for evidence-based medicine. This usually refers to evidence obtained in clinical research. Just as important, if not more so, is the evidence presented every day to those working in and receiving care from the NHS. This is also the best source of evidence of poor standards of practice — a topic which is rarely published or discussed in the journals, but which is of increasing concern to all, including the profession's leading bodies (the General Medical Council and the Royal Colleges in the UK). In contrast to the former Soviet Union, the 'top brass' of medicine are giving a lead. But the former Soviet Union has provided plenty of examples of proclamations and directives from the top which failed to have any impact at the level where it really mattered — amongst those working on the ground. The ground needs to be prepared to receive the seed.

For the NHS to become more self-critical, in a constructive way, it will thus need to become a more 'open society' — a phrase made famous by Karl Popper. He also proposed a mechanism for attaining this state — 'piecemeal social engineering'. This, I think, will be the right method for the NHS, which can build on piecemeal and local initiatives, many of which, I suspect, are happening already. The processes involved in encouraging good practice and detecting and reporting bad practice are just as much ethical as they are social and technical. Students and staff need to be taught to think about and discuss ethical issues and dilemmas in medicine, and the experience should be an enjoyable and stimulating one.

This is why this book is so valuable. It will be clear from my comments that it whets the ethical appetite, and I hope that more volumes will follow, with examples from all types of health care — for the issues with which *In Two Minds* is concerned are not confined to psychiatric practice. The consideration of ethics, informed by philosophy, takes us away from slogans to the very heart of medicine.

References

Birley, J.L.T. (1996) Whistleblowing. *Advances in Psychiatric Treatment*, 2:48–54.

Martin, J.P. (1984) *Hospitals in Trouble*. Oxford. Blackwell.

Smith, A. (1998) 'Sacking threat for lax Community Care' *London Observer*, 28 June 1998.

Thornicroft, G. and Goldberg, O.P. (1998) *Has Community Care Failed?* Maudsley Discussion Paper No. 5. Institute of Psychiatry, London.

CHAPTER 12

Conclusions: psychiatry first

But man He made to serve Him wittily in the tangle of his mind! (Sir Thomas More, in Robert Bolt's play 'A Man for All Seasons')

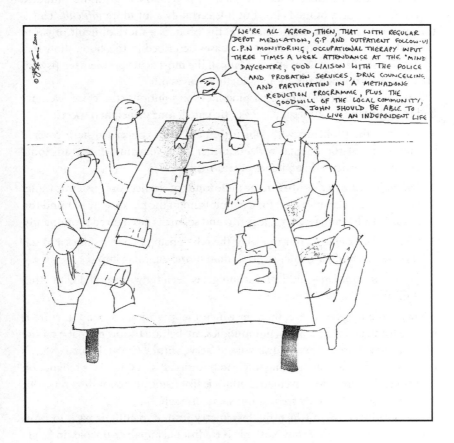

We opened this book with the paradox that psychiatry, although the most deeply value-laden area of medicine, has been relatively neglected by bioethics in favour of more high-tech medical specialties. The reason for this neglect, we argued, has been the stigmatization of psychiatry, by bioethics no less than by biomedicine, as a second-class medical citizen. Psychiatry, according to this 'psychiatry second' picture, is the muddled end of medicine. Hence the problems (ethical and scientific) to which it is subject will be resolved, in due time, by methods and ideas derived from what are taken to be the unmuddled disciplines of physical medicine.

The conclusion we can now draw, as we come to the end of the book, is that the 'psychiatry second' picture is back to front. It is so in two senses — one negative, one positive. The negative sense is that psychiatry, although able to draw on traditional bioethics up to a point, cannot rely on it wholly. This is because, contrary to the 'psychiatry second' picture, psychiatry is no more muddled than any other area of medicine, but it is certainly a lot more *difficult*. This is transparently so in the case of science: the brain is a more difficult organ to study than the liver or the kidney. The cases described in this book show that something similar is true of ethics. Many of the most acute problems in psychiatric ethics start where traditional bioethics leaves off.

Far from looking to traditional bioethics for solutions, therefore, we have had to go beyond bioethics in, as we anticipated, four principal respects:

1 *Scope* — the problems with which we have been concerned have covered each stage of the clinical process rather than focusing, like traditional bioethics, particularly on issues of treatment choice

2 *Philosophical depth* — work in the philosophy of science (on epistemic values in psychiatric classification, for example) and in the philosophy of mind (on rationality, meaning, agency, identity, and so forth) has figured prominently

3 *Closeness to science* — our model of the relationship between ethics and science has been of partnership rather than moral guardianship

4 *Clinical integration* — ethical reasoning has been fully integrated with other clinical practice skills.

This is the negative sense, then, in which the 'psychiatry second' picture is back to front. Genuine tangles, not muddles, are behind the problematic nature of psychiatry. Hence if psychiatrists are to 'serve wittily' (in Sir Thomas More's phrase), it is no use their looking solely to traditional bioethics. Sole reliance on traditional bioethics for psychiatric ethics is like using an abdominal retractor in brain surgery: the tools are just not sharp enough.

The positive sense in which the 'psychiatry second' picture is back to front runs this point the other way. Not only is traditional bioethics unable (in itself) to solve the problems of psychiatric ethics, but psychiatric ethics, to the contrary, has many lessons for bioethics. We will illustrate this in a moment for each of the four respects in which we have gone beyond bioethics. But the essential point, to anticipate a little, is that many of the problems we have considered, although indeed 'writ large' in psychiatry, are not confined to it. They are problems which are also present in other areas of medicine — but in a more covert form. Psychiatric ethics can thus contribute to ethics in medicine generally, first by making these covert problems visible, and then by extension from its experience in dealing with them. In going beyond bioethics, for the purposes of psychiatric ethics, we thus end up with an enriched bioethics for medicine as a whole.

Consider then, first, the scope of ethics. Autonomy of treatment choice — a particular focus of traditional bioethics — was important in the early days of the subject because, at the time, a rapidly expanding technological medicine had resulted in wide disparities between patients' values and those of professionals over questions of treatment. In psychiatry, by contrast, as we have seen, such disparities of value are not confined to treatment but endemic to its very subject matter. Desire, belief, emotion, motivation, and so on, are all, as we noted in Chapter 1, areas in which human values differ widely and legitimately. Hence, we have had to tackle differences of value, not only over issues of treatment choice (Chapter 6), but in balancing medical and moral models of mental disorder (Chapter 3), in differential diagnosis (for example, between spiritual experience and psychosis, Chapter 4), in understanding the meanings which may be aetiologically crucial in psychiatry (Chapter 5), and in weighing the utilities by which (combined with judgements of probability) prognostic assessments of risk are made (Chapter 7).

Analytic ethics — in the work of R.M. Hare, G.J. Warnock, and others — provided us (in Chapter 1) with a clear theoretical framework for understanding this feature of psychiatric ethics. We summed this up at one point in the language of science: in physical medicine, values are (largely) a *constant* (whereas) in psychiatry they are (largely) a *variable*. But of course, values are not *completely* constant even in physical medicine. In the high-tech areas with which traditional bioethics has been concerned there are some constants: a heart attack, renal failure, and so on, are *bad* conditions for *anyone* (they are bad in themselves — though as we noted in Chapter 1, bad conditions may have good consequences). But even in these high-tech areas there may be wide divergencies of values. In reproductive medicine, for example, people's values may differ radically over such procedures as foetal reduction and assisted reproduction. When we move into the area of primary care, the diversity of values is wide indeed. The general practitioner, Roger Higgs, and the philosopher, Alastair Campbell, have described, in a richly detailed case history, how different value perspectives help to structure and guide every aspect of the work of a primary care team (Campbell and Higgs 1982).

It is not only in psychiatry then, but in medicine generally, that all the practical consequences of recognizing the diversity of human values follow. It is not only in psychiatry that patients should have a say in how their problems are understood as well as in how they are treated. It is not only in psychiatry that patients' individual experiences of illness (the meanings of their experiences to them) are as important as objective knowledge of disease processes (Chapter 5). It is not only in psychiatry that utilities are as important as probabilities in judgements of risk (Chapter 7). It is not only in psychiatry that the multidisciplinary team has a key role in offering a balance of value perspectives (Chapter 8). All these practical consequences are writ large in psychiatry — but they are relevant to medicine as a whole.

The second respect in which we have gone beyond bioethics is into its philosophical underpinnings. Ideas from general philosophy, it should be said, already figure prominently in some areas of traditional bioethics. Personal identity, for example (a key issue in our Case 6.2, Ida Harbottle), has been drawn on extensively in relation to the ethical issues surrounding cloning. But there are more subtle philosophical lessons for bioethics from psychiatry, notably in the analysis of consent. Thus we argued (in Chapter 2) that the traditional bioethical account of involuntary treatment in terms of impaired capacities fails to explain the central psychiatric case of loss of autonomy, that of delusion. But one of the founders of traditional bioethics in the UK, the lawyer Ian Kennedy, has made essentially the same point in a commentary on a recent legal case involving consent to a Caesarean section (Kennedy 1997). The judgement in this case, Kennedy concluded, leaves us 'in no doubt, or not much, as to how to proceed. But', he continued, 'the conundrum at the heart of the procedure, the true meaning of capacity, remains unsolved'.

The capacities approach, as we noted in Chapter 2, works well enough for relatively simple cases like unconsciousness and severe dementia. But just as it begs the key questions for consent in the more complex case of the functional psychoses, so too, it seems, does it beg the key questions in more complex cases in physical medicine. Those who favour a capacities approach to consent point to the advantages of psychiatry shadowing physical medicine (Szmukler and Holloway 1998). They believe this could help to reduce stigma, for example. But this is a 'psychiatry second' approach. The lesson the other way, writ large in psychiatry and echoed in Ian Kennedy's commentary, is that the adoption of inappropriate criteria for consent could be highly abusive in effect not only in psychiatry but in physical medicine too.

In both these respects then — in the scope of ethics and in its philosophical underpinnings — going beyond bioethics in pursuit of psychiatric ethics has brought us back to key lessons for medicine as a whole. There are similar lessons, and for similar reasons, from the third and fourth respects in which we have gone beyond bioethics — for the relationship between ethics and science and for the practice skills model of ethical reasoning.

As to the relationship between ethics and science, the moral guardian model of the role of ethics in medicine was no doubt necessary in the early days of bioethics when a strong champion of patient autonomy was needed as a counterbalance to medical paternalism. The moral guardian approach becomes inappropriate, however, once the wider diversity of values, revealed by psychiatric ethics, is recognized to be a feature of medicine generally. For this approach then becomes a case of substituting for the old medical paternalism ('doctor knows best'), a new ethical paternalism ('ethicist knows best').

We have argued that the moral guardian model is particularly inappropriate in research (Chapter 10). The danger here is that it will lead to a culture of 'them and us' between researchers and research ethics committees. So far as medical research is concerned, we are already seeing a backlash amongst researchers against the increasingly legalistic and practically unrealistic criteria for consent to research being promulgated by many ethicists (Osborn 1999). As we noted in Chapter 10, such developments are as likely to inhibit good research as to prevent bad research. There is a need, especially in research, for independent ethical review (arising from the gap between the primary intention of research being to advance knowledge and the best interests principle). But such review should be by a well-balanced research ethics committee, representing different value perspectives (including that of the target group of patients) and operating on a model of partnership. Absent such arrangements, we may not actually kill the goose that lays the golden eggs but we will certainly put it off its lay.

Partnership means communication, of course, and this is at the heart of the practice skills approach to ethical reasoning in medicine. Interestingly, although developed initially for clinical medical students, the approach grew out of theoretical work in psychiatry (Fulford 1989, Chapter 11; Hope and Fulford 1993). Practice skills thus provide a case in point of the way in which psychiatry may lead the way for physical medicine. As we illustrated in Chapter 9 (the re-run of Case 3.1, Elizabeth Orton, as a teaching seminar), ethical reasoning and communication are woven fully together in the problem-solving objectives of good practice skills. This is especially important for the effectiveness of multidisciplinary teams in providing a balance of value perspectives (Chapter 8). Besides values, however, a well-functioning multidisciplinary team may contribute to other key aspects of shared decision making important in physical medicine as well as psychiatry: in exploiting the implicit or craft knowledge which is an essential counterbalance to the explicit knowledge of evidence-based medicine (as in risk assessment, Chapter 7); in understanding meanings (Chapter 5); and in the requirement for attention to process as well as criteria in applying the high-level concepts (such as rationality) on which ethical aspects of clinical decision making often turn (Chapter 8).

The upshot then, of the positive sense in which the 'psychiatry second' picture is back to front, is that, in all these respects the right way round is 'psychiatry first'! Far from psychiatry being dependent on ideas from physical medicine to solve its problems, psychiatry can take the lead, offering key lessons for medicine as a whole.

These lessons, it should be said, will not be universally welcomed. Medicine, after all, is a practical discipline. Replacing muddles with (Sir Thomas More's) tangles, some may say, is all very well; but medicine needs answers, and if the answers we get involve values, this would seem to be leading us down a slippery slope to the chaos of moral relativism. Loose talk, moreover, of implicit (alongside explicit) knowledge, of meanings (alongside causes), and of process (alongside criteria), is hardly conducive to a sense of security, of certainty in stable solutions. Taking our lead from psychiatry then, some may say, is to risk becoming so *en*tangled that we end up unable to 'serve' at all, wittily or otherwise.

This is a casebook; its aims are practical. We have noted several reasons why taking the diversity of human values which guide medicine seriously is not a recipe for ethical chaos: human values, although indeed diverse, are not chaotic; to recognize values is not to exclude facts; and recognizing and learning to work with both facts and values is, like the acquisition of other clinical skills, something to be done in preparation for meeting the demands of clinical work rather than in the heat of an acute clinical situation (recall Hare's distinction between level 1 and level 2 ethical reasoning, Chapter 2).

Improved clinical skills, therefore, not ethical paralysis, is the outcome of recognizing the importance of values in medicine. Mark you, the skills in question will not bring certainty. To the contrary, they are the skills required to act under conditions of uncertainty. Yet this is no bad thing. As we have many times commented, it is from absolutism, not relativism, that we have most to fear in medicine. And slippery slopes, once the legitimate diversity of human values is acknowledged, are as likely to lead to good consequences as to bad. It is, anyway, as Sir Thomas More's aphorism reminds us, in an openness to interpretive possibilities, rather than in the closed following of rules, that our essential freedom as human beings consists. This then is the final lesson of 'psychiatry first' — that being in two minds is the price we pay for our common humanity.

References

Campbell, A.V. and Higgs, R. (1982) *In That Case: Medical Ethics in Everyday Practice.* London, Darton, Longman, and Todd.

Fulford, K.W.M. (1989, reprinted 1995; 2nd edn forthcoming) *Moral Theory and Medical Practice.* Cambridge, Cambridge University Press.

Hope, R.A. and Fulford, K.W.M. (1994) Medical education: patients, principles and practice skills. In *Principles of Health Care Ethics* (ed. Gillon, R.), Chapter 59. Chichester (England), John Wiley and Sons.

Kennedy, I. (1997) Consent: adult, refusal of consent, capacity. Commentary on Re MB [1997] 2 F.L.R. 426. *Medical Law Review*, 5:317–25.

Osborn, D.P.J. (1999) Research and ethics: leaving exclusion behind. *Current Opinion in Psychiatry*, 12:601–4.

Szmukler, G. and Holloway, F. (1998) Mental health legislation is now a harmful anachronism. *Psychiatric Bulletin*, 22:662–5.

Notes

Notes to Chapter 1

1 This is not a strict or linguistic paradox as in the paradox of the liar: 'this statement is a lie' is paradoxical in the sense that if it is true it is false and if it is false it is true. The paradox of the neglect of psychiatry by bioethics is no more than a striking oddity that contradicts expectations. Such contradictions share with strict paradoxes the property of prompting deeper understanding.

2 Not all questions of value are ethical questions. Aesthetic questions, for example, although involving questions of value, are not ethical questions. Equally, empirical questions *about* people's values (in psychology and anthropology, for example) are not in themselves ethical questions. An important tradition in ethics, furthermore, denies the distinction between fact and value (see Reading Guide, Chapter 2). In this book, we assume the distinction between facts and values and use the terms 'scientific' and 'ethical' to mark their respective contributions to medicine (see von Wright, 1963, *The Varieties of Goodness*, for an exhaustive description of the huge variety of different kinds of value judgement).

3 See Fulford (1990). A more detailed theoretical account of the role of values in medicine and psychiatry is given in Fulford's *Moral Theory and Medical Practice* (1989). The link between theory and practice is set out more fully in Fulford and Bloch (forthcoming).

4 This obviously oversimplifies. Recent work in the philosophy and sociology of science shows the extent to which science itself is a deeply value-laden enterprise.

Notes to Chapter 2

1 This case history was first published as 'Mr AB' in Fulford's *Moral Theory and Medical Practice* (1989, Chapter 10). It has also been discussed from different points of view in Fulford 1991 and 1995*a*. (See reference list to this chapter for full details.)

2 We return to the ethical significance of the mismatch between delusion and cognitive criteria of incapacity in Case 5.2

3 A careful philosophical account of the value-free medical model has been developed, for example, by the American philosopher, Christopher Boorse (1975). (We consider the medical and other models in detail in Chapters 3 and 4.)

Notes to Chapter 3

1   Although, as we emphasize elsewhere, there are continuing major concerns about cultural and gender biases (see, for example, Radden (1994) for a recent review).

Notes to Chapter 4

1   Simon's case history is taken from a study of psychosis and religious experience carried out by Dr Mike Jackson in Oxford (see Jackson, 1997; Jackson and Fulford, 1997; and Jackson, 2000). It was first reported in this form in Jackson, M. and Fulford, K.W.M. (1997) 'Spiritual experience and psychopathology', *Philosophy, Psychiatry, and Psychology,* **4/1**:41–66, and is reproduced by kind permission of Mike Jackson and of the Johns Hopkins University Press. Much of the discussion of the case is based on that article and the supporting commentaries by Roland Littlewood (67–74), Francis G. Lu, David Lukoff, and Robert P. Turner (75–8), Andrew Sims (79–82), and Anthony Storr (83–6), together with a response by Jackson and Fulford (87–90). We are grateful to all these authors. The views expressed in this discussion of the case are our own.

2   References to PSE symptoms are all to the 'Present State Examination' as detailed in Wing *et al.* (1974)

Notes to Chapter 5

1   See also the Reading Guide to Chapter 1 for the introductions to modern philosophy of mind.

2   The 'game', although not substantively different, has changed in the *kind* of implication involved. 'Endogenous depression' was actually defined by the (putative) presence of an underlying causal disease process; this is what the term meant. 'Major depression' is defined rather by the presence of one or more particular *symptoms*. It is in this sense that it is a symptomatic rather than causal disease category, albeit that the presence of these symptoms strongly suggests an underlying causal disease process. The difference in implication between 'endogenous depression' and 'major depression', then, is between what in logic is usually called strict implication and ordinary implication. Strict implication is a connection of meaning (as in 'bitch' implies 'female dog'); ordinary implication is a merely contingent connection (as in 'it is raining' implies 'the ground is wet'). Needless to say, this apparently straightforward distinction, useful as it often is (see, for example, Fulford 1989, Chaper 3), is itself the subject of intense philosophical debate!

Notes to Chapter 7

1   Discussed elsewhere in this book, for example, p. 62.

Notes to Chapter 8

1   One reaction to this is to say that time can be defined something along the lines of 'that which is measured by clocks'. So far as the *definition* of time is concerned, this begs the question (since a clock is 'that which measures time'). However, the approach of focusing on the procedures by which time is measured or identified has a good pedigree. It was Einstein's approach, no less! A generalization of the approach led to the idea of operational criteria for defining physical quantities (Bridgman 1927); and this, in turn, inspired a similar approach in psychopathology (Kendell 1975): the criteria in modern classifications of mental disorders are often called 'operational'. The very power of this approach though, is that it gets around the problem of *definition* by relying directly on the shared *use* of the concept in question in a given context.

2   This is of course not to say that biology is *wholly* without conceptual problems.

Notes to Chapter 9

1   This approach is broadly in line with what has become known as problem-based learning — see Reading Guide.

Notes to Chapter 10

1   In England and Wales, community mental health care is provided mainly through National Health Service Trusts.

2   These principles were first set out in this form by Fulford and Howse (1993).

3   A concern often raised by researchers with projects in different parts of the country is the extraordinarily wide variety of opinions they receive on any one application. LRECs need to be independent so that they can reflect local needs and concerns, but a degree of standardization would help to avoid researchers becoming disenchanted with the whole system.

Appendix: glossary of legal cases

This Appendix draws together some of the more important legal cases described in the text. Even in the UK there are many other cases, besides much statute law, bearing on psychiatry, and the law is developing in different ways in different parts of the world.

Bolam v. Friern HMC (1957) 2 All ER 118

Established the standard of care required by the law of negligence in England and Wales: 'A doctor is not guilty of negligence if he has acted in accordance with a practice accepted as proper by a responsible body of medical men skilled in that particular art'. Subsequent case law established that this standard applies not only in matters of treatment, but also diagnosis (*Maynard* v. *West Midlands RHA* (1985) 1 All ER 635) and disclosure of information (see *Sidaway*: details in appendix).

Durflinger v. *Artiles* (1983) 673 P 2d 86 (Kan.)

Established a similar US standard: a physician possesses a duty to exercise due care while treating patients. This duty applies regardless of practitioner's specialization and is judged by standards in that specialization.

Gillick v. *West Norfolk and Wisbech AHA* (1985) 3 All ER 402

Established that a young person under the age of 16 could consent to treatment, even in the absence of parental consent, provided that he/she has 'sufficient understanding and intelligence to enable him or her to understand fully what is proposed'. This includes the consequences of treatment, including possible side-effects, and the consequences of no treatment. '*Gillick* competence', as the standard has become known, must be assessed in respect of each individual child and each individual procedure. However, even a '*Gillick* competent' young person can only consent to treatment, not refuse it, provided that someone with parental responsibility consents (see *Re W*: details in appendix).

Knight v. Home Office (1990) 3 All ER 237

Concerned the admissibility of resource limitation as a justification for failing to provide a given standard of care. Dismissed a negligence action against a prison, which was alleged to have failed to provide sufficient supervision to prevent a prisoner from hanging himself, on the grounds that it was wrong to compare staffing ratios in a prison hospital wing with those in a specialist psychiatric unit. Although the court shrank back from saying that resource limitation would always be an adequate defence against negligence, it ratified the general position in common law that the courts will not intervene in political matters such as resource allocation.

R. v. Hallstrom, ex parte W (1986) 3 All ER 775 and 2 All ER 306

Established that it is not permissible to use Section 3 of the Mental Health Act 1983 to enforce treatment on out-patients. Only applies in England and Wales, not in Scotland.

Re C (1994) 1 All ER 819

Concerned a schizophrenic patient in a secure hospital who refused to give consent to the amputation of a gangrenous leg. Established the following test of mental capacity:

1 Understanding and retaining information about the nature, purpose, and effects of the proposed treatment.
2 Believing that information.
3 Weighing up the information to arrive at a decision about consenting to or rejecting the proposed treatment.

Also established the validity of advance directives insofar as C was also allowed to refuse the amputation in advance; if he became comatose, the hospital was still barred from operating without his consent.

Re E (1993) 1 FLR 386; (1994) 2 FLR 1065

Concerned a 15-year-old Jehovah's Witness, dying of leukaemia, who rejected a proposed blood transfusion. The boy was found not to be 'Gillick competent' because it was held that he did not understand the distress he would suffer. Also illustrates the stability of some adolescents' values: when the boy reached 18, he continued to refuse transfusions and died.

Re R (1991) 4 All ER 177

Concerned a 15-year-old girl who rejected antipsychotic medication on the grounds of the side-effects. The court held that the girl was not '*Gillick* competent', finding that her competence was only intermittent, and that therefore she could not refuse treatment.

Re T (1992) 4 All ER 649

Concerned a 20-year-old woman who refused a blood transfusion after a road accident. Whilst providing a firm statement of adults' absolute right to refuse life-saving treatment, the court held that her refusal was not fully voluntary, in that she was under pressure from her mother, a Jehovah's Witness.

Re W (1992) 4 All ER 627

Concerned a 16-year-old girl diagnosed with anorexia nervosa and receiving treatment in a specialist eating disorders unit. W refused transfer to a second unit at which there was a possibility that she might be force-fed. The local authority, which had parental responsibility for her, sought a court order to require the transfer. In the Court of Appeal, Lord Donaldson MR held that even a 'competent' young person could only consent to treatment, but could not refuse it. Although the trial judge had found W competent, Lord Donaldson also held that her clinical condition undermined her ability to make an informed choice. Thus young people aged 16 and 17 do not have to establish 'Gillick competence', but even so, they may only consent to treatment, not refuse.

Sidaway v. *Bethlem RHG* (1985) 1 All ER 643

The leading English case on consent to treatment. Mrs Sidaway was left partially paralysed after an elective operation to release a trapped spinal nerve. She brought an action in negligence, claiming that the risk of paralysis had not been explained to her and that therefore her consent was not valid. The Law Lords rejected her claim in a judgement which leaves the doctor's duty of disclosure subject only to the '*Bolam test*' (see this appendix for details). Thus, while the US standard for consent is, roughly, what a reasonable patient would want to know, the UK standard remains what a reasonable doctor would disclose. One of the Law Lords went so far as to state that 'informed consent is no part of English law': consent is required, but 'informed' is not, on this reading. However, Lord Scarman did argue for a 'prudent patient' test in *Sidaway*.

Tarasoff v. *Regents of the University of California* (1974), 118 California Reporter 129, 529, P 2d 553

Concerned the extent of the duty of confidentiality owed to a possibly dangerous patient. The patient had confessed to his therapist that he intended to harm Ms Tarasoff, whom he saw as rejecting his advances. When he subsequently killed Ms Tarasoff, her family successfully sued the therapist's employers for failure to disclose the danger. *Tarasoff* concerned a threat to a named individual, but subsequent cases in both the USA and the UK have extended the principle to more general dangerousness (see *W* v. *Egdell*; details in appendix).

W v. *Egdell* (1990) 1 All ER 835

Upheld the right of a psychiatrist to release to the Home Office a confidential report on a patient whom he deemed dangerous. Limits the duty of patient confidentiality in certain cases where the public interest is involved, but also gives legal backing to an implied contract, enjoining confidentiality, between the clinician and his patient.

Wilsher v. *Essex AHA* (1986) 3 All ER 801

Established part of the legal position on the standard of competence expected of a practitioner. A member of a specialist unit will be expected to display a higher standard of competence than someone in an equivalent position in a general ward, but if professionals do not possess the requisite competence, they must refer the patient on to someone properly skilled in order to avoid an action in negligence.

Bibliography

Adshead, G. (1997) 'All in the mind: autonomy, feminism and the self.' Paper presented at the second Turku workshop of the European Biomedical Ethics Practitioner Education Project, June 1997.

Adshead, G. (forthcoming) A different voice in psychiatric ethics. In *Healthcare Ethics and Human Values* (ed. Fulford, K.W.M., Dickenson, D., and Murray, T.H.). Oxford, Blackwell Science.

Agich, G.J. (1993) *Autonomy and Long-Term Care*. Oxford, Oxford University Press.

Alderson, P. (1994) *Children's Consent to Surgery*. Buckingham, Open University Press.

Alderson, P. (1990) *Choosing for Children: Parents' Consent to Surgery*. Oxford, Oxford University Press.

Almond, B. (ed.) (1995) *Introducing Applied Ethics*. Oxford, Blackwell Publishers.

Almond, B. and Hill, D. *Applied ethics: Moral and Metaphysical Issues in Contemporary Debate*. London and New York, Routledge. 1991

American Psychiatric Association (3rd edn, revised, 1987; 4th edn 1994) *Diagnostic and Statistical Manual of Mental Disorders*. Washington DC, American Psychiatric Association.

Anscombe, G.E.M. (1981). Modern moral philosophy. In *The Collected Philosophical Papers of G.E.M. Anscombe. Volume 3: Ethics, Religion and Politics*, pp. 26–42. Oxford, Blackwell. (First published in 1958 in *Philosophy*, **33**.)

Anzia, D.J. and La Puma, J. (1991) An annotated bibliography of psychiatric medical ethics. *Academic Psychiatry*, **15**:1–7.

Attanucci, J. (1988) In whose terms: a new perspective on self, identify and relationship. In *Mapping the Moral Domain* (ed. Gilligan, C., Ward J., and Taylor, J.). Cambridge (Mass.), Harvard University Press.

Austin, J.L. (1956–7) A plea for excuses. *Proceedings of the Aristotelian Society* 57:1–30. Reprinted in White, A.R., ed. (1968) *The Philosophy of Action*. Oxford: Oxford University Press.

Avon Mental Health (1996) *The Avon Mental Health Measure: A User-centred Approach to Assessing Need*. London, MIND Publications.

Baron, M.W., Petit, P., and Slote, M. (1997) *Three Methods of Ethics* Oxford, Blackwell.

Batson, C.P. and Ventis, L.W. (1982). *The Religious Experience*. Oxford, Oxford University Press.

Beauchamp, T. (1999) The philosophical basis of psychiatric ethics. In *Psychiatric Ethics* (3rd edn) (ed. Bloch, S., Chodoff, P., and Green, S.A.), Chapter 3. Oxford, Oxford University Press.

Beauchamp, T.L. and Childress, J.F. (1989) *Principles of Biomedical Ethics* (3rd edn). New York, Oxford University Press.

Beauchamp, T.L. and Childress, J.F. (1994) *Principles of Biomedical Ethics* (4th edn). Oxford, Oxford University Press.

Ben-Arie, O., Koch, A., Welman, M., and Teggin, A.F. (1990) The effect of research on readmission to a psychiatric hospital. *British Journal of Psychiatry*, **156**:37–9.

Bhugra, D. (ed.) (1996) *Psychiatry and Religion*. Context, Consensus and Controversies. London and New York: Routledge.

Bhui, K. and Olajide, D. (ed.) (1999) *Mental Health Service Provision for a Multi-Cultural Society*. London, W.B. Saunders Ltd.

Binns, P. (1994) Affect, agency and engagement: conceptions of the person in philosophy, neuropsychiatry, and psychotherapy. *Philosophy, Psychiatry and Psychology*, **1**:11–26. (Commentary by Caws, P.).

Birchwood, M., Cochrane, R., Macmillan, F., *et al.* (1992) The influence of ethinicity and family structure on relapse in first episode schizophrenia. *British Journal of Psychiatry*, **161**:783–90).

Birley, J.L.T. (1996) Whistleblowing. *Advances in Psychiatric Treatment*, **2**:48–54.

Bloch, M., Adam, S., Fuller, A., *et al.* (1993) Diagnosis of Huntington's disease: a model for the stages of psychological response based on experience of a predictive testing program. *American Journal of Medical Genetics*, **47**:368–74.

Bloch, S. (1991) The political misuse of psychiatry in the Soviet Union. In *Psychiatric Ethics* (2nd edn) (ed. Bloch, S. and Chodoff, P.), pp. 493–515. Oxford, Oxford University Press.

Bloch, S. and Chodoff, P. (1991) Introduction. In *Psychiatric Ethics* (2nd edn) (ed. Bloch, S. and Chodoff, P.), pp. 1–13. Oxford, Oxford University Press.

Bloch, S., Chodoff, P., and Green S.A. (1999) *Psychiatric Ethics* (3rd edn; 1st edn 1981). Oxford, Oxford University Press.

Bloch, S. and Reddaway, P. (1997) *Russia's Political Hospitals: The Abuse of Psychiatry in the Soviet Union*. London, Gollancz. (Also published in the USA in 1997 as *Psychiatric Terror*. New York, Basic Books.)

Blum, L.A. (1980) *Friendship, Altruism and Morality*. London, Routledge and Kegan Paul.

BMA (1993) *Mental Ethics Today: Its Practice and Philosophy*. London, BMA.

BMA (1999) *Confidentiality and Disclosure of Health Information*. London, BMA.

BMA (1998) *Human Genetics: Choice and Responsibility*. Oxford, Oxford University Press.

BMA and the Law Society (1995) *Assessment of Mental Capacity. Guidance for Doctors and Lawyers*. London, BMA.

Bolam v. Friern HMC (1957) 2 All ER 118.

Bolton, D. (1997) Encoding of meaning: deconstructing the meaning/causality distinction. *Philosophy, Psychiatry, and Psychology*, **4/4**:255–68.

Bolton, D. and Hill, J. (1996) *Mind, Meaning and Mental Disorder: the Nature of Causal Explanation in Psychology and Psychiatry.* Oxford, Oxford University Press.

Boorse, C. (1975) On the distinction between disease and illness. *Philosophy and Public Affairs,* 5: 49–68.

Boorse, C. (1976) What a theory of mental health should be. *Journal of Theory and Social Behaviour,* 6:61–84.

Boyd, R., Gasper, P., and Trout, J.D. (ed.) (1991) *The Philosophy of Science.* Cambridge (Mass.), The MIT Press.

Bracken, P.J. (1995) Beyond liberation: Michael Foucault and the notion of a critical psychiatry. *Philosophy, Psychiatry, and Psychology,* 2:1–14.

Brandt, J. (1994) Ethical considerations in genetic testing: an empirical study of presymptomatic diagnosis of Huntington's disease. In *Medicine and Moral Reasoning* (ed. Fulford, K.W.M., Gillett, G.R., Soskice, J.M.) pp. 41–59. Cambridge, Cambridge University Press.

Braude, S.E. (1991; 2nd edn, 1995) *First Person Plural: Multiple Personality and the Philosophy of Mind.* London, Routledge.

Braude, S.E. (1996) Multiple personality and moral responsibility. *Philosophy, Psychiatry and Psychology,* 3:37–54. (Commentary by Clark, S.R.L., 55–8 and Shuman, D.W., 59–60.)

Brazier, M. (1992) *Medicine, Patients and the Law.* London, Penguin Books.

Brazier, M. and Miola, J. (2000) Bye-bye Bolam: a medical litigation revolution? *Medical Law Review,* 8:85–114.

Bridgman, P.W. (1927) *The Logic of Modern Physics.* New York, Macmillan.

Brody, H. (1992). *The Healer's Power.* New Haven, Yale University Press.

Brown, G.W. (1989) Life events and measurement. In *Life Events and Illness* (ed. Brown, G.W. and Harris, T.O.), pp. 49–94. New York, Guildford Press; London, Unwin and Hyman.

Brown, G.W. and Harris, T.O. (1978) *Social Origins of Depression: a Study of Psychiatric Disorders in Women.* London, Tavistock Publications, New York, Free Press.

Burgess, S. and Hawton, K. (1998) Suicide, euthanasia, and the psychiatrist. *Philosophy, Psychiatry, and Psychology,* 5/2:113–26.

Butler, the Rt. Hon., Lord (1975) *Report of the Committee on Mentally Abnormal Offenders, Cmnd., 6244.* London, Her Majesty's Stationery Office.

Callahan, D. (1996) Can the moral commons survive autonomy? *Hastings Center Report,* vol. 26, no. 6, pp. 41–7.

Calman, K.C. (1996) Cancer: science and society and the communication of risk. *BMJ,* 313:799–802.

Campbell, A.B. and Higgs, R. (1982) *In That Case: Medical Ethics in Everyday Practice.* London, Darton, Longman and Todd.

Campbell, P. (1996) What we want from crisis services. In *On Speaking Our Minds: Anthology* (ed. Read, J. and Reynolds, J.), pp. 180–4. London, MacMillan Press Ltd. (for The Open University).

Caplan, A. L., Engelhardt, T., and McCartney, J. (ed.) (1981) *Concepts of Health and Disease, Interdisciplinary Perspectives.* Addison–Wesley Publishing Company.

Carroll, R.S., Miller, A., Ross, B., and Simpson, G.M. (1980) Research as an impetus to improved treatment. *Archives of General Psychiatry,* **37**:377–80.

Chadwick, R. (1994) Kant, thought insertion and mental unity. *Philosophy, Psychiatry, and Psychology,* **1**:105–14. (Commentary by Stephens, G. Lynn and Graham, G., 115–16.)

Chadwick, R. (ed.) (1995) *Ethics and the Professions.* Aldershot (England), Avebury Press.

Chadwick, R. and Levitt, M. (1995) 'The ethics of community health care.' Paper presented at the Riverside Mental Health Trust, 30 January.

Charland, L.C. (1998) Is Mr Spock mentally competent? Competence to consent and emotion. *Philosophy, Psychiatry, and Psychology,* **5/1**:67–82.

Children Act (1989). London, HMSO.

Chodoff, P. (1999) Misuse and abuse of psychiatry: an overview. In *Psychiatric Ethics* (3rd edn) (ed. Bloch, S., Chodoff, P., and Green, S.), Chapter 4. Oxford, Oxford University Press.

Clare, A. (1979) The disease concept in psychiatry. In *Essentials of Postgraduate Psychiatry* (ed. Hill, P., Murray, R., and Thorley, A.) New York, Academic Press, Grune and Stratton.

Clark, S.R.L. (1996) Minds, memes and multiples. *Philosophy, Psychiatry and Psychology,* **3**:21–8. (Commentary by Bavidge, M., 29–30 and Sprigge, T., 31–6.)

Clinical Genetics Society (1994) The genetic testing of children: report of a working party. *Journal of Medical Genetics,* **31**:785–97.

Clunis *v* Camden and Islington Health Authority (1988) 2 WLR 902.

Cohen, J. and Stewart, I. (1997) *Figments of Reality.* Cambridge: Cambridge University Press.

Collard, D. (1978) *Altruism and Economy: A Study in Non-Selfish Economics.* Oxford, Martin Robertson.

Colombo, A. (1997) *Understanding Mentally Disordered Offenders: a Multi-Agency Perspective.* Aldershot (England), Ashgate.

Cooper, D. (1967) *Psychiatry and Anti-Psychiatry.* London, Tavistock.

Cooper, J.E., Kendell, R.E., Gurland, B.J., Sharpe, L., Copeland, J.R.M., and Simon, R. (1972) *Psychiatric Diagnosis in New York and London.* London, Oxford University Press.

Cox, J.L. (1999) Psychiatry and religion: a general psychiatrist's perspective. In *Religion and Psychiatry* (ed. Bhugra, D.), Chapter 11. London, Routledge.

Crisp, R. (1994) Quality of life and health care. In *Medicine and Moral Reasoning* (ed. Fulford, K.W.M., Gillett, G., and Soskice, J.M.), Chapter 13. Cambridge, Cambridge University Press.

CSAG (1995) Report of the Clinical Standards Advisory Group on Schizophrenia (Volume 1). London, HMSO.

Dancy, J. (1993) *Moral Reasons.* Oxford, Blackwell.

Daniels, N. (1985) *Just Health Care.* Cambridge, Cambridge University Press.

Davidson, D. (1980) *Essays on Actions and Events.* Oxford, Oxford University Press.

Davidson, D. (1982) Paradoxes of irrationality. In *Philosophical Essays on Freud* (ed. Hopkins, J. and Wollheim, R. Cambridge, Cambridge University Press.

Davidson, D. (1984) Belief and the basis of meaning. In *Inquiries into Truth and Interpretation* (ed. Donaldson, D.) Oxford, Clarendon Press.

Davis, M.H. and Harden, R.M. (1999) Problem-based learning: a practical guide. *Medical Teacher,* **21**:130–40.

Davis, G., Sullivan, B., and Yeatman, A. (1997) *The New Contractualism?* Melbourne, Macmillan Education Australia.

Declaration of Helsinki (1964, rev. 1975, 1983 and 1989). In: Department of Health, *Local Research Ethics Committees,* App. C. London, DOH, 1991 (HSG (91)5).

Department of Health (1991). *Working Together under the Children Act 1989.* London, HMSO.

Department of Health (1994) *Draft Guide to Arrangements for Inter-Agency Working for the Care and Protection of Severely Mentally Ill People.* London, DoH.

Department of Health (1999) *Modernising the Care Programme Approach — a Policy Booklet.* London, DoH.

Devereux, J.A., Jones, D.P.H., and Dickenson, D.L. (1993) Can children withhold consent to treatment? *BMJ,* **306**:1459–61.

Dickenson, D. (1991) *Moral Luck in Medical Ethics and Practical Politics* (1st edn). Aldershot, Gower Publishers. (2nd edn (forthcoming), published as *Risk and Luck in Medical Ethics.* Cambridge, Polity Press.)

Dickenson, D. (1994) Children's informed consent to treatment: is the law an ass? Guest Editorial, *Journal of Medical Ethics,* **20/4**:205–6.

Dickenson, D. (1995) Is efficiency ethical? Resource issues in health care. In *Introducing Applied Ethics* (ed. Almond, B.) Oxford, Blackwell.

Dickenson, D. (1997) *Property, Women and Politics: Subjects or Objects?* Cambridge, Polity Press.

Dickenson, D. (1997) Ethical issues in long-term psychiatric care. *Journal of Medical Ethics,* **23/5**:300–4.

Dickenson, D. (1998) Consent in children. *Current Opinion in Psychiatry,* **11/4**.

Dickenson, D. (1999) Can medical criteria settle priority-setting debates? The need for ethical analysis. *Health Care Analysis,* **7**:1–7.

Dickenson, D. (1999) Can children and young people consent to testing for adult-onset genetic disorders? *BMJ,* **381**:1003–5.

Dickenson, D. and Jones, D. (1995) True wishes: The philosophy and developmental psychology of children's informed consent. *Philosophy, Psychiatry, and Psychology,* **2**:287–304.

Duff, R.A. (1986) *Trials and Punishments.* Cambridge: Cambridge University Press.

Duff, R.A. (1990) *Intention, Agency and Criminal Liability.* Oxford, Blackwell.

Durflinger v. Artiles (1983) 673 P 2d.

Dworkin, R. (1993). *Life's Dominion.* London, Harper Collins.

Earle, W.J. (1992) *Introduction to Philosophy.* New York, McGraw–Hill.

Eastman, N.L.G. (1996) Inquiry into homicides by psychiatric patients: systematic audit should replace mandatory inquiries. *BMJ,* **313**:1069–71.

Eastman, N.L.G. and Hope, R.A. (1988) Ethics of enforced medical treatment: the balance model. *Journal of Applied Philosophy,* **5**:49–59.

Eastman, N. and Peay, J. (1999) *Law Without Enforcement: Integrating Mental Health and Justice.* Oxford and Portland (Oregon), Hart Publishing.

Edwards, R.B. (ed.) (1982) *Psychiatry and Ethics: Insanity, Rational Autonomy, and Mental Health Care.* New York, Prometheus Books.

Eekelaar, J. and Dingwall, R. (1990) *The Reform of Child Care Law: A Practical Guide to the Children Act 1989.* London, Tavistock/Routledge.

Elliott, C. (1999) *A Philosophical Disease: Bioethics, Culture and Identity.* London, Routledge.

Engelhardt, H.T. Jr. (1988) Medicine and the concept of person. In *What is a Person?* (ed. Goodman, M.F.) Clifton, N.J., The Humana Press Inc.

Ersser, S. (1995) Ethnography and the development of patient-centred nursing. In *Essential Practice in Patient-Centred Care* (ed. Fulford, K.W.M., Ersser, S., and Hope, T.), Chapter 1. Oxford, Blackwell Science.

Evans, M. (1996) Commentary on Fitzpatrick, R. 'Patient-centred approaches to the evaluation of healthcare'. In *Essential Practice in Patient-Centred Care* (ed. Fulford, K.W.M., Ersser, S., and Hope, T.), pp. 240–3. Oxford, Blackwell Science.

Evans, D. and Evans, M. (1996) *A Decent Proposal: Ethical Review of Clinical Research.* Chichester (England), John Wiley.

Feinberg, J. (1986) *Harm to Self: The Moral Limits of the Criminal Law.* Oxford, Oxford University Press.

Ferriman, A. (1996) 'A cruel inheritance', *Guardian,* 11 June.

Fitzpatrick, R. (1996) Patient-centred approaches to the evaluation of healthcare. In *Essential Practice in Patient-Centred Care* (ed. Fulford, K.W.M., Ersser, S., and Hope, T.), Chapter 15. Oxford, Blackwell Science.

Flew, A. (1973) *Crime or Disease?* New York, Barnes and Noble.

Flew, A. (1979). *A Dictionary of Philosophy.* London, Pan Books.

Foreman, D.M. (1990) The ethical use of paradoxical interventions in psychotherapy. *Journal of Medical Ethics,* **16**(4):200–5.

Foreman, D.M. (1999) The family rule: a framework for obtaining consent for medical interventions from children. *Journal of Medical Ethics,* **25**:491–6.

Foreman, D.M. and Farsides, C. (1993) Ethical use of covert videoing techniques in detecting Munchausen syndrome by proxy [see comments]. *BMJ,* **307**:611–13.

Foucault, M. (1973) *Madness and Civilization: a History of Insanity in the Age of Reason.* New York, Randon House.

Freedman, A.M. and Halpern, A.L. (1999) The psychiatrist's dilemma: a conflict of roles in executions. *Australian and New Zealand Journal of Psychiatry*, 33:629–35.

Fulford, K.W.M. (1987) Insanity. In *Dictionary of Philosophy and Psychology* (ed. Harré, R. and Lamb, D.). Oxford, Blackwells.

Fulford, K.W.M. (1989, reprinted 1995; 2nd edn forthcoming) *Moral Theory and Medical Practice*. Cambridge, Cambridge University Press.

Fulford, K.W.M. (1990) Philosophy and medicine: the Oxford connection. *British Journal of Psychiatry*, 157:111–15. Reprinted in translation in 1995 as 'Filosofin och läkekonsten: förbindelsen över Oxford' in *Begrepp om Hälsa. Filosofiska och etiska perspektiv på livskvalitet, hälsa och vård* (*Concepts of Health. Philosophical and Ethical Perspectives on Quality of Life, Health and Care*) (translated by Utbildning L.) (ed. Klockers, C and Österman B), Chapter 7. Stockholm (Sweden), Liber Utbildning.

Fulford, K.W.M. (1991). The potential of medicine as a resource for philosophy. *Theoretical Medicine*, 12:81–5.

Fulford, K.W.M. (1991) The concept of disease. In *Psychiatric Ethics* (2nd edn) (ed. Bloch, S. and Chodoff, P.), Chapter 6. Oxford, Oxford University Press.

Fulford, K.W.M. (1993) Value, action, mental illness and the law. In *Action and Value in Criminal Law* (ed. Shute, S., Gardner, J., and Horder, J.), pp. 279–310. Oxford, Oxford University Press.

Fulford, K.W.M. (1993) Bioethical blind spots: four flaws in the field of view of traditional bioethics. *Health Care Analysis*, 1:155–62.

Fulford, K.W.M. (1993) Thought insertion and insight: disease and illness paradigms of psychotic disorder. In *Phenomenology, Language and Schizophrenia* (ed. Spitzer, M., Uehlein, F., Schwartz, M.A., and Mundt, C.). New York, Springer–Verlag.

Fulford, K.W.M. (1994) Medical education: knowledge and know-how. In *Ethics and the Professions* (ed. Chadwick, R.), Chapter 2. Aldershot (England), The Avebury Press.

Fulford, K.W.M. (1994) Closet logics: hidden conceptual elements in the DSM and ICD classifications of mental disorders. In *Philosophical Perspectives on Psychiatric Diagnostic Classification* (ed. Sadler, J.Z., Wiggins, O.P., and Schwartz, M.A.), Chapter 9. Baltimore, Johns Hopkins University Press.

Fulford, K.W.M. (1995) Introduction: just getting started. Introduction to *Philosophy, Psychology, and Psychiatry* (ed. A. Phillips Griffiths). Cambridge, Cambridge University Press (for the Royal Institute of Philosophy).

Fulford, K.W.M. (1995) Mind and madness: new directions in the philosophy of psychiatry. In *Philosophy, Psychology, and Psychiatry* (ed. A. Phillips Griffiths), Chapter 1. Cambridge, Cambridge University Press (for the Royal Institute of Philosophy).

Fulford, K.W.M. (1995) Psychiatry, compulsory treatment and a value-based model of mental illness. In *Introducing Applied Ethics* (ed. Almond, B.), Chapter 10. Oxford, Blackwell.

Fulford, K.W.M. (1995) Concepts of disease and the meaning of patient-centred care. In *Essential Practice in Patient-Centred Care* (ed. Fulford, K.W.M., Ersser, S., and Hope, T.), Chapter 1. Oxford, Blackwell Science.

Fulford, K.W.M. (1996) Responsibility, mental illness and psychiatric experts. In *Punishment, Excuses and Moral Development* (ed. H. Tam). Aldershot (England), Avebury Press.

Fulford, K.W.M. (1996) Modern conceptions of health and illness. In *Coping with Sickness: Perspectives on Healthcare Past and Present* (ed. Woodward, J. and Jütte R.). Sheffield, European Association for History of Medicine and Health Publications

Fulford, K.W M. (1996) Religion and psychiatry: extending the limits of tolerance. In *Religion and Psychiatry: Context, Consensus and Controversies* (ed. Bhugra, D.), Chapter 1. London, Routledge and Kegan Paul.

Fulford, K.W.M. (1998) Mental health legislation is now a harmful anachronism. *Psychiatric Bulletin*, **22**:666–8.

Fulford, K.W.M. (1998) Mental illness. In *Encylopaedia of Applied Ethics* (ed. Chadwick, R.). San Diego, Academic Press.

Fulford, K.W.M. (1999) Philosophy and cross-cultural psychiatry. In *Mental Health Service Provision for a Multi-Cultural Society* (ed. Bhui, K. and Olajide, D), Chapter 2. London, W.B. Saunders, Ltd.

Fulford, K.W.M. (2000a) Philosophy Meets Psychiatry in the Twentieth Century — Four Loorks Back and a Brief Look Forward. In Louhiala, P., Stenman, S. (eds.): *Philosophy Meets Medicine*. Helsinki: Helsinki University Press; p. 116–34

Fulford, K.W.M. (2000b) Disordered Minds, Diseased Brains and Real People in *Philosophy, Psychiatry and Psychopathy: Personal identity in mental disorder.* (ed. Heginbotham, C.), Chapter 4 Avebury Series in Philosophy in association with The Society for Applied Philosophy. Aldershot (England): Ashgate Publishing Ltd.

Fulford, K.W.M. and **Bloch, S.** (forthcoming). Psychiatric ethics: codes, concepts and clinical practice skills. In *New Oxford Textbook of Psychiatry* (ed. Gelder, M., Andreasen, N., and Lopez–Ibor, J.), Chapter 17. Oxford, Oxford University Press.

Fulford, K.W.M. and **Hope, R.A.** (1993) Psychiatric ethics: a bioethical ugly duckling? In *Principles of Health Care Ethics* (ed. Gillon, R. and Lloyd, A.), Chapter 58. Chichester (England), John Wiley and Sons.

Fulford, K.W.M. and **Hope, T.** (1996) Informed consent in psychiatry: comparative assessment of Section 5 of the National Reports — Report for Biomed 1 project (published as Control and Practical Experience).In *Informed Consent in Psychiatry: European Perspectives on Ethics, Law and Clinical Practice* (ed. Koch, H.-G., Reiter–Theil, S., and Helmchen, H.), pp. 349–77. Baden–Baden, Nomos Verlagsgesellschaft.

Fulford, K.W.M. and **Howse, K.** (1993) Ethics of research with psychiatric patients: principles, problems and the primary responsibilities of researchers, *Journal of Medical Ethics*, **19**:85–91.

Fulford, K.W.M., Dickenson, D.L., and Murray, T.H. (forthcoming) (eds.) *Healthcare Ethics and Human Values*. Oxford, Blackwells.

Fulford, K.W.M., Smirnoff, A.Y.U., and E. Snow. (1993) Concepts of disease and the abuse of psychiatry in the USSR. *British Journal of Psychiatry*, **162**:801–10. Reprinted in 1996 in *Medical Ethics* (ed. Downie, R.S.), volume in *The International Research Library of Philosophy* series (series ed. J. Skorupski). Aldershot (England), Dartmouth.

Gardner, S. (1993) *Irrationality and the Philosophy of Psychoanalysis*. Cambridge, Cambridge University Press.

Garety, P. A. and Freeman, D. (1999) Cognitive approaches to delusions: a critical review of theories and evidence. *British Journal of Clinical Psychology*, **38**:113–54.

Gauthier, D. (1990) *Moral Dealing: Contract, Ethics and Reason*. Ithaca and London, Cornell University Press.

Gelder, M.G., Gath, D., and Mayou, R. (1989) *The Oxford Textbook of Psychiatry* (2nd edn). Oxford, Oxford University Press.

Genetics Interest Group (1994) *GIG Response to the Clinical Genetics Society Report, 'The Genetic Testing of Children'*. GIG, London.

Gibbard, A. (1990) *Wise Choices, Apt Feelings: A Theory of Normative Judgment*. Oxford, Clarendon Press.

Gillett, G.R. (1986) Multiple personality and the concept of a person. *New Ideas in Psychology*, **4** (2):173–84.

Gillett, G. (1989) *Reasonable Care*. Bristol (England), The Bristol Press.

Gillett, G. (1999) *The Mind and its Discontents*. Oxford, Oxford University Press.

Gillick *v* West Norfolk and Wisbech Area Health Authority (1986) 1 Appeal Cases 112.

Gilligan, C. (1982; 2nd edn, 1993) *In a Different Voice: Psychological Theory and Women's Development*. Cambridge (Mass.), Harvard University Press.

Gillon, R. (1985) *Philosophical Medical Ethics*. Chichester (England), John Wiley and Sons.

Gillon, R. (1994) (ed.) *Principles of Health Care Ethics*. Chichester (England), John Wiley and Sons.

Gindro, S. and Mordini, E. (1998) Ethical, legal and social issues in brain research. *Current Opinion in Psychiatry*, **11**:575–80.

Glover, J. (1970) *Responsibility*. London, Routledge and Kegan Paul.

Glover, J. (1988) *I: The Philosophy and Psychology of Personal Identity*. London, The Penguin Group.

Glover, J. (1997) *Causing Death and Saving Lives*. Harmondsworth, Penguin Books, 2nd ed.

GMC (1995) *Confidentiality: Guidance from the General Medical Council*. London, GMC.

GMC (1995) *Good Medical Practice*. London, GMC.

Goldie, J. (2000) Review of ethics curricula in undergraduate medical education. *Medical Education,* **34**:108–19.

Goodman, M.F. (ed.) (1988) *What is a Person?* New Jersey, The Humana Press Inc.

Gordon, S. (ed.) (1996) *Care, Autonomy and Justice: Feminism and the Ethic of Care.* Boulder, Co, Westview Press.

Graham, G. (1993) *Philosophy of Mind: An Introduction.* Oxford, Blackwell Publishers.

Graham, G. and Stephen, G. Lynn (1994) *Philosophical Psychopathology.* Cambridge (Mass.), The MIT Press.

Green, K. (1995) *The Woman of Reason: Feminism, Humanism and Political Thought.* Cambridge, Polity Press.

Grisso, T. and Appelbaum, P.S. (1995) The MacArthur Treatment Competence Study: III. Abilities of patients to consent to medical and psychiatric treatments. *Law and Human Behaviour,* **19**:149–74.

Grof, S. and Grof, C. (1986) Spiritual emergency: the understanding and treatment of transpersonal crises. *Re-vision,* **8**:7–20.

Group for the Advancement of Psychiatry (1976) *Mysticism: Spiritual Quest or Psychic Disorder?* New York, G.A.P. Publications.

Grubin, D. (1998) *Sex Offending Against Children: Understanding the Risk.* Home Office Policing and Reducing Crime Unit, Research Development and Statistics Directorate.

Hacking, I. (1995) *Rewriting the Soul.* Princeton, Princeton University Press.

Harding, T. (1991) Ethical issues in the delivery of mental health services: abuses in Japan. In *Psychiatric Ethics* (2nd edn) (ed. Bloch, S. and Chodoff, P.), pp. 473–91. Oxford, Oxford University Press.

Hare, R.M. (1952) *The Language of Morals.* Oxford University Press.

Hare, R.M. (1963) Descriptivism. *Proceedings of the British Academy,* **49**:115–34. Reprinted in 1972 in *Essays on the Moral Concepts.* London, The Macmillan Press Ltd.

Hare, R.M. (1981) *Moral Thinking: Its Levels, Method and Point.* Oxford, Clarendon Press.

Hare, R.M. (1993) Medical ethics, can the moral philosopher help? In *Essays on Bioethics,* pp. 1–14. Oxford, Clarendon Press.

Hare, R.M. (1997) *Sorting out Ethics.* Oxford, Oxford University Press.

Harré, R. (1993) *Laws of Nature.* London, Duckworth.

Harré, R. (1997) Pathological autobiographies. *Philosophy, Psychiatry, and Psychology,* **4**:99–110.

Harré, R. and Gillett, G. (1994) *The Discursive Mind.* London, Sage.

Harris, J. (1980) *Violence and Responsibility.* London, Routledge and Kegan Paul.

Harris, J. (1991) Unprincipled QALYs: a response to Cubbon. *Journal of Medical Ethics,* **17**:185–8.

Harrison, G. and Bartlett, P. (1994) Supervision registers for mentally ill people: medicolegal issues seem likely to dominate decisions by clinicians. *BMJ*, **309**:591–2.

Hart, H.L.A. (1968) *Punishment and Responsibility: Essays in the Philosophy of Law*. Oxford, Oxford University Press.

Hay, D. (1987) *Exploring Inner Space* (2nd edn). Harmondsworth, Penguin Books.

Heil, J. and Mele, A. (1993) *Mental Causation*. Oxford, Oxford University Press.

Held, V. (1993) *Feminist Morality: Transforming Culture, Society and Politics*. Chicago, University of Chicago Press.

Hempel, C.G. (1961) Introduction to problems of taxonomy. In *Field Studies in the Mental Disorders* (ed. Zubin, J.), pp. 3–22. New York, Grune and Stratton. Reproduced in 1994 in *Philosophical Perspectives on Psychiatric Diagnostic Classification* (ed. Sadler, J.Z., Wiggins, O.P., and Schwartz, M.A.), pp. 315–31. Baltimore, The Johns Hopkins University Press.

Hendin, H. and Klerman, G. (1994) Comment: 'Physician-assisted suicide: the dangers of legalization'. *American Journal of Psychiatry*, **150/1**:143–5.

Heyd, D. and Bloch, S. (1991) The ethics of suicide. In *Psychiatric Ethics* (2nd edn) (ed. Bloch, S. and Chodoff, P.), pp. 242–64. Oxford, Oxford University Press.

Hindler, C. (1999) The Supervision Register: 19 months after its introduction. *Psychiatric Bulletin*, **23**:15–19.

Hinshelwood, R.D. (1995) The social relocation of personal identity as shown by psychoanalytic observations of splitting, projection and introjection. *Philosophy, Psychiatry, and Psychology*, **2**:185–204.

Hinshelwood, R.D. (1995) Commentary on 'Psychoanalysis. Science, and commonsense'. *Philosophy, Psychiatry, and Psychology*, **2/2**:115–18.

Hinshelwood, R.D. (1997) Primitive mental processes: psychoanalysis and the ethics of integration. *Philosophy, Psychiatry, and Psychology*, **4/2**:121–44.

Hinshelwood, R.D. (1997) *Therapy or Coercion? Does Psychoanalysis Differ from Brainwashing?* London, Karnac Books Ltd.

Hollis, M. (1985, reprinted 1992) *Invitation to Philosophy*. Oxford, Blackwell.

Holm, U. and Aspergen, K. (1999) Pedagogical methods and affect tolerance in medical students. *Medical Education*, **33**:14–18.

Holmes J. (1993) *John Bowlby and Attachment Theory*. London, Routlege.

Holmes J. (1999) Ethical aspects of the psychotherapies. In *Psychiatric Ethics* (3rd edn) (ed. Bloch, S., Chodoff, P., and Green, S.A.). Oxford, Oxford University Press.

Holmes, J. and Lindley, R. (1989). *The Values of Psychotherapy*. Oxford, Oxford University Press.

Hope, R.A. (1990) Ethical philosophy as applied to psychiatry. *Current Opinion in Psychiatry*, **3**: 673–6.

Hope, R.A. (1990) Ethics and psychiatry. In *Essential Psychiatry* (ed. Rose, N.D.B.), Chapter 4. Oxford, Blackwells.

Hope, R.A. and Fulford, K.W.M. (1993) Medical education: patients, principles and practice skills. In *Principles of Health Care Ethics* (ed. Gillon, R.), Chapter 59. Chichester (England), John Wiley and Sons.

Hope, T. (1994) Personal identity and psychiatric illness In *Philosophy, Psychology and Psychiatry*, (ed. Phillips Griffiths, A.). *Royal Institute of Philosophy Supplement*, **37**:131–43. Cambridge, Cambridge University Press.

Hope, T. and Oppenheimer, C. (1997) Ethics and the psychiatry of old age. In *Psychiatry in the Elderly* (2nd edn) (ed. Jacoby, R. and Oppenheimer, C.). Oxford, Oxford University Press.

Hope, T., Fulford, K.W.M., and Yates, A. (1996) *Manual of the Oxford Practice Skills Project*. Oxford, Oxford University Press.

Hudson Jones, A. (1999) Narrative in medical ethics. *BMJ*, **318**:253–6.

Hume, D. (1740) *A Treatise of Human Nature* (ed. Selby Bigge, L.A., 1978). Oxford, Oxford University Press.

Hundert, E.M. (1989) *Philosophy, Psychiatry and Neuroscience*. Oxford, Clarendon Press.

Hurley, S.L. (1989) *Natural Reasons: Personality and Polity*. Oxford, Oxford University Press.

IHA (International Huntington Association) and WFN (World Federation of Neurology Research Group on Huntington's Chorea) (1994). Guidelines for the Molecular Genetics Predictive Test in Huntington's disease. *Neurology*, **44**:1533–6.

In Re F (Mental Patient: Sterilisation) (1990) 2 A.C.1.

Jackson, M.C. (1991) A study of the relationship between spiritual and psychotic experience. Unpublished D.Phil thesis, Oxford University.

Jackson, M.C. (1997) Benign schizotypy? The case of spiritual experience. In *Schizotypy. Relations to Illness and Health* (ed. Claridge, G.S.). Oxford, Oxford University Press.

Jackson, M. and Fulford, K.W.M. (1997) Spiritual experience and psychopathology. *Philosophy, Psychiatry, and Psychology*, **4**:41–66. Commentaries by Littlewood, R.; Lu, F.G. *et al.*; Sims, A.; and Storr, A.; and response by authors, pp. 67–90.

James, W. (1902) *The Varieties of Religious Experience*. New York, Longmans.

Jaspers, K. (1913) *Allgemeine Psychopathologie*. Berlin, Springer. In translation in 1963 as *General Psychopathology* (translated by Hoenig, J. and Hamilton, M.W.). Manchester, Manchester University Press. New edition in 1997, with a new foreword by McHugh, Paul R. Baltimore, The Johns Hopkins University Press.

Jaspers, K. (1913) Causal and meaningful connexions between life history and psychosis. Reprinted in 1974 in *Themes and Variations in European Psychiatry* (ed. Hirsch, S.R. and Shepherd, M.), Chapter 5. Bristol, John Wright and Sons Ltd.

Jochemsen, H. (1994) Euthanasia in Holland: an ethical critique of the new law. *Journal of Medical Ethics*, **20/4**:212–17.Jonsen, A.R. and Toulmin, S. (1988) *The Abuse of Casuistry: a History of Moral Reasoning.* University of California Press.

Karasu, T. (1991). Ethical aspects of psychotherapy. In *Psychiatric Ethics* (2nd edn) (ed. Bloch, S. and Chodoff, P.), pp. 135–66. Oxford, Oxford University Press.

Kemshall, H. and Pritchard, J. (ed.) (1997) *Good Practice in Risk Assessment II: Key Themes for Protection, Rights and Responsibilities.* London, Jessica Kingsley Publishers.

Kendell, R.E. (1975) The concept of disease and its implications for psychiatry. *British Journal of Psychiatry*, **127**:305–15.

Kendell, R.E. (1975) *The Role of Diagnosis in Psychiatry.* Oxford, Blackwells Scientific Publications.

Kendell, R.E. (1986) The Mental Health Act Commission's 'guidelines': a further threat to psychiatric research. *BMJ*, **292**:1249–50.

Kennedy, I. (1992) Consent to treatment: the capable person. In *Doctors, Patients and the Law* (ed. Dyer, C.), pp. 58–62. Oxford, Blackwell.

Kennedy, I. (1997) Consent: adult, refusal of consent, capacity. Commentary on Re MB [1997] 2 F.L.R. 426. *Medical Law Review*, **5**:317–25.

Kennedy, I. and Grubb, A. (1994) *Medical Law: Text with Materials.* London, Butterworths.

Kennedy, I. and Grubb, A. (1998) *Principles of Medical Law.* Oxford, Oxford University Press.

Kenny, A.J.P. (1969) Mental health in Plato's Republic. *Proceedings of the British Academy*, **5**: 229–53.

Kitamura, F., Tomoda, A., Tsukuda, K., Tanaka, M., Kawakami, I., and Mishima, S. (1998) Method for assessment of competency to consent in the mentally ill. *International Journal of Law and Psychiatry*, **21**:223–44.

Kleinig, J. (1985). *Ethical Issues in Psychosurgery.* London, George Allen and Unwin.

Knight *v* Home Office (1990) 3 All ER 237.

Knight, A., Mumford, D., and Nichol, B. (1998) Supervised discharge order: the first year in the South and West Region. *Psychiatric Bulletin*, **22**:418–20.

Komrad, M.S. (1993) A defence of medical paternalism: maximising patients' autonomy. *Journal of Medical Ethics*, **9/2**:38–44.

Kopelman, L.M. (1989) Moral problems in psychiatry. In *Medical Ethics* (ed. Veatch, R.). Massachusetts, Jones and Bartlett Publishing Company.

Kopelman, L.M. (ed.) (1992) Philosophical issues concerning psychiatric diagnosis. *Journal of Medicine and Philosophy*, **17/2**.

Kopelman, L.M. (1994) Normal grief: good or bad? Health or disease? *Philosophy, Psychiatry and Psychology*, **1**:209–20 (with commentaries by Dominian, J. and Wise, T.N. 221–4; response by Kopelman, 226–7.)

Kopelman, L.M. (1994) Case method and casuistry: the problem of bias. *Theoretical Medicine,*. **15(1)**:21–38.

Kris, E. (1952) *Psychoanalytic Explorations in Art.* New York, International Universities Press.

Laing, R.D. (1960) *The Divided Self.* London, Tavistock.

Laing, R.D. (1967) *The Politics of Experience.* Harmondsworth, Penguin Books.

Laing, R.D. and Esterson, A. (1964) *Sanity, Madness and the Family.* London, Tavistock. (Also (1970) Harmondsworth, Penguin.)

Laor and Agassi (1990) *Diagnosis: Philosophical and Medical Perspectives.* Volume 15 of the *Episteme* book series. The Netherlands, Kluwer.

Law Commission (1993) *Mentally Incapacitated Adults and Decision-Making: Medical Treatment and Research.* Consultation Paper No. 129. London, HMSO.

Law Commission (1995) *Mental Incapacity.* Report no. 231. London, HMSO.

Leff, J., Vearnals, S., and Brewin, C. (1999) The London depression intervention trial: an RCT of antidepressants versus couple therapy in the treatment and mainte-nance of depressed people with a partner: clinical outcome and costs. *British Journal of Psychiatry.*

Lidz, C.W., Meisel, A., Zerubavel, E., Carter, M., Sestak, R.M., and Roth, L.H. (ed.) (1984) *Informed Consent: A Study of Decision Making in Psychiatry.* London, The Guildford Press.

Lindemann Nelson, H. (1997) *Stories and their Limits: Narrative Approaches to Bioethics.* London, Routledge.

Lindemann Nelson, H. and Lindemann Nelson, J. (1995) *The Patient in the Family: An Ethics of Medicine and Families.* London, Routledge.

Lindley, R. (1986) *Autonomy.* Houndmills, Macmillan.

Littlewood, R. (1993) *Pathology and Identity: The Work of Mother Earth in Trinidad.* Cambridge, Cambridge University Press.

Littlewood, R. (1997) Commentary on Jackson and Fulford's 'Spiritual experience and psychopathology'. *Philosophy, Psychiatry, and Psychology,* **4/1**:67–74.

Lloyd, G. (1993) *The Man of Reason: 'Male' and 'Female' in Western Philosophy.* University of Minnesota Press.

Locke, J. (1979) *An Essay Concerning Human Understanding* (ed. Nidditch, P.H.) Oxford, Clarendon Press.

Lord Chancellor's Department (1997) *Who Decides? Making Decisions on Behalf of Mentally Incapacitated Adults. CM 3803.* London, The Stationery Office Ltd.

Loughlin M. (1996) Rationing, barbarity and the economist's perspective. *Health Care Analysis,* **4**: 146–56.

Lowe–Ponsford, F. L., Wolfson, P., and Lindesay, J. (1998) Consultant psychiatrists' views on the Supervision Register. *Psychiatric Bulletin,* **22**:409–11.

Lu, F.G., Lutcoff, D., and Turner, R.P. (1997) Commentary on 'Spiritual experience and psychopathology'. *Philosophy, Psychiatry, and Psychology,* **4/1**:75–8.

Lucas, F.R. (1993) *Responsibility*. Oxford, Clarendon Press.

MacIntyre, A. (1981) *After Virtue*. London, Duckworth.

MacIntyre, A. (1988) *Whose Justice? Which Rationality?* Notre Dame, University of Notre Dame Press.

Macklin, R. (1973) The medical model in psychoanalysis and psychotherapy. *Comprehensive Psychiatry*, **14**:49–69.

Maden, A. (1998) Risk assessment and management in psychiatry. *CPD Psychiatry* (Rila Publications), **1/1**:8–11.

Marshall, M. (1994) How should we measure need? Concept and practice in the development of a standardised assessment schedule. *Philosophy, Psychiatry, and Psychology*, **1**:27–36. (Commentaries by Crisp, R. and Morgan, J., 37–40.)

Martin, J.P. (1984) *Hospitals in Trouble*. Oxford. Blackwell.

Mason, J.K. and McCall–Smith, R.A. (1991) *Law and Medical Ethics*. London, Butterworth–Heinemann, 3rd edn.

Mathews, E. (1995) Moralist or therapist? Foucault and the critique of psychiatry. *Philosophy, Psychiatry, and Psychology*, **2**:19–30.

Matthew, E. (1996) *Twentieth Century French Philosophy*. Oxford, Oxford University Press.

May, W. F. (1994) The virtues in a professional setting. In *Medicine and Moral Reasoning* (ed. Fulford, K.W.M., Gillett, G.R., and Soskice, J.M.), Chapter 6. Cambridge, Cambridge University Press.

McGinn, C. (1982) *The Character of Mind*. Oxford, Oxford University Press.

McHugh, P.R. and Slaveney, P.R. (1983) *The Perspectives of Psychiatry*. Baltimore (USA), The Johns Hopkins University Press.

Mechanic, D. (1981). The social dimension. In *Psychiatric Ethics* (1st edn) (ed. S. Bloch and P. Chodoff), pp. 46–59. Oxford, Oxford University Press.

Medical Defence Union (1997) *Consent to Treatment* (rev. edn). London, MDU.

Medical Research Council (1998) *Guidelines for Good Clinical Practice in Clinical Trials*. London, Medical Research Council.

Melden, A.I. (1958) *Free Action*. London, Routledge and Kegan Paul.

Mele, A.R. (1995) *Autonomous Agents: From Self-Control to Autonomy*. Oxford, Oxford University Press.

Mental Health Act Commission (1998) *The Threshold for Admission and the Relapsing Patient*. Nottingham, Mental Health Act Commission.

Milton, J. (1998) Section 17 of the Mental Health Act. *Psychiatric Bulletin*, **22**:415–18.

Mohan, D., Thompson, C., and Mullee, M.A. (1998) Preliminary evaluation of supervised discharge order in the South and West Region. *Psychiatric Bulletin*, **22**:421–3.

Monahan, J. and Steadman, H. (1994) *Violence and Mental Disorder: Developments in Risk Assessment*. Chicago, University of Chicago Press.

Montandon, G. and Harding, T. (1984) The reliability of dangerous assessments: a decison-making exercise. *British Journal of Psychiatry,* **144**:149.

Montgomery, J. (1995) Patients first: the role of rights. In *Essential practice in patient-centred care* (ed. Fulford, K.W.M., Ersser, S., and Hope, T.), Chapter 9. Oxford, Blackwell Science.

Montgomery, J. (1997) *Health Care Law.* Oxford, Oxford University Press.

Moore, M. (1984) *Law and Psychiatry: Rethinking the Relationships.*

Moore, A., Hope, T., and Fulford, K.W.M. (1994) Mild mania and well-being. *Philosophy, Psychiatry and Psychology,* **1**:165–92 (with commentaries by Nordenfelt, L. and Seedhouse, D.)

Müller–Hill, B. (1991) Psychiatry in the Nazi era. In *Psychiatric Ethics* (2nd edn) (ed. Bloch, S. and Chodoff, P.), pp. 461–71. Oxford, Oxford University Press.

Murray, T. H. (1994) Medical ethics, moral philosophy and moral tradition. In *Medicine and Moral Reasoning* (ed. Fulford, K.W.M., Gillett, G.R., and Soskice, J.M.), Chapter 8. Cambridge, Cambridge University Press.

Murray, T.H. (1995) Attending to particulars. In Does clinical ethics distort the discipline? *Hastings Center Report,* **26**:28–34.

Nagel, T. (1976, reprinted 1979). Moral luck. In *Mortal Questions* (Nagel, T.) Cambridge, Cambridge University Press.

Nagel, T. (1986) *The View from Nowhere.* Oxford, Oxford University Press.

Nagel, T. (1987) *What Does It All Mean? A Very Short Introduction to Philosophy.* Oxford, Oxford University Press.

National Health Service Management Executive (1993) *Guidance for Staff on Relations with the Public and the Media.* London, HMSO.

Newton, A.Z. (1997) *Narrative Ethics.* Cambridge (Mass.), Harvard University Press.

Noddings, N. (1984) *Caring: A Feminine Approach to Ethics and Moral Education.* Berkeley, University of California Press.

Nussbaum, M.C. (1986) *The Fragility of Goodness.* Oxford, Oxford University Press.

Nussbaum, M.C. (1992) *Love's Knowledge.* Oxford, Oxford University Press.

Ogilvie, A.D. and Potts, S.G. (1994) Assisted suicide for depression: the slippery slope in action? Learning from the Dutch experience. *BMJ,* **309**:492–3.

O'Hagan, K. and Dillenburger, K. (1995). *The Abuse of Women within Childcare Work.* Buckingham, Open University Press.

O'Hear, A. (1985) *What Philosophy Is.* Harmondsworth (England), Penguin.

O'Hear, A. (1989 and 1991) *An Introduction to the Philosophy of Science.* Oxford, Clarendon Press.

Oppenheimer, C. (1991) Ethics and psychogeriatrics. In *Psychiatric Ethics* (2nd edn) (ed. Bloch, S. and Chodoff, P.), pp. 365–90. Oxford, Oxford University Press.

Oppenheimer, C. (1999) Ethical problems in old age psychiatry. In *Psychiatric Ethics*

(3rd edn) (ed. Bloch, S., Chodoff, P., and Green, S.A.). Oxford, Oxford University Press.

Osborn, D.P.J. (1999) Research and ethics: leaving exclusion behind. *Current Opinion in Psychiatry*, 12:601–4.

Palmer *v* Tees Health Authority and Another (1998) Court of Appeal. *Times* Law Report, 1 June.

Parfit, D. (1984) *Reasons and Persons*. Oxford, Clarendon Press.

Parker, M. (1996) Communitarianism and its problems. *Cogito*, 10:3.

Parker, M. (ed.) (1999) *Ethics and Community in the Health Care Professions*. London, Routledge.

Parker, M. and Dickenson, D. (2000) *The Cambridge Medical Ethics Workbook*. Cambridge, Cambridge University Press.

Parsons, T. (1951) *The Social System*. Glencoe (Illinois), Free Press.

Pateman, C. (1988) *The Sexual Contract*. Cambridge, Polity Press.

Peacocke, A. and Gillett, G. (ed.) (1987) *Persons and Personality*. Oxford, Basil Blackwell Ltd.

Peele, R. (1991) The ethics of deinstitutionalization. In *Psychiatric Ethics* (2nd edn) (ed. Bloch, S. and Chodoff, P.), pp. 291–311. Oxford, Oxford University Press.

Perkins, R. and Repper, J. (1998) *Dilemmas in Community Mental Health Practice: Choice or Control*. Aberdeen, Radcliffe Medical Press.

Perneger, T.V., Giner, F., del Rio, M., and Mino, A. (1998) Randomised trial of heroin maintenance programme for addicts who fail in conventional drug treatments. *BMJ*, 317:13–18.

Persinger, M.A. (1983). Religious and mystical experiences as artefacts of temporal lobe function: A general hypothesis. *Perception and Motor Skills*, 57, 1255–1262.

Phillips Griffiths, A. (ed.) (1989) *Key Themes in Philosophy*. Cambridge, Cambridge University Press.

Phillips Griffiths, A. (ed.) (1995) *Philosophy, Psychology and Psychiatry*. Cambridge, Cambridge University Press (for the Royal Institute of Philosophy).

Pinfold, V., Bindman, J., Friedl, K., Beck, A., and Thornicroft, G. (1999) Supervised discharge orders in England. Compulsory care in the community. *Psychiatric Bulletin*, 23:199–203.

Protagoras. In *The Collected Dialogues of Plato*. (1961) (ed. Hamilton, E. and Huntington, C.). New York, Pantheon Books.

Quine, W. (1948) On what there is. *Review of Metaphysics*, 2. Reprinted in 1953 in *From a Logical Point of View* (Quine, W.). Cambridge (Mass.), Harvard University Press.

Quinton, A. (1985) Madness. In *Philosophy and Practice* (ed. Griffiths, A.P.), Chapter 2. Cambridge, Cambridge University Press.

R. *v*. Bournewood Community and Mental Health NHS Trust, *ex parte* L (1998) 2 WLR 764.

R. *v*. Hallstrom, *ex parte* W (No. 2) (1986), 2 All ER 306.

Rachels, J. (1999) *The Elements of Moral Philosophy*. McGraw–Hill.

Radden, J. (1994) Recent criticisms of psychiatric nosology: a review. *Philosophy, Psychiatry, & Psychology*, 1/3: 193–200.

Radden, J. (1996) *Divided Minds and Successive Selves: Ethical Issues in Disorders of Identity and Personality*. Cambridge (Mass.), The MIT Press.

Raphael, D.D. (1994) *Moral Philosophy* (2nd edn). Oxford, Oxford University Press.

Rawls, J. (1971) *A Theory of Justice*. Cambridge (Mass.), Harvard University Press. (Published in 1972 by Oxford University Press.)

Re C (Adult: Refusal of medical treatment) (1994) 1 All ER 819.

Re E (1993) 1 FLR 386; (1994) 2 FLR 1065, 1075.

Re Jobes (1987) 108 NJ 394.

Re Quinlan (1976) 70 NJ 10.

Re R (1991) 4 All ER 177.

Re T (1992) 4 All ER 649.

Re W (1992) 4 All ER 627.

Reich, W. (1991). Psychiatric diagnosis as an ethical problem. In *Psychiatric Ethics* (2nd edn) (ed. Bloch, S. and Chodoff, P.), pp. 101–34. Oxford, Oxford University Press.

Reilly, R.B., Teasdale, T.A., and McCullough, L.B. (1994) Projecting patients' preferences from living wills: an invalid strategy for management of dementia with life-threatening illness. *Journal of the American Geriatric Society*, 42:997–1003.

Remmelink Commissie onderzoek medische praktijk inszke euthanasie (1991) *Rapport Medische Besslissingen rond het Levenseinde* (Report on Euthanasia and Other Medical Decisions concerning the End of Life). Den Haag,SDU-Uitgeverij.

Reset, J.L. and Gracia, D. (1992) *The Ethics of Diagnosis*. Volume 40 in *Philosophy and Medicine* series (series ed. Engelhardt, T. and Spicker, S.). The Netherlands, Kluwer.

Reznek, L. (1991). *The Philosophical Defence of Psychiatry*. London, Routledge.

Reznek, L. (1997) *Evil or Ill? Justifying the Insanity Defence*. London and New York, Routledge.

Ricoeur, P. (1970) *Freud and Philosophy* (trans. Savage, D.). London, Yale University Press.

Robson, P. (1992) Opiate misusers: are treatments effective? In *Practical Problems in Clinical Psychiatry* (ed. Hawton, K. and Cowen, P.). Oxford, Oxford University Press.

Robson, P. (1999) Drug policy — a time for change? In *Forbidden Drugs* (2nd edn). Oxford, Oxford University Press.

Robertson, D.W. (1996) Ethical theory, ethnography and differences between doctors and nurses in approaches to patient care. *Journal of Medical Ethics*, 22:292–9.

Robinson, D. (1996) *Wild Beasts and Idle Humours*. Cambridge (Mass.), Harvard University Press.

Robinson, G. and Merar, A. (1983) Informed consent: recall by patients tested post-operatively. In *Moral Problems in Medicine* (2nd edn) (ed. Gorovitz, S. *et al.*). Englewood Cliffs (New Jersey), Prentice–Hall.

Rogers, A., Pilgrim, D., and Lacey, R. (1993) *Experiencing Psychiatry: Users' Views of Services.* London, The Macmillan Press.

Rosenhan, D. (1973) On being sane in insane places. *Science,* **179**:250–8.

Roth, L.H. and Meisel, A. (1977) Dangerousness, confidentiality, and the duty to warn. *American Journal of Psychiatry,* **126**:508–11.

Roth, M. and Kroll, J. (1986) *The Reality of Mental Illness.* Cambridge, Cambridge University Press.

Rouf, K. (1997) Child protection issues within the mental health setting: a forgotten problem. *Clinical Psychology Forum,* **99**:23–7.

Royal College of Physicians (1996) *Guidelines on the Practice of Ethics Committees in Medical Research Involving Human Subjects.* London, Royal College of Physicians.

Royal College of Psychiatrists Research Unit (1998) *Management of Imminent Violence: Clinical Practice Guidelines to Support Mental Health Services.* London, Royal College of Psychiatrists.

Royal College of Psychiatrists (1996) *The Responsibilities of Consultant Psychiatrists. Council Report No. 51.* London, Royal College of Psychiatrists.

Sabat, S.R. and Harré, R. (1997) The Alzheimer's Disease sufferer as semiotic subject. *Philosophy, Psychiatry, and Psychology,* **4/2**:145–60.

Sadler, J.Z. (1996) Epistemic value commitments in the debate over categorical vs. dimensional personality diagnosis. *Philosophy, Psychiatry, and Psychology,* **3**:203–22.

Sadler, J.Z. and Agich, G.J. (1995) Dysfunction as a value-free concept: a reply to Sadler and Agich. *Philosophy, Psychiatry, and Psychology,* **2**:233–46.

Sadler, J.Z., Wiggins, O.P., and Schwartz, M.A. (ed.) (1994) *Philosophical Perspectives on Psychiatry Diagnostic Classification.* Baltimore, Johns Hopkins University Press.

Sandel, M. (1998) *Liberalism and the Limits of Justice* (2nd edn). Cambridge, Cambridge University Press.

Savulescu, J. and Dickenson, D. (1998) The time frame of preferences, dispositions, and the validity of advance directives for the mentally ill. *Philosophy, Psychiatry, and Psychology,* **5/3**:225–46.

Savulescu, J., Crisp, R., Fulford, K.W.M., and Hope, T. (1999) Evaluating ethics competence in medical education. *Journal of Medical Ethics,* **25**:367–74.

Sayce, L. (1998) Mental health legislation is now a harmful anachronism. *Psychiatric Bulletin,* **22**: 669–70.

Scheff, T. J. (1963) The role of the mentally ill and the dynamics of mental disorder: a research framework. *Sociometry,* **26**:436–53.

Scheff, T. (1966) *Being Mentally Ill: A Sociological Theory.* Chicago, Aldine.

Scourfield, J., Soldan, J., Gray, J., Houlihan, G., and Harper, P.S. (1997) Huntington's disease: psychiatric practice in molecular genetic prediction and diagnosis. *British Journal of Psychiatry*, **178**:144–9.

Semler *v.* Psychiatric Institute of Washington DC (1976) 538 F 2d 121.

Sensky, T., Hughes, T., and Hirsch, S. (1991) Compulsory psychiatric treatment in the community, part 1. A controlled study of compulsory community treatment with extended leave under the Mental Health Act: special characteristics of patients treated and impact of treatment. *British Journal of Psychiatry*, **158**:792.

Shapiro, J. (1989) *Ourselves, Growing Older: Women Ageing with Knowledge and Power.* London, Fontana/Collins. (British version of original text by Doress, P.B., Siegal, D.L., and the Midlife and Older Women Book Project in co-operation with the Boston Women's Health Book Collective.)

Sherer, D.G. and Repucci, N.D. (1988) Adolescents' capacities to provide voluntary informed consent. *Law and Human Behaviour*, **12**:123–41.

Sherlock, R. (1983). Contribution to symposium on 'Consent, competence and ECT'. *Journal of Medical Ethics*, **9/3**.

Sherwin, S. (1993) *No Longer Patient: Feminist Ethics and Health Care.* Philadelphia, Temple University Press.

Shorter, E. (1997) *A History of Psychiatry.* New York, John Wiley and Sons.

Sidaway *v.* Bethlem RHG (1985) 1 All ER 643.

Sims, A. (1988) *Symptoms in the Mind: An Introduction to Descriptive Psychopathology.* London, Baillière Tindall.

Sims, A. (1997) Commentary on 'Spiritual experience and psychopathology'. *Philosophy, Psychiatry, and Psychology*, **4/1**:79–82.

Singer, P. (ed.) (1993) *A Companion to Ethics* (2nd edn). Oxford, Blackwell.

Smart, J.J.C. and Williams, B. (1973) *Utilitarianism: For and Against.* Cambridge, Cambridge University Press.

Smith, A. (1998) 'Sacking threat for lax community care' *London Observer*, 28 June 1998.

Snowdon, C., Garcia, J., and Elbourne, D. (1997) Making sense of randomization; responses of parents of critically ill babies to random allocation of treatment in a clinical trial. *Social Science and Medicine*, **45/9**:1337–55.

Spitzer, M. and Maher, B. (1990) *Philosophy and Psychopathology.* New York, Springer–Verlag Inc.

Spitzer, M., Uehlein, F., Schwartz, M. A., and Mundt, C. (ed.) (1993) *Phenomenology, Language and Schizophrenia.* New York, Springer–Verlag.

Statman, D. (1994) Introduction to *Moral Luck* (ed. Statman, D.). State University of New York.

Stephens, G.L. and Graham, G. (1994) Self-consciousness, mental agency, and the clinical psychopathology of thought insertion. *Philosophy, Psychiatry, and Psychology*, **1**:1–10. (Commentary by Wiggins, O.P.)

Stiles, W.B., Meshot, C.M., Anderson, T.M., and Sloan, W.W. (1992). Assimilation of problematic experiences: the case of John Jones. *Psychotherapy Research*, 2:81–101.

Stone, A.A. (1984) *Law, Psychiatry, and Morality*. Washington, American Psychiatric Press.

Storr, A. (1997) Commentary on Jackson and Fulford's 'Spiritual experience and psychopathology'. *Philosophy, Psychiatry, and Psychology*, 4/1:83–6.

Sunday Times (1997) 'Anorexia trigger found in the brain', 13 April.

Sutherland, S. (1992) *Irrationality: The Enemy Within*. Harmondsworth, Penguin Books.

Szasz, T. (1960) The myth of mental illness. *American Psychologist*, 15: 113–18.

Szasz, T. (1961) *The Myth of Mental Illness*. New York, Harper and Row.

Szasz, T. (1963). *Law, Liberty and Psychiatry*. New York, Macmillan.

Szasz, T. (1986). The case against suicide prevention. *American Psychologist*, 41:806–12.

Szasz, T. (1987) *Insanity: The Idea and Its Consequences*. John Wiley and Sons.

Szmukler, G. and Holloway, F. (1998) Mental health legislation is now a harmful anachronism. *Psychiatric Bulletin*, 22:662–5.

Tam, H. (1996) *Punishment, Excuses and Moral Development*. Aldershot, Avebury Press.

Tarasoff *v.* Regents of the University of California (1974), 118 California Reporter 129, 529, P 2d 553.

Taylor, C. (1989) *Sources of the Self: The Making of the Modern Identity*. Cambridge, Cambridge University Press.

Taylor, P. (1995) Schizophrenia and the risk of violence. In *Schizophrenia* (ed. Hirsch, S. and Weinberger, D.), pp. 163–83. Oxford, Blackwell Science.

Taylor, P. J. and Gunn, J. (1999) Homicides by people with mental illness: myth and reality. *British Journal of Psychiatry*, 174:9–14.

Thornicroft, G. and Goldberg, O.P. (1998) *Has Community Care Failed?* Maudsley Discussion Paper No. 5. Institute of Psychiatry, London.

Thornton, T. (1997) Reasons and causes in philosophy and psychopathology. *Philosophy, Psychiatry, and Psychology*, 4/4: 307.

Thornton, T. (1998) *Wittgenstein on Language and Thought*. Edinburgh, Edinburgh University Press.

Tyrer, P. and Steinberg, D. (1993) *Models for Mental Disorder: Conceptual Models in Psychiatry* (2nd edn). Chichester (England), John Wiley & Sons.

Tyrer, P., Smith, J., and Adshead, G. (1994) Ethical dilemmas in drug treatments. *Psychiatric Bulletin*, 18:203–4.

Urmson, J.O. (1950) On grading. *Mind*, 59:145–69.

Van der Maas, P.J., Van Delden J.J.M., and Pijnenborg, I., (1992) Euthanasia and other medical decisions concerning the end of life. *Health Policy*, 22(1/2):1–262.

van Lysebetten, T. and Igodt, P. (2000) Compulsory psychiatric admission. A comparison of English and Belgian legislation. *Psychiatric Bulletin*, 24:66–8.

Vaughan, P.J. (1998) Supervision register in practice. *Psychiatric Bulletin*, 22:412–15.

Vesey, G. (ed.) (1986) *Philosophers Ancient and Modern*. Cambridge, Cambridge University Press.

Vesey, G. (1987) Personal identity. In *The Oxford Companion to the Mind* (ed. Gregory, R.L.). Oxford, Oxford University Press.

von Wright, H.G. (1963) *The Varieties of Goodness*. London, Routledge and Kegan Paul. New York, The Humatics Press.

W *v.* Egdell (1990) 1 All ER 835.

Wakefield, J.C. (1995) Dysfunction as a value-free concept: a reply to Sadler and Agich. *Philosophy, Psychiatry, and Psychology*, 2:233–46.

Waldron, J. (1988) *The Right to Private Property*. Oxford, Clarendon Press.

Walker, N. (1967) *Crime and Insanity in England*. Edinburgh, Edinburgh University Press.

Wallace, J. and Ball, C. J. (1998) Use of the Care Programme Approach register by an inner-city old age psychiatry team. *Psychiatric Bulletin*, 22:489–91.

Wallace, C., Mullen, C., Burgess, P., Palmer, S., Ruschena, D., and Braune, C. (1998) Serious criminal offending and mental disorder. *British Journal of Psychiatry*, 172: 477–84.

Warnock, G.J. (1967) *Contemporary Moral Philosophy*. London and Basingstoke, The Macmillan Press Ltd.

Warnock, G.J. (1971) *The Object of Morality*. London, Methuen & Co. Ltd.

Warnock, M. (1978) *Ethics Since 1900* (3rd edn). Oxford, Oxford University Press.

Warnock, M. (1992) *The Uses of Philosophy*. Oxford, Blackwell Publishers.

Warnock, M. (1998) *An Intelligent Person's Guide to Ethics*. London, Duckworth.

Wear, S. (1993) Empirical studies of informed consent. *Informed Consent: Patient Autonomy and Physician Beneficence Within Clinical Medicine*, Chapter 3, Subsection II. Dordrecht (Netherlands), Kluwer Academic Publishers.

Weiss, B.D. (1982) Confidentiality in expectations of patients, physicians, and medical students. *JAMA*, 247(19):2695–7.

Wertz, D.C., Fanos, J.H., and Reilly, P.R. (1997) Genetic testing for children and adolescents: who decides? *Journal of the American Medical Association*, 272/11:875–81.

White, R., Carr, P., and Lowe, N. (1990) *A Guide to the Children Act 1989*. London, Butterworths.

Widdershoven, G. (forthcoming) Alternatives to principlism. In *Healthcare Ethics and Human Values* (ed. Fulford, K.W.M., Dickenson, D.L., and Murray, T.H.). Oxford, Blackwell Science.

Wilkes, K.V. (1988) *Real People: Personal Identity Without Thought Experiments*. Oxford, Clarendon Press.

Wilkinson, G. *et al.* (1995) Case reports and confidentiality: opinion is sought, medical and legal. *British Journal of Psychiatry*, 166:555–8.

Williams, A. (1995), Economics, QALYs and medical ethics — a health economist's perspective. *Health Care Analysis*, **3(3)**:221–6.

Williams, B. (1981) *Moral Luck*. Cambridge, Cambridge University Press.

Williams, B. (1994) Postscript to *Moral Luck* (ed. Statman, D.), pp. 251–8. State University of New York.

Wilsher *v*. Essex AHA (1986) 3 All ER 801, 834.

Wing, J.K. (1978) *Reasoning about Madness*. Oxford, Oxford University Press.

Wing, J.K., Cooper, J.E., and Sartorius, N. (1974) *Measurement and Classification of Psychiatric Symptoms*. Cambridge, Cambridge University Press.

Wirshing, D., Wirshing, W., Marder, S., Liberman, R.P., and Mintz, J. (1998) Informed consent; assessment of comprehension. *American Journal of Psychiatry*, **155**:1503–11.

Wittgenstein, L. (1999) *Philosophical Investigations* (2nd edn) (trans. Anscombe, G.E.M. and Rhees, R.). Oxford, Blackwells.

Wolfensberger, W. (1972) *The Principle of Normalization in Human Services*. Toronto, NIMR.

Wolfensberger, W. (1983) Social role valorization: a proposed new term for the principle of normalization. *Mental Retardation*, **21**:234–9.

Wolpert, L. (1999) *Malignant Sadness*. London, Faber & Faber.

Wong, J.G., Clare, I.C.H., Holland, A.J., Watson, P.C., and Gunn, M. (forthcoming) The capacity of people with a 'mental disability' to make a health carer decision. *Psychological Medicine*.

World Health Organisation (1967) *Manual of the International Statistical Classification of Diseases, Injuries and Causes of Death (ICD–8)*. Geneva, WHO.

World Health Organisation (1973) *The International Pilot Study of Schizophrenia. Volume 1*. Geneva, WHO.

World Health Organisation (1992) *The ICD–10 Classification of Mental and Behavioural Disorders: Clinical Descriptions and Diagnostic Guidelines*. Geneva, WHO.

World Medical Association (September/October 1981; updated September 1995) *Declaration of Lisbon on the Rights of the Patient*. WMA.

World Psychiatric Association, Geneva (1996) Declaration of Madrid. (Reproduced with a brief commentary in 1999 in *Psychiatric Ethics* (3rd edn) (Bloch, S., Chodoff P., and Green S.A.), Appendix — Codes of Ethics, pp. 511–31. Oxford, Oxford University Press.)

Index

Page numbers in *italics* refer to figures and tables, those in **bold** indicate main discussion.

abuses of psychiatry
  and casuistry, 33–4
  diagnosis, 53–4, 71
  former USSR, 55, 57, 88, 122, 328, 330,
    332–3
  medical model, 34, 56–7
  see also case histories: Elizabeth Orton, Tom
    Benbow
addiction
  case history, 179–88
  management strategies, 181–6
  and rationality, 186–7
  and values, 175
adolescents, 205–7
aetiology, 133–9
  biological, 142, 143–4, 145–9
  biopsychosocial, 150
  social, 144–5
Aftercare Under Supervision Orders, 241, 242,
  245–6, 255, 271
agency, 54, 55
  see also case histories: Elizabeth Orton, Jane
    Gillespie
akrasia, 102–4
Alzheimer's disease, *see* dementia
Alzheimer's Disease Society, 261
analytical ethics, 39–41, 138–9, 337
  Oxford, 4–6, 9–11, 40–1, 337
antipsychiatry, 5–6, 9, *10*, 20, 34, 54–5, 257
Association of Local Research Ethics
  Committees, 305
attitudes, 22, 29
  staff, 329–30
  teaching seminar, 285–7, 291, 297
audit, 304, 305
autonomy, 27, 185–6
  and beneficence, 31, 32, 37–8, 262
  and control of adolescents, 205–6
  criteria, 31–2
  and duty of care, 241, 244, 273
  and multiple selves, 193
  and paternalism, 4, 31
  and relationship, 174, 272–3
  and 'sick role', 270
  see also case histories: 'Captain Ahab', Jane
    Gillespie, Tom Benbow
awareness, 21–2, 29, 285–7, 291, 297
  staff, 330

balance of utilities, 38–9, 221, 224–5
beneficence, 27
  and autonomy, 31, 32, 37–8, 262
'best interests', 174–5, 195, 196
  of children, 201–2
bioethics, 3–4, 8, 11
  approaches in psychiatry, 27–9
  advantages and disadvantages, 29–30, 174–5
  lessons from psychiatry, 336–40
  see also medical model; physical medicine vs.
    psychiatry; science and ethics
BMA, *see* British Medical Association
'Bolam principle', 221–2, 311, **347**
British Medical Association (BMA), 204
Butler Committee, 25–6, 82

capacity, 8–9, 31, 32
  criteria for involuntary treatment, 87–8
  and delusion, 87–8, 159–60
  to consent, 206–7, 263–4, 311, 320
  to form criminal intent (*mens rea*), 101–3
case histories:
  Alan Masterson, 226
    discussion, 219–20, 221, 222, 225, **227–33**
    practitioner commentary, 233–6
  'Captain Ahab' (George), 179–80
    discussion, 174–5, 178, **180–6**, 190–1
    practitioner commentary, 186–7
  Delia Jarrett, 98
    discussion, 85, **98–105**
    practitioner commentary, 105–8
  Elizabeth Orton, 58–9
    discussion, 53, 56, 57, **59–65**, 100–1
    practitioner commentary, 65–6
    problem-solving seminar, 291–9
  Francesca Gindro, 155
    discussion, 136, 137, 138, **155–66**
    practitioner commentary, 166–9
  Gilbert Ryan, 259
    discussion, 253, 254, 255, **259–65**
    practitioner commentary, 265–6
  Ida Harbottle, 188
    discussion, 175–6, 178, **188–94**, 261–2
    practitioner commentary, 195–6
  Jane Gillespie, 140
    discussion, 135, 138, **140–51**, 220
    practitioner commentary, 151–3
  Martin McKendrick, 91

case histories (*continued*):
    discussion, 85, **91–6**
    practitioner commentary, 96–7
    Mr Able, 19–20
        discussion, 20–2, 27–9, 32, 33, 34, 36, 37,
          39–40
    Philip Caversham, 237–8
        discussion, 220, 221, 222, **237–44**, 242,
          330
        practitioner commentary, 244–7
    research ethics, 302–22
    Robin and Alex, 197–8
        discussion, 176, 178, **198–208**
        practitioner commentary, 208–10
    Sam Mason, 267
        discussion, 253–5, **267–73**
        practitioner commentary, 273–5
    Simon Greer, 109
        discussion, 85, **109–22**, 258
        practitioner commentary, 123–4
    in teaching, 282–3
    Tom Benbow, 67–8
        discussion, 53–4, 56, **68–74**, 240
        practitioner commentary, 74–5
casuistry, 27–8
    advantages and disadvantages, 30
    inductive approach, 190
    and values, 33–4
causality, 223–4
    see also meanings, and causes
CGS, *see* Clinical Genetics Society
character, weakness of, 104–5
children
    adolescents, 205–7
    adults abused as, 140, 144, 155, 156, 163
    'best interests', 201–2
    consent, 176–7, 199–200, 271
    genetic screening
        case history, 197–210
        professional guidelines, 202–4
    legal mechanisms for intervention, 271–2
    protection of, 228–9, 230–2
    see also case histories: Alan Masterson,
        Elizabeth Orton
Children Act (1989), 176–7, 182, 184–5,
    200–1, 274
    Section 2(7), 271
    Section 8, 271
Clinical Genetics Society (CGS), 202–3, 205,
    209
clinical governance, 332–3
cognition and delusion, 32, 159–60
cognitive—behavioural therapy, 141–2, 150,
    151, 152
communication, 57, 149, 166, 339
'community treatment orders', 56
competence
    'Gillick', 72, 199–200, 203, 204, 206, **347**
    patient, *see* capacity

staff, 329–30
confidentiality, 331–2
    'commercial', 332
    and disclosure, 219–20, 221, 222, 225,
        230–1, 235
    GMC guidance, 61–2, 230
    see also case histories: Alan Masterson
consciousness
    identity of, 193–4
    unity of, 164–6
consensus, 122
consent
    adolescents, 206–7
    children, 176–7, 199–200, 271
    dementia, 263–4
    and disclosure, 235
    informed, 231
    moral luck dilemmas, 243
    psychotherapy, 176
    receiving care at home, 265
    research ethics, 311–16, *317*, 320, 321
    see also involuntary treatment
consequentialist ethics, 37
    limitations in psychiatry, 38–9, 234
contracts, 232
    limit-setting, 181, 184–5
    philosophical definition, 185
cultural formulations, 119–22

'dangerousness'
    case histories, 226–48
    and hospitalization, 233–4
    and supervision, 330–1
    see also risk assessment
delusion
    and capacity, 87–8, 159–60
    and cognition, 32, 159–60
    difficulties in defining, 157–61
    form and content, 136–8
    and involuntary treatment, 36
    and practical reasoning, 160–1
    and self–deception, 162–3
    vs. motivated self–deception (case history),
        155–70
    vs. religious experience (case history),
        109–26
dementia
    case histories, 188–97, 259–67
    consent, 32, 263–4
    management, 191
    and personal identity, 190, 191, 196
depression, 219–20
    causes, social and biological, 144–9
    'endogenous' and 'reactive', 142, 143
    'major' and 'minor', 143–4
    postnatal, *see* case histories: Elizabeth Orton
    see also case histories: Alan Masterson, Jane
        Gillespie, Mr Able
descriptive psychopathology, 133–8

determinism, 223–4
deviance, 53, 54, 55
diagnosis, 81–9
  abuses of psychiatry, 53–4, 71
  differential, 111–13, 118–19
  and distributive justice (case history),
    67–75
  in elderly, 71, 191
  and incapacity criteria, 87–8
  and meanings, 84–5, 118–19
  'operational criteria', 83–4
  value judgements in, 6–7, 32, 82–3, 86,
    114–22
  see also case histories: Delia Jarrett,
    Elizabeth Orton, Martin McKendrick,
    Simon Greer, Tom Benbow
Diagnostic and Statistical Manual
DSM-III, 84, 115
DSM-IV 'Criterion B' for schizophrenia, 86,
  114–15, 117, 121, 256
DSM-IV cultural formulation, 119, 121–2
disclosure, confidentiality and, 219–20, 221,
  222, 225, 230–1, 235
disease
  as harmful dysfunction, 116–18
  and illness, 116, 118, 146–8
dissociation, 163–4
distributive justice, 56, 262–3
  and diagnosis (case history), 67–75
doctrine of double effect, 264–5
DSM, see Diagnostic and Statistical Manual
dual role psychiatry (case history), 179–88
Dutch Medical Council, 94
duty of care, 231–3, 245–5
  and autonomy, 241, 244, 273
duty-based ethics, 37, 38

electrotherapy (ECT), 141, 151, 152, 153
'empirical ethics', 23
ethical reasoning, levels of, 40–1, 282
ethical theory, psychiatric, 36–8
  aims of, 20–4
  lessons for bioethics, 336–40
  scope of, 3–8, 337–8
  see also bioethics, approaches in psychiatry
eudaimonia, 175
euthanasia, 93–5
evidence-based practice, 301

family, 270, 274–5
  genetic information, 207–8
Family Reform Act (1969), 199

General Medical Council (GMC)
  guidance on confidentiality, 61–2, 230
  staff 'competence assessment', 330
Genetic Interest Group (GIG), 203–4, 205,
  209
genetic screening of children

case history, 197–210
  professional guidelines, 202–4
Geneva Initiative on Psychiatry, 328
'Gillick competence', 72, 199–200, 203, 204,
  206, **347**
guardianship, 63, 271–2

homicide, 222–3, 224, 241, 330, 331

ICD, see International Classification of
  Diseases
identity, see consciousness, identity of;
  personal identity
illness, 257
  and disease, 116, 118, 146–8
incapacity, see capacity
integration principle, 176
  psychotherapeutic ethics, 165–6
International Classification of Diseases
  ICD-8, 84
  ICD-10, 112, 114
involuntary treatment
  applied principles, 31–2, 34
  bioethical approach, 8–9
  casuistry, 34, 35–6
  conceptual issues, 39–40
  incapacity criteria for, 87–8
  legal perspective, 24–6, 56
  perspectives approach, 34, 36
  for suicidally depressed, 20–1
  see also consent

justice, 27
  see also distributive justice

knowledge, 22–3, 29
  research ethics, 308–9
  teaching seminar, 285–7, 291, 298

law
  on assisted suicide, Holland, 93–5
  criminal, 101–3
  mechanisms for intervention, 24–6, 271–2
  mental health, Denmark, 26
  see also specific Acts
Law Commission, 321
learning disability (case history), 67–75
legal cases
  A-G v. Guardian (1990), 230
  Bolam (1957), 221–2, 311, **347**
  Dr Charbot, 93–4, 97
  Gillick, 72, 199–200, 203, 204, 206, **347**
  Re C (1994), 86–8, 95, 103, **348**
  Re E (1993), 206–7, **348–9**
  Re R (1991), 71–3, 271, **348–9**
  Re T (1992), 206, **349**
  Re W (1992), 271, **349**
  Tarasoff (1974), 219, 222, **349–50**
  W v. Egdell, 62, **350**

legal cases (*continued*):
  Wilsher v. Essex AHA (1986), 261, **350**
linguistic analysis, 39–40
loss of control (case history), 135, 140–55
'loss of insight', 36, 136

meanings
  and causes, 134–5, 136, 138–9, 144–5,
    149–50
  and diagnosis, 84–5, 118–19
medical model, 53–6, 63–4
  abuses of psychiatry, 34, 56–7
  'brain trumps mind', 133–5, 146, 147,
    148–9
  'disease trumps illness', 146–8
  and moral conceptions, 54–5
  neuroscience, 54–5, 56, 113, 135, 145–6,
    161
  of suicide, 92–4
  see also bioethics; physical medicine vs.
    psychiatry; science and ethics
Medical Research Council (MRC), 320–1
mens rea, 101–3
mental disorder
  models/definitions, 53–7, 81–2, 88–9,
    113–14, 257–8
    antipsychiatry, 5–6, 9, *10*, 20, 34, 54–5,
      257
    fact + value, 5, 9–11, 120–1, 122, 255–6
    see also medical model
  over-diagnosis in elderly, 71, 191
  public perception of, 38–9, 56, 222–3
  and rationality, 103
  see also specific disorders
Mental Health Act (1983)
  Butler Committee, 25–6, 82
  'community treatment orders', 56
  guardianship procedures, 271–2
  and research, 320
  reviews, 87, 255, 331
  Section 2, 24, 240–1, 246
  Section 3, 240, 245
  Section 4, 240
Mental Health (Patients in the Community)
    Act (1985), 241, 271
MIND (National Association for Mental
    Health), 34, 241
mind, philosophy of, 134–5, 161, 175–6,
    195–6
mind-brain relationship, 133–5, 146, 147,
    148–9
moral luck, risk assessment and, 225–6,
    229–31, 242–3, 263
motivated self-deception, 161–2
  case history, 155–70
  and delusion, 162–3
  and dissociation, 163–4
MRC, *see* Medical Research Council
multidisciplinary teams, 55, 120–1, 255–6, 258

communication, 57, 166
confidentiality, 331
conflict of purposes, 266
partnerships, 11, 339
see also case histories: Gilbert Ryan, Sam
    Mason
multiple selves
  and autonomy, 193
  personal identity, 192–4
myths
  of the amazing coincidence, 222–3
  of billiard-ball causality, 223–4
  of value-free risk, 224–6

National Association for Mental Health
    (MIND), 34, 241
needs assessment, 254
negligence, 201–2, 203, 261
neuroscience, 54–5, 56, 113, 135, 145–6, 161
non-maleficence, 27, 205
normalization, 68, **74–75**

objective judgements, 223–4
open societies, 329–30, 332–3
ownership of individual, 207–8

partnerships, 11, 339
paternalism, 194, 204–5
  shift away from, 4, 31
patient perspectives, 23, 34–6, 122
patient rights, 38
personal identity, 165–6, 175–6
  case history, 188–97
  and dementia, 190, 191, 196
  multiple selves, 192–4
  'successive selves', 164–5
personality disorder, 86
  case study, 98–109
perspectives, 28–9
  advantages and disadvantages, 30
  patient, 23, 34–6, 122
  Research Ethics Committees, 319–21
philosophy, 8–11, 336, 338
  definitions
    contract, 185
    delusions, 159, 161
    rationality, 183–4
  and medicine, 8, 9
  of mind, 134–5, 161, 175–6, 195–6
physical environment, 329
physical medicine vs. psychiatry, 12, 32, 34,
    87, 257
  values, 5–8, 337–8
  see also bioethics; medical model; science
    and ethics
practical reasoning, impaired, 160–1
'practice skills', application of, 12–13, 21–4, 41
principles, 27
  advantages and disadvantages, 29–30
  applied to involuntary treatment, 31–2, 34

applied to research, 308–16
    summary, 316–18
    and casuistry, 28
problem-solving approach, 283–5
    key elements, 284
    stages, 283–5
    see also teaching, problem–solving seminar
psychosis
    definitions, 25–6, 82
    and homicide, 222–3, 224, 241, 330, 331
    and involuntary treatment, 25–6, 36
    psychoanalytical explanations, 136, 163
    see also schizophrenia
psychotherapy
    consent, 176
    ethics, 151–3, 163
        integration principle, 165–6
    relationship, 166–9

QALYS (Quality–Adjusted Life Year), 38, 39
quality of physical environment, 329

rationality, 81–2, 85–6, 182–4
    and addiction, 186–7
    case study, 91–8
    and mental disorder, 103
    see also capacity; cognition and delusion;
        practical reasoning, impaired
reflection on practice, 41, 282
'reflective equilibrium', 190
relationship(s), 183
    and autonomy, 174, 185–6, 272–3
    breakdown of therapeutic alliance (case
        history), 267–76
    ethics, 236, 245–5
    psychotherapy, 166–9
relativism, 30, 35, 122
religious experience vs. delusion (case
    history), 109–26
research ethics, 11–12, 339
    case history, 302–22
        background (initial letter), 302–3
        definition of research, 303–5
        proposals, 305–8
        appraisal, 308–18
        action plan, 318
        follow-up, 318–19
    stages, 302, 305–19, 321–2
Research Ethics Committees, 303, 304, 305,
    310
    role, 11–12, 319–21
resource allocation, 261, 262–3
responsibility, 25, 81–3, 86
    case study, 98–109
    professional, 231–3, 259
        dual role of psychiatrist (case history),
            179–88
rights
    patient, 38

to genetic information, 207–8
risk assessment, 222
    benefits of research, 310
    clinicians' responsibility, 225–6, 259
    'getting it wrong', 224, 242–4
        see also 'Bolam principle'
    legal perspective, 24–6
    and moral luck, 225–6, 229–31, 242–3, 263
    objective, 223–4
    subjective, 222–3
    value–free, 224–6
    see also case histories: Gilbert Ryan, Tom
        Benbow; children, protection of;
        'dangerousness'; suicide, risk assessment
        (case history)
Royal College of Physicians, 303–5, 311
Royal College of Psychiatrists, 241, 304–5,
    311–12
Russia, see USSR, former
Russian Psychiatric Society, 328

schizophrenia
    case histories, 220, 237–48
        child, 267–76
    DSM-IV 'Criterion B', 86, 114–15, 117, 121,
        256
science and ethics, 11–12, 84–5, 336, 339
sexual offences, 220, 237, 238–9, 244
'sick role', 270
'significant harm', 200–1
social coercion, 53, 54, 55
    see also case histories: Delia Jarrett,
        Elizabeth Orton
Social Services, 219, 220, 225, 228, 229, 231,
    260–1, 266
staff, 329–30, 331
substantive theory, 36–8
    and conceptual problems, 39–40
'successive selves', 164–5
suicide
    assisted, 93–5
    risk assessment (case history), 91–7
        see also case histories: Alan Masterson,
            Jane Gillespie, Mr Able
Suicide Act, Section 2, 93
supervision order, see Aftercare Under
    Supervision Orders
supervision of potentially dangerous patients,
    330–1
Supervision Register, 220, 221, 222, 241
    case history, 237–48

tagging and tracking (case history), 259–67
teaching
    case histories, building on, 283
    case material in, 282–3
    case vignettes, 283
    issue-based, 282
    model, 281–2

teaching (*continued*):
    problem-solving seminar
        examples, 286, 291–9
        stages, 285–90
thinking skills, *12–13*, 23–4, 29
    learning and doing, 40–1
    teaching seminar, 285–7, 291, 298
tracking and tagging (case history), 259–67
true wishes, 191, 194, 210
    case history, 188–97

unity of consciousness, 164–6
USSR, former
    abuses of psychiatry, 55, 57, 88, 122, 328,
        330, 332–3
    confidentiality, 331
    'Register', 331
utilities, balance of, 38–9, 221, 224–5

value judgements in diagnosis, 6–7, 32, 82–3,
    86, 114–22

value-free risk, myth of, 224–6
value-ladenness of psychiatry, 4–8
values, 148–9, 150–1
    balance of, 30
    and casuistry, 33–4
    concept of eudaimonia, 175
    diverse, 4–5, 11, 12, 310, 322
        and shared, 5–8, 30, 33, 34, 88
    fact + value model of psychiatry, 5, 9–11,
        120–1, 122, 255–6
    patient perspectives, 23, 34–6, 122
    physical medicine vs. psychiatry, 5–8,
        337–8
    professional
        and client, 23
        and personal, 22
'virtue ethics', 22, 41, 183

weakness of character, 104–5
weakness of will (akrasia), 102–4